Teen Health Series

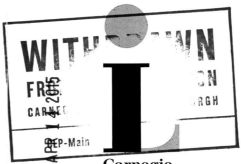

Women's Health Concerns

SOURCEBOOK

Fourth Edition

Health Reference Series

Fourth Edition

Women's Health Concerns

SOURCEBOOK

Basic Consumer Health Information about Breast and Gynecological Conditions, Menopause, Sexuality and Female Sexual Dysfunction, Birth Control, Infertility, Pregnancy, Common Cancers in Women, Cardiovascular Disease, Mental Health, and Chronic Disorders that Affect Women Disproportionally, Including Gastrointestinal Disorders, Thyroid Disease, Urinary Tract Disorders, Osteoporosis, Chronic Pain, and Migraines

Along with an Introduction to the Female Body, Information on Maintaining Wellness and Avoiding Risk Factors for Disease, a Glossary, and a Directory of Resources for Additional Help and Information

Edited by
Laura Larsen

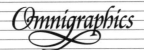

155 W. Congress, Suite 200, Detroit, MI 48226

Bibliographic Note

Because this page cannot legibly accommodate all the copyright notices, the Bibliographic Note portion of the Preface constitutes an extension of the copyright notice.

Edited by Laura Larsen

Health Reference Series
Karen Bellenir, *Managing Editor*
David A. Cooke, MD, FACP, *Medical Consultant*
Elizabeth Collins, *Research and Permissions Coordinator*
EdIndex, Services for Publishers, *Indexers*

* * *

Omnigraphics, Inc.
Matthew P. Barbour, *Senior Vice President*
Kevin M. Hayes, *Operations Manager*

* * *

Peter E. Ruffner, *Publisher*
Copyright © 2013 Omnigraphics, Inc.
ISBN 978-0-7808-1303-8
E-ISBN 978-0-7808-1304-5

Library of Congress Cataloging-in-Publication Data

Women's health concerns sourcebook : basic consumer health information about breast and gynecological conditions, menopause, sexuality and female sexual dysfunction, birth control, infertility, pregnancy, common cancers in women, cardiovascular disease, mental health, and chronic disorders that affect women disproportionally, including gastrointestinal disorders, thyroid disease, urinary tract disorders, osteoporosis, chronic pain, and migraines; along with an introduction to the female body, information on maintaining wellness and avoiding risk factors for disease, a glossary, and a directory of resources for additional help and information / edited by Laura Larsen. -- Fourth edition.
    pages cm. -- (Health reference series)
  Includes bibliographical references and index.
  Summary: "Provides basic consumer health information about conditions and disorders that affect women, along with facts about recommended health screenings and tips on avoiding risk factors to maintain wellness. Includes index, glossary of related terms, and other resources"-- Provided by publisher.
  ISBN 978-0-7808-1303-8 (hardcover : alk. paper) 1. Women--Health and hygiene. 2. Women--Diseases. I. Larsen, Laura.
  RA778.W7543 2013
  613'.04244--dc23
                                                                2013013430

Table of Contents

Visit www.healthreferenceseries.com to view *A Contents Guide to the Health Reference Series*, a listing of more than 16,000 topics and the volumes in which they are covered.

Part II: Maintaining Women's Health and Wellness

Part III: Breast and Gynecological Concerns

Part IV: Sexual and Reproductive Concerns

ix

Part VI: Other Health Conditions with Issues of Significance to Women

Part VII: Additional Help and Information

Preface

About This Book

Statistics indicate that women—on average—live approximately five years longer than men, but this longevity is not linked to better overall health. According to the Health Resources and Services Administration, part of the U.S. Department of Health and Human Services, women experience more physically and mentally unhealthy days than men. Part of this disparity is related to age. Because of their longer life expectancy, women are at greater risk for age-related conditions, like Alzheimer disease. Irrespective of their age, however, women experience gender-related health care needs and are more likely than men to have certain conditions, including asthma, arthritis, migraine headaches, osteoporosis, thyroid disorders, chronic pain, and activity limitations.

Women's Health Concerns Sourcebook, Fourth Edition, provides updated information about the medical issues of most significance to women. It explains female anatomy and reports on women's health and wellness topics, including vaccination and screening recommendations, fitness and nutrition guidelines, and tips for healthy aging. It also discusses breast health, sexual and reproductive issues, conditions that disproportionately affect women, and the leading causes of death and disability in women, including heart disease, stroke, and diabetes. The book concludes with a glossary of terms related to women's health and a directory of resources for additional information.

How to Use This Book

This book is divided into parts and chapters. Parts focus on broad areas of interest. Chapters are devoted to single topics within a part.

Part I: Introduction to Women's Health provides basic information about female anatomy and physiology, including the reproductive system, menstruation, puberty, and menopause. Statistics related to women's health are included, and special concerns among specific female populations are addressed.

Part II: Maintaining Women's Health and Wellness provides guidelines for pursuing a healthy lifestyle. It includes nutrition and exercise recommendations, facts about obesity and weight management, and tips for handling sleep problems, stress, and common concerns associated with aging. It also discusses ways to prevent or mitigate risk factors for the leading causes of death among women. These tactics include following recommended health screenings, receiving appropriate immunizations, controlling high blood pressure and cholesterol, and avoiding the use of tobacco products.

Part III: Breast and Gynecological Concerns describes female-specific health matters, including breast disorders and changes, menstrual irregularities, and menopause. Disorders of the reproductive organs and pelvic floor are also explained, and the part concludes with information about common gynecological procedures.

Part IV: Sexual and Reproductive Concerns presents information about sexuality and sexual dysfunction from a female perspective. It also looks at topics related to fertility and pregnancy, including birth control methods, infertility treatments, abortion, prenatal and postnatal care, and labor and delivery. Other topics related to maternal health, such as breastfeeding, postpartum depression, and dealing with pregnancy loss, are also addressed.

Part V: Gynecological and High-Prevalence Cancers in Women takes a look at cancers that are of special significance to women. These include cervical, ovarian, uterine, and other cancers of the female reproductive system. Cancers that occur more often in women than in men—such as breast cancer and thyroid cancer—and other cancers that are among those most frequently diagnosed in women—including lung, colon, rectal, and skin cancers—are also discussed.

Part VI: Other Health Conditions with Issues of Significance to Women focuses on disorders with a high or disproportionate incidence among women, including Alzheimer disease, arthritis, autoimmune disorders, migraine headaches, osteoporosis, and thyroid disease. It also looks at the ways in which women experience some common disorders differently from men, and it describes special issues related to women's mental well-being.

Part VII: Additional Help and Information provides resources for readers seeking further assistance. It includes glossary of women's health terms and a directory of organizations related to women's health care needs.

Bibliographic Note

This volume contains documents and excerpts from publications issued by the following U.S. government agencies: Centers for Disease Control and Prevention (CDC); Health Resources and Services Administration (HRSA); National Cancer Institute (NCI); National Heart, Lung, and Blood Institute (NHLBI); National Institute of Allergy and Infectious Diseases (NIAID); National Institute of Arthritis and Musculoskeletal and Skin Diseases (NIAMS); National Institute of Child Health and Human Development (NICHD); National Institute of Diabetes and Digestive and Kidney Diseases (NIDDK); National Institute of Neurological Disorders and Stroke (NINDS); National Institute on Aging (NIA); National Institutes of Health (NIH); Office on Women's Health; U.S. Department of Veterans Affairs; U.S. Food and Drug Administration (FDA); and U.S. Preventive Services Task Force.

In addition, this volume contains copyrighted documents from the following organizations: About.com; A.D.A.M., Inc.; American Heart Association; American Pregnancy Association; Immunization Action Coalition; National Women's Health Resource Institute; Nemours Foundation; Northwestern University; Planned Parenthood; Skin Cancer Foundation; and University of Michigan Health System.

Full citation information is provided on the first page of each chapter or section. Every effort has been made to secure all necessary rights to reprint the copyrighted material. If any omissions have been made, please contact Omnigraphics to make corrections for future editions.

Acknowledgements

Thanks go to the many organizations, agencies, and individuals who have contributed materials for this *Sourcebook* and to medical consultant Dr. David Cooke and prepress services provider WhimsyInk.

Special thanks go to managing editor Karen Bellenir and research and permissions coordinator Liz Collins for their help and support.

About the Health Reference Series

The *Health Reference Series* is designed to provide basic medical information for patients, families, caregivers, and the general public. Each volume takes a particular topic and provides comprehensive coverage. This is especially important for people who may be dealing with a newly diagnosed disease or a chronic disorder in themselves or in a family member. People looking for preventive guidance, information about disease warning signs, medical statistics, and risk factors for health problems will also find answers to their questions in the *Health Reference Series*. The *Series*, however, is not intended to serve as a tool for diagnosing illness, in prescribing treatments, or as a substitute for the physician/patient relationship. All people concerned about medical symptoms or the possibility of disease are encouraged to seek professional care from an appropriate health care provider.

A Note about Spelling and Style

Health Reference Series editors use *Stedman's Medical Dictionary* as an authority for questions related to the spelling of medical terms and the *Chicago Manual of Style* for questions related to grammatical structures, punctuation, and other editorial concerns. Consistent adherence is not always possible, however, because the individual volumes within the Series include many documents from a wide variety of different producers and copyright holders, and the editor's primary goal is to present material from each source as accurately as is possible following the terms specified by each document's producer. This sometimes means that information in different chapters or sections may follow other guidelines and alternate spelling authorities. For example, occasionally a copyright holder may require that eponymous terms be shown in possessive forms (Crohn's disease vs. Crohn disease) or that British spelling norms be retained (leukaemia vs. leukemia).

Locating Information within the Health Reference Series

The *Health Reference Series* contains a wealth of information about a wide variety of medical topics. Ensuring easy access to all the fact sheets, research reports, in-depth discussions, and other material contained within the individual books of the *Series* remains one of our highest priorities. As the *Series* continues to grow in size and scope, however, locating the precise information needed by a reader may become more challenging.

A *Contents Guide to the Health Reference Series* was developed to direct readers to the specific volumes that address their concerns. It presents an extensive list of diseases, treatments, and other topics of general interest compiled from the Tables of Contents and major index headings. To access *A Contents Guide to the Health Reference Series*, visit www.healthreferenceseries.com.

Medical Consultant

Medical consultation services are provided to the *Health Reference Series* editors by David A. Cooke, MD, FACP. Dr. Cooke is a graduate of Brandeis University, and he received his M.D. degree from the University of Michigan. He completed residency training at the University of Wisconsin Hospital and Clinics. He is board-certified in Internal Medicine. Dr. Cooke currently works as part of the University of Michigan Health System and practices in Ann Arbor, MI. In his free time, he enjoys writing, science fiction, and spending time with his family.

Our Advisory Board

We would like to thank the following board members for providing guidance to the development of this *Series*:

- Dr. Lynda Baker, Associate Professor of Library and Information Science, Wayne State University, Detroit, MI

- Nancy Bulgarelli, William Beaumont Hospital Library, Royal Oak, MI

- Karen Imarisio, Bloomfield Township Public Library, Bloomfield Township, MI

- Karen Morgan, Mardigian Library, University of Michigan-Dearborn, Dearborn, MI

- Rosemary Orlando, St. Clair Shores Public Library, St. Clair Shores, MI

Health Reference Series *Update Policy*

The inaugural book in the *Health Reference Series* was the first edition of *Cancer Sourcebook* published in 1989. Since then, the *Series* has been enthusiastically received by librarians and in the medical community. In order to maintain the standard of providing high-quality health information for the layperson the editorial staff at Omnigraphics felt it was necessary to implement a policy of updating volumes when warranted.

Medical researchers have been making tremendous strides, and it is the purpose of the *Health Reference Series* to stay current with the most recent advances. Each decision to update a volume is made on an individual basis. Some of the considerations include how much new information is available and the feedback we receive from people who use the books. If there is a topic you would like to see added to the update list, or an area of medical concern you feel has not been adequately addressed, please write to:

Editor
Health Reference Series
Omnigraphics, Inc.
155 W. Congress, Suite 200
Detroit, MI 48226
E-mail: editorial@omnigraphics.com

Part One

Introduction to Women's Health

Chapter 1

The Female Body

Chapter Contents

Section 1.1

Breast Anatomy

Excerpted from SEER Training Modules, Breast Cancer. U.S. National
Institutes of Health, National Cancer Institute. 25 February 2013
<http://training.seer.cancer.gov/>.

The breasts of an adult woman are milk-producing, tear-shaped
glands. They are supported by and attached to the front of the chest
wall on either side of the breast bone or sternum by ligaments. They
rest on the major chest muscle, the pectoralis major.

The breast has no muscle tissue. A layer of fat surrounds the glands
and extends throughout the breast.

The breast is responsive to a complex interplay of hormones that
cause the tissue to develop, enlarge, and produce milk. The three major
hormones affecting the breast are estrogen, progesterone, and prolactin, which cause glandular tissue in the breast and the uterus to
change during the menstrual cycle.

Each breast contains 15 to 20 lobes arranged in a circular fashion.
The fat (subcutaneous adipose tissue) that covers the lobes gives the
breast its size and shape. Each lobe is comprised of many lobules, at the
end of which are tiny bulblike glands, or sacs, where milk is produced
in response to hormonal signals.

Ducts connect the lobes, lobules, and glands in nursing mothers.
These ducts deliver milk to openings in the nipple. The areola is the
darker-pigmented area around the nipple.

Section 1.2

The Female Reproductive System

About Human Reproduction

All living things reproduce. Reproduction—the process by which organisms make more organisms like themselves—is one of the things that sets living things apart from nonliving matter. But even though the reproductive system is essential to keeping a species alive, unlike other body systems, it's not essential to keeping an individual alive.

In the human reproductive process, two kinds of sex cells, or gametes, are involved. The male gamete, or sperm, and the female gamete, the egg or ovum, meet in the female's reproductive system to create a new individual.

Both the male and female reproductive systems are essential for reproduction. The female needs a male to fertilize her egg, even though it is she who carries offspring through pregnancy and childbirth.

Humans, like other organisms, pass certain characteristics of themselves to the next generation through their genes, the special carriers of human traits. The genes that parents pass along are what make their children similar to others in their family, but also what make each child unique. These genes come from the male's sperm and the female's egg.

Most species have two sexes: male and female. Each sex has its own unique reproductive system. They are different in shape and structure, but both are specifically designed to produce, nourish, and transport either the egg or sperm.

Components of the Female Reproductive System

Unlike the male, the human female has a reproductive system located entirely in the pelvis. The external part of the female reproductive organs is called the vulva, which means covering. Located between the legs, the vulva covers the opening to the vagina and other reproductive organs located inside the body.

The fleshy area located just above the top of the vaginal opening is called the mons pubis. Two pairs of skin flaps called the labia (which means lips) surround the vaginal opening. The clitoris, a small sensory organ, is located toward the front of the vulva where the folds of the labia join. Between the labia are openings to the urethra (the canal that carries urine from the bladder to the outside of the body) and vagina. Once girls become sexually mature, the outer labia and the mons pubis are covered by pubic hair.

A female's internal reproductive organs are the vagina, uterus, fallopian tubes, and ovaries.

The vagina is a muscular, hollow tube that extends from the vaginal opening to the uterus. The vagina is about 3 to 5 inches (8 to 12 centimeters) long in a grown woman. Because it has muscular walls, it can expand and contract. This ability to become wider or narrower allows the vagina to accommodate something as slim as a tampon and as wide as a baby. The vagina's muscular walls are lined with mucous membranes, which keep it protected and moist.

The vagina serves three purposes:

- It's where the penis is inserted during sexual intercourse.

- It's the pathway that a baby takes out of a woman's body during childbirth, called the birth canal.

- It provides the route for the menstrual blood (the period) to leave the body from the uterus.

A thin sheet of tissue with one or more holes in it called the hymen partially covers the opening of the vagina. Hymens are often different from female to female. Most women find their hymens have stretched or torn after their first sexual experience, and the hymen may bleed a little (this usually causes little, if any, pain). Some women who have had sex don't have much of a change in their hymens, though.

The vagina connects with the uterus, or womb, at the cervix (which means neck). The cervix has strong, thick walls. The opening of the cervix is very small (no wider than a straw), which is why a tampon can never get lost inside a girl's body. During childbirth, the cervix can expand to allow a baby to pass.

The uterus is shaped like an upside-down pear, with a thick lining and muscular walls—in fact, the uterus contains some of the strongest muscles in the female body. These muscles are able to expand and contract to accommodate a growing fetus and then help push the baby out during labor. When a woman isn't pregnant, the uterus is only about 3 inches (7.5 centimeters) long and 2 inches (5 centimeters) wide.

At the upper corners of the uterus, the fallopian tubes connect the uterus to the ovaries. The ovaries are two oval-shaped organs that lie to the upper right and left of the uterus. They produce, store, and release eggs into the fallopian tubes in the process called ovulation. Each ovary measures about 1 1/2 to 2 inches (4 to 5 centimeters) in a grown woman.

There are two fallopian tubes, each attached to a side of the uterus. The fallopian tubes are about 4 inches (10 centimeters) long and about as wide as a piece of spaghetti. Within each tube is a tiny passageway no wider than a sewing needle. At the other end of each fallopian tube is a fringed area that looks like a funnel. This fringed area wraps around the ovary but doesn't completely attach to it. When an egg pops out of an ovary, it enters the fallopian tube. Once the egg is in the fallopian tube, tiny hairs in the tube's lining help push it down the narrow passageway toward the uterus.

The ovaries are also part of the endocrine system because they produce female sex hormones such as estrogen and progesterone.

What the Female Reproductive System Does

The female reproductive system enables a woman to:

- produce eggs (ova);
- have sexual intercourse;
- protect and nourish the fertilized egg until it is fully developed;
- give birth.

Sexual reproduction couldn't happen without the sexual organs called the gonads. Although most people think of the gonads as the male testicles, both sexes actually have gonads: In females the gonads are the ovaries. The female gonads produce female gametes (eggs); the male gonads produce male gametes (sperm). After an egg is fertilized by the sperm, the fertilized egg is called the zygote.

When a baby girl is born, her ovaries contain hundreds of thousands of eggs, which remain inactive until puberty begins. At puberty, the pituitary gland, located in the central part of the brain, starts making hormones that stimulate the ovaries to produce female sex hormones, including estrogen. The secretion of these hormones causes a girl to develop into a sexually mature woman.

Toward the end of puberty, girls begin to release eggs as part of a monthly period called the menstrual cycle. Approximately once a month, during ovulation, an ovary sends a tiny egg into one of the fallopian tubes.

Unless the egg is fertilized by a sperm while in the fallopian tube, the egg dries up and leaves the body about two weeks later through the uterus—this is menstruation. Blood and tissues from the inner lining of the uterus combine to form the menstrual flow, which in most girls lasts from three to five days. A girl's first period is called menarche.

It's common for women and girls to experience some discomfort in the days leading to their periods. Premenstrual syndrome (PMS) includes both physical and emotional symptoms that many girls and women get right before their periods, such as acne, bloating, fatigue, backaches, sore breasts, headaches, constipation, diarrhea, food cravings, depression, irritability, or difficulty concentrating or handling stress. PMS is usually at its worst during the seven days before a girl's period starts and disappears once it begins.

Many girls also experience abdominal cramps during the first few days of their periods caused by prostaglandins, chemicals in the body that make the smooth muscle in the uterus contract. These involuntary contractions can be either dull or sharp and intense.

It can take up to two years from menarche for a girl's body to develop a regular menstrual cycle. During that time, her body is adjusting to the hormones puberty brings. On average, the monthly cycle for an adult woman is 28 days, but the range is from 23 to 35 days.

Fertilization

If a female and male have sex within several days of the female's ovulation, fertilization can occur. When the male ejaculates (when semen leaves a male's penis), between 0.05 and 0.2 fluid ounces (1.5 to 6.0 milliliters) of semen is deposited into the vagina. Between 75 and 900 million sperm are in this small amount of semen, and they "swim" up from the vagina through the cervix and uterus to meet the egg in the fallopian tube. It takes only one sperm to fertilize the egg.

About a week after the sperm fertilizes the egg, the fertilized egg (zygote) has become a multicelled blastocyst. A blastocyst is about the size of a pinhead, and it's a hollow ball of cells with fluid inside. The blastocyst burrows itself into the lining of the uterus, called the endometrium. The hormone estrogen causes the endometrium to become thick and rich with blood. Progesterone, another hormone released by the ovaries, keeps the endometrium thick with blood so that the blastocyst can attach to the uterus and absorb nutrients from it. This process is called implantation.

As cells from the blastocyst take in nourishment, another stage of development, the embryonic stage, begins. The inner cells form a flattened circular shape called the embryonic disk, which will develop into a baby. The outer cells become thin membranes that form around the baby. The cells multiply thousands of times and move to new positions to eventually become the embryo.

After approximately eight weeks, the embryo is about the size of an adult's thumb, but almost all of its parts—the brain and nerves, the heart and blood, the stomach and intestines, and the muscles and skin—have formed.

During the fetal stage, which lasts from nine weeks after fertilization to birth, development continues as cells multiply, move, and change. The fetus floats in amniotic fluid inside the amniotic sac. The fetus receives oxygen and nourishment from the mother's blood via the placenta, a disk-like structure that sticks to the inner lining of the uterus and connects to the fetus via the umbilical cord. The amniotic fluid and membrane cushion the fetus against bumps and jolts to the mother's body.

Pregnancy lasts an average of 280 days—about nine months. When the baby is ready for birth, its head presses on the cervix, which begins to relax and widen to get ready for the baby to pass into and through the vagina. The mucus that has formed a plug in the cervix loosens, and with amniotic fluid, comes out through the vagina when the mother's water breaks.

When the contractions of labor begin, the walls of the uterus contract as they are stimulated by the pituitary hormone oxytocin. The contractions cause the cervix to widen and begin to open. After several hours of this widening, the cervix is dilated (opened) enough for the baby to come through. The baby is pushed out of the uterus, through the cervix, and along the birth canal. The baby's head usually comes first; the umbilical cord comes out with the baby and is cut after the baby is delivered.

The last stage of the birth process involves the delivery of the placenta, which at that point is called the afterbirth. After it has separated from the inner lining of the uterus, contractions of the uterus push it out, along with its membranes and fluids.

Problems of the Female Reproductive System

Some girls might experience reproductive system problems, such as:

Problems of the Vulva and Vagina

- **Vulvovaginitis** is an inflammation of the vulva and vagina. It may be caused by irritating substances (such as laundry soaps

9

or bubble baths) or poor personal hygiene (such as wiping from back to front after a bowel movement). Symptoms include redness and itching in the vaginal and vulvar areas and sometimes vaginal discharge. Vulvovaginitis also can be caused by an overgrowth of *Candida*, a fungus normally present in the vagina.

- **Nonmenstrual vaginal bleeding** is most commonly due to the presence of a vaginal foreign body, often wadded-up toilet paper. It may also be due to urethral prolapse, in which the mucous membranes of the urethra protrude into the vagina and form a tiny, doughnut-shaped mass of tissue that bleeds easily. It also can be due to a straddle injury (such as when falling onto a gymnastics beam or bicycle frame) or vaginal trauma from sexual abuse.

- **Labial adhesions**, the sticking together or adherence of the labia in the midline, usually appear in infants and young girls. Although there are usually no symptoms associated with this condition, labial adhesions can lead to an increased risk of urinary tract infection. Sometimes topical estrogen cream is used to help separate the labia.

Problems of the Ovaries and Fallopian Tubes

- **Ectopic pregnancy** occurs when a fertilized egg, or zygote, doesn't travel into the uterus, but instead grows rapidly in the fallopian tube. A woman with this condition can develop severe abdominal pain and should see a doctor because surgery may be necessary.

- **Endometriosis** occurs when tissue normally found only in the uterus starts to grow outside the uterus—in the ovaries, fallopian tubes, or other parts of the pelvic cavity. It can cause abnormal bleeding, painful periods, and general pelvic pain.

- **Ovarian tumors**, although they're rare, can occur. Girls with ovarian tumors may have abdominal pain and masses that can be felt in the abdomen. Surgery may be needed to remove the tumor.

- **Ovarian cysts** are noncancerous sacs filled with fluid or semi-solid material. Although they are common and generally harmless, they can become a problem if they grow very large. Large cysts may push on surrounding organs, causing abdominal pain. In most cases, cysts will disappear on their own and treatment is unnecessary. If the cysts are painful, a doctor may prescribe birth control pills to alter their growth or they may be removed by a surgeon.

- **Polycystic ovary syndrome** is a hormone disorder in which too many male hormones (androgens) are produced by the ovaries. This condition causes the ovaries to become enlarged and develop many fluid-filled sacs, or cysts. It often first appears during the teen years. Depending on the type and severity of the condition, it may be treated with drugs to regulate hormone balance and menstruation.

- **Ovarian torsion**, or the twisting of the ovary, can occur when an ovary becomes twisted because of a disease or a developmental abnormality. The torsion blocks blood from flowing through the blood vessels that supply and nourish the ovaries. The most common symptom is lower abdominal pain. Surgery is usually necessary to correct it.

Menstrual Problems

A variety of menstrual problems can affect girls, including:

- **Dysmenorrhea** is when a girl has painful periods.

- **Menorrhagia** is when a girl has a very heavy periods with excess bleeding.

- **Oligomenorrhea** is when a girl misses or has infrequent periods, even though she's been menstruating for a while and isn't pregnant.

- **Amenorrhea** is when a girl has not started her period by the time she is 16 years old or three years after starting puberty, has not developed signs of puberty by age 14, or has had normal periods but has stopped menstruating for some reason other than pregnancy.

Infections of the Female Reproductive System

- **Sexually transmitted infections (STIs):** These include infections and diseases such as pelvic inflammatory disease (PID), human immunodeficiency virus/acquired immunodeficiency syndrome (HIV/AIDS), human papillomavirus (HPV, or genital warts), syphilis, chlamydia, gonorrhea, and genital herpes (HSV). Most are spread from one person to another by sexual contact.

- **Toxic shock syndrome:** This uncommon illness is caused by toxins released into the body during a type of bacterial infection that is more likely to develop if a tampon is left in too long. It can produce high fever, diarrhea, vomiting, and shock.

If you think your daughter may have symptoms of a problem with her reproductive system or if you have questions about her growth and development, talk to your doctor—many problems with the female reproductive system can be treated.

Section 1.3

Menstruation and the Menstrual Cycle

Excerpted from "Menstruation and the Menstrual Cycle Fact Sheet," U.S. Department of Health and Human Services Office on Women's Health (www.womenshealth.gov), October 21, 2009.

What is menstruation?

Menstruation is a woman's monthly bleeding. When you menstruate, your body sheds the lining of the uterus (womb). Menstrual blood flows from the uterus through the small opening in the cervix and passes out of the body through the vagina. Most menstrual periods last from three to five days.

What is the menstrual cycle?

When periods (menstruations) come regularly, this is called the menstrual cycle. Having regular menstrual cycles is a sign that important parts of your body are working normally. The menstrual cycle provides important body chemicals, called hormones, to keep you healthy. It also prepares your body for pregnancy each month. A cycle is counted from the first day of one period to the first day of the next period. The average menstrual cycle is 28 days long. Cycles can range anywhere from 21 to 35 days in adults and from 21 to 45 days in young teens.

The rise and fall of levels of hormones during the month control the menstrual cycle.

What happens during the menstrual cycle?

In the first half of the cycle, levels of estrogen (the "female hormone") start to rise. Estrogen plays an important role in keeping you healthy, especially by helping you to build strong bones and to help keep them strong as you get older. Estrogen also makes the lining of the uterus (womb) grow and thicken. This lining of the womb is a place that will nourish the embryo if a pregnancy occurs. At the same time the lining of the womb is growing, an egg, or ovum, in one of the ovaries starts to mature. At about day 14 of an average 28-day cycle, the egg leaves the ovary. This is called ovulation.

After the egg has left the ovary, it travels through the fallopian tube to the uterus. Hormone levels rise and help prepare the uterine lining for pregnancy. A woman is most likely to get pregnant during the three days before or on the day of ovulation. Keep in mind, women with cycles that are shorter or longer than average may ovulate before or after day 14.

A woman becomes pregnant if the egg is fertilized by a man's sperm cell and attaches to the uterine wall. If the egg is not fertilized, it will break apart. Then, hormone levels drop, and the thickened lining of the uterus is shed during the menstrual period.

What is a typical menstrual period like?

During your period, you shed the thickened uterine lining and extra blood through the vagina. Your period may not be the same every month. It may also be different than other women's periods. Periods can be light, moderate, or heavy in terms of how much blood comes out of the vagina. This is called menstrual flow. The length of the period also varies. Most periods last from three to five days. But, anywhere from two to seven days is normal.

For the first few years after menstruation begins, longer cycles are common. A woman's cycle tends to shorten and become more regular with age. Most of the time, periods will be in the range of 21 to 35 days apart.

What kinds of problems do women have with their periods?

Women can have a range of problems with their periods, including pain, heavy bleeding, and skipped periods.

Amenorrhea is the lack of a menstrual period. This term is used to describe the absence of a period in the following:

- Young women who haven't started menstruating by age 15

- Women and girls who haven't had a period for 90 days, even if they haven't been menstruating for long

13

Causes can include the following:

- Pregnancy
- Breastfeeding
- Extreme weight loss
- Eating disorders
- Excessive exercising
- Stress
- Serious medical conditions in need of treatment

When your menstrual cycles come regularly, this means that important parts of your body are working normally. In some cases, not having menstrual periods can mean that your ovaries have stopped producing normal amounts of estrogen. Missing these hormones can have important effects on your overall health. Hormonal problems, such as those caused by polycystic ovary syndrome (PCOS) or serious problems with the reproductive organs, may be involved. It's important to talk to a doctor if you have this problem.

Dysmenorrhea is painful periods, including severe cramps. Menstrual cramps in teens are caused by too much of a chemical called prostaglandin. Most teens with dysmenorrhea do not have a serious disease, even though the cramps can be severe. In older women, the pain is sometimes caused by a disease or condition such as uterine fibroids or endometriosis.

For some women, using a heating pad or taking a warm bath helps ease their cramps. Some over-the-counter pain medicines can also help with these symptoms. If these medicines don't relieve your pain or the pain interferes with work or school, you should see a doctor. Treatment depends on what's causing the problem and how severe it is.

Abnormal uterine bleeding is vaginal bleeding that's different from normal menstrual periods. It includes the following:

- Bleeding between periods
- Bleeding after sex
- Spotting anytime in the menstrual cycle
- Bleeding heavier or for more days than normal
- Bleeding after menopause

Abnormal bleeding can have many causes. Your doctor may start by checking for problems that are most common in your age group. Some of them are not serious and are easy to treat. Others can be more serious. Treatment for abnormal bleeding depends on the cause.

In both teens and women nearing menopause, hormonal changes can cause long periods along with irregular cycles. Even if the cause is hormonal changes, you may be able to get treatment. You should keep in mind that these changes can occur with other serious health problems, such as uterine fibroids, polyps, or even cancer. See your doctor if you have any abnormal bleeding.

When does a girl usually get her first period?

In the United States, the average age for a girl to get her first period is 12. This does not mean that all girls start at the same age. A girl can start her period anytime between the ages of 8 and 15. Most of the time, the first period starts about two years after breasts first start to develop. If a girl has not had her first period by age 15, or if it has been more than two to three years since breast growth started, she should see a doctor.

How long does a woman have periods?

Women usually have periods until menopause. Menopause occurs between the ages of 45 and 55, usually around age 50. Menopause means that a woman is no longer ovulating (producing eggs) or having periods and can no longer get pregnant. Like menstruation, menopause can vary from woman to woman and these changes may occur over several years.

The time when your body begins its move into menopause is called the menopausal transition. This can last anywhere from two to eight years. Some women have early menopause because of surgery or other treatment, illness, or other reasons. If you don't have a period for 90 days, you should see your doctor. He or she will check for pregnancy, early menopause, or other health problems that can cause periods to stop or become irregular.

When should I see a doctor about my period?

See your doctor about your period if any of the following are true of you:

- You have not started menstruating by the age of 15.

15

- You have not started menstruating within three years after breast growth began, or if breasts haven't started to grow by age 13.

- Your period suddenly stops for more than 90 days.

- Your periods become very irregular after having had regular, monthly cycles.

- Your period occurs more often than every 21 days or less often than every 35 days.

- You are bleeding for more than seven days.

- You are bleeding more heavily than usual or using more than one pad or tampon every one to two hours.

- You bleed between periods.

- You have severe pain during your period.

- You suddenly get a fever and feel sick after using tampons.

How often should I change my pad and/or tampon?

You should change a pad before it becomes soaked with blood. Each woman decides for herself what works best. You should change a tampon at least every four to eight hours. Make sure to use the lowest absorbency tampon needed for your flow, which decreases your risk for toxic shock syndrome (TSS). TSS is a rare but sometimes deadly disease. TSS is caused by bacteria that can produce toxins. If your body can't fight the toxins, your immune (body defense) system reacts and causes the symptoms of TSS.

Young women may be more likely to get TSS. Using any kind of tampon puts you at greater risk for TSS than using pads. If you have any of the following symptoms of TSS while using tampons, take the tampon out and contact your doctor right away:

- Sudden high fever (over 102 degrees)

- Muscle aches

- Diarrhea

- Vomiting

- Dizziness and/or fainting

- Sunburn-like rash

- Sore throat

- Bloodshot eyes

Section 1.4

Puberty

"Puberty," Eunice K. Shriver National Institute of Child Health
and Human Development (www.nichd.nih.gov), January 22, 2007.

What is puberty?

Puberty is the time in life when a person becomes sexually mature.
It is a physical change that usually happens between ages 10 and 14 for
girls and ages 12 and 16 for boys. Some African American girls start puberty earlier than white girls, making their age range for puberty 9 to 14.

Puberty starts when a part of the brain called the hypothalamus
begins releasing a hormone called gonadotropin releasing hormone
(GnRH). GnRH then signals the pituitary gland to release two more
hormones—luteinizing hormone (LH) and follicle-stimulating hormone
(FSH)—to start sexual development.

A study has identified a gene that appears to be the crucial signal
for the beginning of puberty. Without a functioning copy of the gene,
known as GPR54, humans appear unable to enter puberty normally.

What are the signs of puberty?

Puberty affects boys and girls differently. Puberty in females follows
these characteristics:

- The first sign of puberty is usually breast development.
- Other signs are the growth of hair in the pubic area and
  armpits, and acne.
- Menstruation (or a period) usually happens last.

Puberty in males has these characteristics:

- Puberty usually begins with the testicles and penis getting bigger.
- Then hair grows in the pubic area and armpits.
- Muscles grow, the voice deepens, and acne and facial hair
  develop as puberty continues.

Both boys and girls usually have a growth spurt (a rapid increase in height) that lasts for about two or three years along with the signs listed here. This brings them closer to their adult height, which they reach after puberty.

Does everyone go through puberty the same way?

Puberty can have different patterns, so everyone may not go through puberty in the same way. For example:

- Some children may begin puberty earlier than normal, a condition called precocious puberty. If signs of puberty occur early (before age seven or eight for girls and before age nine for boys), parents and caregivers should talk to their child's health care provider to see if treatment is needed.

- Other children may have delayed puberty, meaning the process begins later than normal. Sometimes there is a reason for puberty starting late; for example, many young girls who are gymnasts start puberty later than those who are not gymnasts. But in many cases, there is no known reason for the delay.

If development is later than normal, parents and caregivers should talk to a health care provider, who can make sure there is not a medical condition causing the delay. But most kids with delayed puberty need no treatment and begin puberty on their own body's time.

Section 1.5

Perimenopause and Menopause

Excerpted from "Menopause Basics,"
U.S. Department of Health and Human Services Office on
Women's Health (www.womenshealth.gov), September 29, 2010.

What is menopause?

Menopause is the point in time when a woman's menstrual periods stop. Menopause happens because the ovaries stop producing the hormones estrogen and progesterone. Once you have gone through menopause, you can't get pregnant anymore. Some people call the years leading up to a woman's last period menopause, but that time actually is the menopausal transition, or perimenopause.

During the time of the menopausal transition, your periods can stop for a while and then start again. Therefore, the only way to know if you have gone through menopause is if you have not had your period for one year. (And it's not menopause if your periods stop for some other reason, like being sick.) The average age of menopause is 51, but for some women it happens as early as 40 or as late as 55.

After you go through menopause, you are considered in the postmenopausal stage of your life. Your female hormones won't go up and down the way they used to with your periods. They will stay at very low levels.

Some women worry about menopause, and it can cause uncomfortable symptoms. But there are many ways to treat symptoms and stay active and strong.

Usually, menopause is natural. That means it happens on its own, and you don't need medical treatment unless your symptoms bother you. Sometimes, though, menopause is medically induced, which means it's caused by an operation or medication. If so, you should work closely with your doctor to feel comfortable and take good care of your health.

What is perimenopause?

Perimenopause, or the menopausal transition, is the time leading up to a woman's last period. Periods can stop and then start again, so you are in perimenopause until a year has passed since you've had a period. During perimenopause a woman will have changes in her levels of estrogen and progesterone, two female hormones made in the ovaries. These changes may lead to symptoms like hot flashes. Some symptoms can last for months or years after a woman's period stops.

There is no way to tell in advance how long it will take you to go through the menopausal transition. It could take between two and eight years.

Sometimes it's hard to tell if you are in the menopausal transition. Symptoms, a physical exam, and your medical history may provide clues to you and your doctor. Your doctor also could test the amount of hormones in your blood. But because hormones change during your menstrual cycle, these tests alone can't tell for sure that you have gone through menopause or are getting close to it. Unless there is a medical reason to test, doctors usually don't recommend it.

If you're still having periods, even if they are not regular, you can get pregnant. Talk to your doctor about birth control.

What are the symptoms of menopause?

Menopause affects every woman differently. Some women have no symptoms, but some women have changes in several areas of their lives. It's not always possible to tell if these changes are related to aging, menopause, or both.

Some changes that might start in the years around menopause include the following:

- **Irregular periods:** Your periods can come more often or less, last more days or fewer, and be lighter or heavier. Do not assume that missing a couple of periods means you are beginning the menopausal transition. Check with your doctor to see if you are pregnant or if there is another medical cause for your missed periods. Also, if you have not had a period for a year and start "spotting," see your doctor. Spotting could be caused by cancer or another health condition.

- **Hot flashes:** These are a sudden feeling of heat in the upper part or all of your body. Your face and neck may become red. Red blotches may appear on your chest, back, and arms. Heavy sweating and cold shivering can follow.

- **Trouble sleeping:** You may find it hard to sleep through the night. You may have night sweats, which are hot flashes that make you perspire while you sleep. You may also feel extra tired during the day.

- **Vaginal and urinary problems:** These problems may start or increase in the time around menopause. The walls of your vagina may get drier and thinner because of lower levels of the hormone estrogen. Estrogen also helps protect the health of your bladder and urethra, the tube that empties your urine. With less estrogen, sex may become less comfortable. You also could have more vaginal infections or urinary tract infections. Some women find it hard to hold their urine long enough to get to the bathroom (which is called urinary urge incontinence). Urine might also leak out when you sneeze, cough, or laugh (called urinary stress incontinence).

- **Mood changes:** You could have mood swings, feel crabby, or have crying spells. If you had mood swings before your monthly periods or if you had depression after giving birth, you may have more mood issues around the time of menopause. Mood changes at this time also could be coming from stress, family changes, or feeling tired. Mood swings are not the same as depression.

- **Changing feelings about sex:** Some women feel less aroused, while others feel more comfortable with their sexuality after menopause. Some women may be less interested in sex because sex can be more physically uncomfortable. Learn about what you can do to address any concerns about sex.

- **Osteoporosis:** This is a condition in which your bones get thin and weak. It can lead to loss of height and broken bones.

- **Other changes:** You might become forgetful or have trouble focusing. Your waist could become larger. You could lose muscle and gain fat. Your joints and muscles also could feel stiff and achy. Experts do not know if some of these changes are a result of the lower estrogen levels of menopause or are a result of growing older.

How does menopause affect your health?

Changes in your body in the years around menopause increase your chances of having certain health problems. Lower levels of estrogen and other changes related to aging (like possibly gaining weight) increase women's risk of heart disease, stroke, and osteoporosis.

There are many important steps you can take to build your health in the years around menopause:

- Eat well. Keep some key points in mind:
  - Older people need just as many nutrients but tend to need fewer calories for energy. Make sure you have a balanced diet.

21

- Women over 50 need 2.4 micrograms (mcg) of vitamin B12 and 1.5 milligrams of vitamin B6 each day. Ask your doctor if you need a vitamin supplement.

- After menopause, a woman's calcium needs go up to maintain bone health. Women 51 and older should get 1,200 milligrams (mg) of calcium each day. Vitamin D also is important to bone health. Women 51 to 70 should get 600 international units (IU) of vitamin D each day. Women ages 71 and older need 800 IU of vitamin D each day.

- Women past menopause who are still having vaginal bleeding because they are using menopausal hormone therapy might need extra iron.

- Be active. Exercise can help your bones, heart, mood, and more. Ask your doctor about what activities are right for you. Aim to do the following:

  - At least 2 hours and 30 minutes a week of moderate aerobic physical activity or 1 hour and 15 minutes of vigorous aerobic activity or some combination of the two

  - Exercises that build muscle strength on two days each week

- Quit smoking. Smoking hurts your health in many ways, including by damaging your bones. Stay away from secondhand smoke and get help quitting if you need it.

- Take care of your gynecological health. You will still need certain tests like a pelvic exam after menopause. Most women need a Pap test every three years. Depending on your health history, you may need a Pap test more often, so check with your doctor. Also, remember to ask how often you need mammograms (breast X-rays).

- Ask your doctor about immunizations and screenings. Discuss blood pressure, bone density, and other tests. Find out about flu and other shots.

Chapter 2

Women's Health Statistics

Women's Health USA 2011

In 2009, females represented 50.7% of the 307 million people residing in the United States. In most age groups, women accounted for approximately half of the population, with the exception of people aged 65 years and older; within this age group, women represented 57.5% of the population. The growing diversity of the U.S. population is reflected in the racial and ethnic distribution of women across age groups. Non-Hispanic black and Hispanic women accounted for 8.9% and 6.9% of the female population aged 65 years and older, but they represented 13.8% and 22.4% of females under 18 years of age, respectively. Non-Hispanic whites accounted for 79.7% of women aged 65 years and older, but only 55.0% of those under 18 years of age. Hispanic women now account for a greater proportion of the female population than they did in 2000, when they made up 17.0% of the population under age 18 and only 4.9% of those 65 years and older.

America's growing diversity underscores the importance of examining and addressing racial and ethnic disparities in health status and the use of health care services. From 2007–2009, 58.1% of non-Hispanic white women reported themselves to be in excellent or very good health, compared to only 40% or less of Hispanic, non-Hispanic

Excerpted from "Women's Health USA 2011," U.S. Department of Health and Human Services, Health Resources and Services Administration (www.hrsa.gov), October 2011, and "FastStats: Women's Health," Centers for Disease Control and Prevention (www.cdc.gov), August 20, 2012.

American Indian/Alaska Native, and non-Hispanic black women. Minority women are disproportionately affected by a number of diseases and health conditions, including HIV/AIDS, sexually transmitted infections, diabetes, and asthma. For instance, in 2009, rates of new HIV cases were highest among non-Hispanic black, non-Hispanic multiple race, non-Hispanic Native Hawaiian/Pacific Islander, and Hispanic females (47.8, 13.4, 13.3, and 11.9 per 100,000 females, respectively), compared to just 2.4 cases per 100,000 non-Hispanic white females.

Hypertension, or high blood pressure, was also more prevalent among non-Hispanic black women than women of other races. From 2005–2008, 39.4% of non-Hispanic black women were found to have high blood pressure, compared to 31.3% of non-Hispanic white, 16.3% of Mexican American, and 19.9% of other Hispanic women.

Diabetes is a chronic condition and a leading cause of death and disability in the United States and is especially prevalent among minority and older adults. From 2007–2009, 14.0% of non-Hispanic American Indian/Alaska Native women and 11.9% of non-Hispanic Native Hawaiian/Other Pacific Islander women reported having been diagnosed with diabetes compared to 6.4% of non-Hispanic white women. Hispanic and non-Hispanic black women also have higher rates of diabetes.

As indigenous populations that share similar histories of disenfranchisement, American Indian/Alaska Natives and Native Hawaiian/Other Pacific Islanders have some health disparities in common related to substance abuse and chronic conditions, like diabetes. However, American Indian/Alaska Native women have especially high rates of injury, while Native Hawaiian/Other Pacific Islanders have higher cancer incidence and mortality.

In addition to race and ethnicity, income and education are important factors that contribute to women's health and access to health care. Regardless of family structure, women are more likely than men to live in poverty. In 2009, poverty rates were highest among women who were heads of their households with no spouse present (27.1%). Poverty rates were also high among non-Hispanic American Indian/Alaska Native, non-Hispanic black, and Hispanic women (25.5%, 24.3%, and 23.8%, respectively). Women in these racial and ethnic groups were also more likely to be heads of households than their non-Hispanic white, non-Hispanic Asian, and non-Hispanic Native Hawaiian/Pacific Islander counterparts.

Many conditions and health risks are more closely linked to education and family income than to race and ethnicity, and differences in poverty tend to explain a large portion of racial and ethnic health differences. For example, healthy choices for diet and exercise may not be as accessible to those with lower incomes and may contribute to higher obesity levels among minority women. From 2005–2008, 40.0% of women with household incomes less than 100% of poverty were obese, compared to 31.1% of women with incomes of 300% or more of poverty.

Sleep disorders, such as insomnia and sleep apnea, were also more common among women with lower household incomes. From 2005–2008, 10.5% of women with household incomes below 100% of poverty had been diagnosed with a sleep disorder, compared to 5.5% of women with incomes of 300% or more of poverty. Oral health status and receipt of oral health care among women also varied dramatically with household income. From 2005–2008, women with household incomes below poverty were three times more likely to have untreated dental decay than women living in households with incomes of 300% or more of poverty (30.3% versus 10.3%, respectively). Less than half of women with incomes below 100% of poverty had received a dental visit in the past year (43.2%), compared to 77.7% of women with household incomes of 400% or more of poverty.

In addition to race and ethnicity and income, disparities in health status and behaviors, as well as health care access, are also observed by sexual orientation. From 2006–2008, only 37.4% of lesbian women received a Pap smear in the past year compared to over 60% of heterosexual and bisexual women. Bisexual women were also less likely than heterosexual women to have health insurance or report excellent or very good health status. Both lesbian and bisexual women reported high rates of smoking and binge drinking.

Although women can expect to live five years longer than men on average, women experience more physically and mentally unhealthy days than men. From 2007–2009, women reported an average of 4.0 days per month that their physical health was not good and 3.9 days per month that their mental health was not good, compared to an average of 3.2 physically unhealthy and 2.9 mentally unhealthy days per month reported among men. Due to their longer life expectancy, women are more likely than men to have certain age-related conditions like Alzheimer disease. Regardless of age, however, women are more likely to have asthma, arthritis, osteoporosis, and activity limitations. For example, 9.2% of women had asthma in 2007–2009, compared to 5.5% of men.

Men, nonetheless, bear a disproportionate burden of other health conditions, such as HIV/AIDS, high blood pressure, and coronary heart disease. In 2008, for instance, the rate of newly reported HIV cases among adolescent and adult males was more than three times the rate among females (32.7 versus 9.8 per 100,000, respectively). Despite the greater risk, however, a smaller proportion of men had ever been tested for HIV than women (36.1% versus 41.0%, respectively). In addition, men were more likely than women to lack health insurance and less likely to have received a preventive checkup in the past year.

Many diseases and health conditions can be avoided or minimized through good nutrition, regular physical activity, and preventive health care. In 2009, 65.8% of women aged 65 years and older reported receiving a flu vaccine; however, this percentage ranged from about 50% of non-Hispanic black and Hispanic women to 69.0% of non-Hispanic white women.

Regular physical activity and a healthy diet have numerous health benefits, such as helping to prevent obesity and chronic conditions like diabetes, heart disease, and certain types of cancer. From 2007–2009, only 14.7% of women participated in at least 2.5 hours of moderate intensity physical activity per week or 1.25 hours of vigorous intensity activity per week in addition to muscle-strengthening activities on two or more days per week. The majority of women (83.1%) also exceeded the recommended daily maximum intake of sodium—a contributor to high blood pressure and cardiovascular and kidney disease.

Not smoking or quitting smoking is another important component to disease prevention and health promotion. Smoking during pregnancy is particularly harmful for both mother and infant. Women with lower incomes and less education are more likely to smoke and less likely to quit, both overall and during pregnancy. Past month smoking rates are also highest among non-Hispanic American Indian/Alaska Native women (41.8%) and lowest among non-Hispanic Asian women (8.3%).

Women's Health Statistics

U.S. Population

- Number of residents (all ages): 155.6 million (2009)

Health Status

- Percent of women 18 years and over in fair or poor health: 13.5%

Health Risk Factors

- Percent of women 18 years and over who met the 2008 federal physical activity guidelines for aerobic activity through leisure-time aerobic activity: 44.6%

- Percent of women 18 years and over who currently smoke: 16.5%
- Percent of women 18 years and over who had five or more drinks in one day at least once in the past year: 13.6%
- Percent of women 20 years and over who are obese: 35.9% (2007–2010)
- Percent of women 20 years and over with hypertension: 32.8% (2007–2010)

Health Insurance Coverage

- Percent of females under 65 years without health insurance coverage: 15.6%

Preventive Care

- Percent of women 40 years and over who had a mammogram within the past two years: 67.1% (2010)
- Percent of women 18 years and over who had a Pap smear within the past three years: 73.2% (2010)

Mortality

- Number of deaths (all ages): 1,219,784
- Deaths per 100,000 population: 784.1
- Leading causes of death:
  - Heart disease
  - Cancer
  - Stroke

Chapter 3

Health Concerns of Women with Disabilities

Even though having a disability sometimes makes it harder to get and stay healthy, do your best to live a healthy lifestyle.

Eating Well

Adopting a healthy eating plan can help you feel better, control your weight, and help prevent illnesses such as heart disease that can cause further disability. Still, eating well isn't always easy. Depending on the type of disability a person has, some of the barriers to eating well might include the following:

- **Difficulty shopping:** Limited mobility can make it hard for some people to get to a grocery store or reach products that are stacked or on high shelves.

- **Difficulty preparing healthy meals:** Washing and preparing fresh produce and meats can be hard for people with certain physical limitations or a condition that causes shakiness. Cooking also can take a lot of time. Some people might lack the energy needed to prepare and cook a healthy meal.

- **Problems chewing or swallowing**

Excerpted from "Staying Healthy," U.S. Department of Health and Human Services Office on Women's Health (www.womenshealth.gov), September 22, 2009.

People who rely on others for food shopping and cooking face additional barriers. Caregivers must know how and be willing to plan and prepare healthy meals. People who live in a group residence that provides dining services might not be able to choose the foods that are served. People who rely on a personal caregiver might also have limited say over the types of food served. For instance, rather than prepare fresh foods, a caregiver might use less healthy, ready-to-serve products because they can be prepared in advance and then easily reheated when the caregiver is no longer there.

The good news is that even small changes can affect the quality of the food you eat. Here are some examples:

- Simple changes in the home can make cooking safer and easier. Some examples are hanging a mirror above stove burners so you can watch cooking while sitting; using a rolling utility cart to move things without fear of spilling or breaking; and using knives, plates, and other products designed for single-handed use.

- Attend classes to learn how to shop for healthy foods and stretch your food dollar.

- Learn to cook simple recipes that involve only a few ingredients.

- Ask your caregiver to prepare more fruits and vegetables and fewer unhealthy foods.

Physical Activity

Being physically active is an important part of a healthy lifestyle for all women, including women with disabilities. If you have a disability, getting regular physical activity can help you stay independent by preventing illnesses such as heart disease that can make it more difficult to take care of yourself. Being physically active also can help you to tone the muscles you use less often because of your disability. For instance, if you're in a wheelchair, you probably have strong arms from pushing yourself around. But it's also important to exercise your other muscles, including your leg muscles. Being active also can improve your mood and help you feel better about yourself.

According to the *2008 Physical Activity Guidelines for Americans*, adults with disabilities, who are able to, should do the following each week:

- 2 hours and 30 minutes of moderate-intensity aerobic physical activity **or**

- 1 hour and 15 minutes of vigorous-intensity aerobic physical activity **or**

- a combination of moderate and vigorous-intensity aerobic physical activity **and**

- muscle-strengthening activities on two or more days.

Try to spread aerobic activity throughout the week and make sure you spend at least ten minutes in a session.

If you are not able to meet these guidelines, try to engage in regular physical activity according to your abilities and avoid inactivity.

But before you start, talk to your doctor about the amount and types of physical activity that are okay for you to do. With your doctor's okay, start slowly and work your way up to a more intense routine as you become more physically fit.

Mental Health

Between family life and work life, today's woman can feel pulled in many directions. Living with a disability can make coping with everyday life even harder. It also can put you at risk for depression. Learning healthy ways of coping will help you handle day-to-day stress, as well as any tough times you face. Healthy ways of coping include the following:

- Take time each day to relax and unwind. This could be as simple as enjoying a cup of coffee and a good book.

- Work out, which in addition to physical benefits can relieve tension and boost your mood.

- Have someone outside the home to talk to. Healthy relationships can serve as a source of encouragement and also protect you against isolation and loneliness. Support groups can put you in touch with people who face similar challenges.

- Volunteering is a great way to get involved and help others in need.

If you find that emotional problems interfere with daily living or your ability or desire to care for yourself, talk to your doctor. Treatment such as talk therapy or medicine can help you to feel good again.

Substance Abuse

The rates of substance abuse among people with disabilities are about two to four times greater than that of the general population.

Some reasons people with disabilities might abuse alcohol or drugs are the following:

- To cope with social isolation
- To ease frustration
- To lessen long-lasting pain

Alcohol and drug abuse can be very harmful to a woman's health and well-being. Women who abuse these substances are at higher risk of the following:

- Sexual assault
- Unprotected sex
- Unplanned pregnancies
- Sexually transmitted infections, including HIV/AIDS
- Infertility

Alcohol and drugs also can cause dangerous interactions with prescription drugs a woman might be using. Substance abuse also is a major reason that most adults with disabilities are unemployed.

If you have a substance abuse problem, be sure to talk to your doctor and get into a treatment program. Many substance abuse treatment programs can accommodate people with disabilities.

Healthy Aging

Well over half of all women older than 65 are living with a disability that limits to some extent what they can do. This means that as you age, you might need to learn new ways of doing things or need more help from others.

People with long-term disabilities also have special health concerns as they age. Many people with long-term disabilities face problems common in aging people sooner than other aging adults. This means that people with long-term disabilities might face problems in their forties that other adults don't usually face until their sixties. New problems with pain, fatigue, and weakness also can come up, making it harder to work, get around, or take care of routine household chores and personal care. Although changes in function are common, they are not always normal. Functional changes should always be checked out by a doctor. Often, new problems are the cause of new pain, fatigue, and weakness and can be treated.

Caregiving is another concern for aging people with long-term disabilities. People who were once living independently might need more help than a spouse or other family member can provide. Aging adults with some long-term disabilities, such as intellectual disability or cerebral palsy, often outlive their primary caregivers. Thinking about future caregiving needs and advanced planning is especially important for people with disabilities.

Abuse

Research has shown that women with disabilities have a higher risk of emotional, physical, and sexual abuse than do women without disabilities. Along with common types of abuse such as verbal abuse or rape, women with disabilities can also face disability-related abuse, such as withholding of wheelchairs or refusal to help with personal tasks. Research also shows that women with disabilities who have been abused are more likely to be abused longer and by multiple people than women who do not have disabilities.

Get help if you are a victim of assault or if you are being abused by someone you rely on for help with daily living. You are not at fault. You did not cause the abuse to occur. If you can, reach out to someone close to you, such as a family member, a caretaker, a good friend, or a neighbor, and ask for help. Or call the National Domestic Violence Hotline at 800-799-SAFE (7233).

Chapter 4

Lesbian and Bisexual Health Concerns

What does it mean to be a lesbian or bisexual?

A lesbian is a woman who is sexually attracted to another woman or who has sex with another woman, even if it is only sometimes. A lesbian is currently only having sex with a woman, even if she has had sex with men in the past. A bisexual person is sexually attracted to, or sexually active with, both men and women.

What are important health issues that lesbians and bisexual women should discuss with their health care professionals?

All women have specific health risks and can take steps to improve their health through regular medical care and healthy living. Research tells us that lesbian and bisexual women are at a higher risk for certain problems than other women.

- **Heart disease:** Heart disease is the number one killer of all women. The more risk factors you have, the greater the chance that you will develop heart disease. There are some risk factors that you cannot control, such as age, family health history, and race. But you can protect yourself from heart disease by not smoking, by controlling your blood pressure and cholesterol, by

Excerpted from "Lesbian and Bisexual Health Fact Sheet," U.S. Department of Health and Human Services Office on Women's Health (www.womenshealth.gov), February 17, 2011.

exercising, and by eating well. Lesbians and bisexual women have a higher rate of obesity, smoking, and stress.

- **Cancer:** The most common cancers for all women are breast, lung, colon, uterine, and ovarian. Several factors put lesbian and bisexual women at higher risk for developing some cancers:

  - Lesbians are less likely than heterosexual women to have had a full-term pregnancy. Hormones released during pregnancy and breastfeeding are thought to protect women against breast, endometrial, and ovarian cancers.

  - Lesbians and bisexual women are less likely to get routine screenings, such as a Pap test, which can prevent or detect cervical cancer.

  - Lesbians and bisexual women are less likely than other women to get routine mammograms and clinical breast exams.

  - Lesbians are more likely to smoke than heterosexual women are, and bisexual women are the most likely to smoke.

- **Depression and anxiety:** Lesbian and bisexual women report higher rates of depression and anxiety than other women do. Depression and anxiety in lesbian and bisexual women may be due to the following:

  - Social stigma
  - Rejection by family members
  - Abuse and violence
  - Unfair treatment in the legal system
  - Stress from hiding some or all parts of one's life
  - Lack of health insurance

- **Polycystic ovary syndrome (PCOS):** PCOS is the most common hormonal problem of the reproductive system in women of childbearing age. PCOS affects 5% to 10% of women of childbearing age. Lesbians may have a higher rate of PCOS than heterosexual women.

What factors put lesbians' and bisexual women's health at risk?

There are a lot of things that can cause health problems for lesbians and bisexual women. Some of these may be outside of your control.

Other things you can work to improve upon:

- **Lack of fitness:** Being obese and not exercising can raise your risk of heart disease, some cancers, and early death. Many studies show that lesbians and bisexual women have a higher body mass index (BMI) than other women. Some studies also suggest that lesbians think less about weight issues than heterosexual women do.

- **Smoking:** Smoking can lead to heart disease and cancers of the lung, throat, stomach, colon, and cervix. The group of women most likely to smoke is bisexual women.

- **Alcohol and drug abuse:** Substance abuse is a serious health problem for all people in the United States. Recent data suggests that substance use among lesbians—mostly alcohol use—has gone down over the past two decades. But heavy drinking and drug abuse appear to be more common among lesbians (especially young women) than heterosexual women. Lesbian and bisexual women are also more likely to drink alcohol and smoke marijuana in moderation than other women are. Bisexual women are the most likely to have injected drugs, putting them at a higher risk for sexually transmitted infections (STIs).

- **Domestic violence:** Domestic violence can occur in lesbian relationships (as it does in heterosexual ones). But lesbian victims are more likely to stay silent about the violence. There are many resources available to women who are victims of domestic violence.

Are lesbian and bisexual women at risk of getting sexually transmitted infections?

Women who have sex with women are at risk for STIs. Lesbian and bisexual women can transmit STIs to each other through the following:

- Skin-to-skin contact
- Mucosa contact (e.g., mouth to vagina)
- Vaginal fluids
- Menstrual blood
- Sharing sex toys

Some STIs are more common among lesbians and bisexual women and may be passed easily from woman to woman (such as bacterial vaginosis). Other STIs are much less likely to be passed from woman to woman through sex (such as HIV). When lesbians get these less common STIs, it may be because they also have had sex with men, especially when they were younger. It is also important to remember that some of the less common STIs may not be passed between women during sex, but through sharing needles used to inject drugs. Bisexual women may be more likely to get infected with STIs that are less common for lesbians, since bisexuals have typically had sex with men in the past or are presently having sex with a man.

What challenges do lesbian and bisexual women face in the health care system?

Lesbians and bisexual women face unique problems within the health care system that can hurt their health. Many health care professionals have not had enough training to know the specific health issues that lesbians and bisexuals face. They may not ask about sexual orientation when taking personal health histories. Things that can stop lesbians and bisexual women from getting good health care include the following:

- Being scared to tell your doctor about your sexuality or your sexual history

- Having a doctor who does not know your disease risks or the issues that affect lesbians and bisexual women

- Not having health insurance (many lesbians and bisexuals don't have domestic partner benefits, which means that one person does not qualify to get health insurance through the plan the partner has)

- Not knowing that lesbians are at risk for STIs and cancer

For these reasons, lesbian and bisexual women often avoid routine health exams. They sometimes even delay seeking health care when feeling sick. It is important to be proactive about your health, even if you have to try different doctors before you find the right one. Early detection—such as finding cancer early before it spreads—gives you the best chance to do something about it.

What can lesbian and bisexual women do to protect their health?

Find a doctor who is sensitive to your needs and will help you get regular checkups: The Gay and Lesbian Medical Association provides online health care referrals. You can access its provider directory (at www.glma.org) or contact the association at 202-600-8037.

Get a Pap test: The Pap test finds changes in your cervix early, so you can be treated before a problem becomes serious.

Get an HPV test: Combined with a Pap test, an HPV test helps prevent cervical cancer. It can detect the types of HPV that cause cervical cancer.

Talk to your doctor or nurse about other screening tests you may need: You need regular preventive screenings to stay healthy.

Practice safer sex: Get tested for STIs before starting a sexual relationship. If you are unsure about a partner's status, practice methods to reduce the chances of sharing vaginal fluid, semen, or blood.

Eat a balanced, healthy diet: Your diet should include a variety of whole grains, fruits, and vegetables. These foods give you energy, plus vitamins, minerals, and fiber. Reduce the amount of sodium you eat to less than 2,300 mg per day.

Drink moderately: If you drink alcohol, don't have more than one drink per day.

Get moving: An active lifestyle can help any woman. You will benefit most from about 2 hours and 30 minutes of moderate-intensity aerobic physical activity each week.

Don't smoke: If you do smoke, try to quit. Avoid secondhand smoke as much as you can.

Try different things to deal with your stress: Stress from discrimination and from loneliness is hard for every lesbian and bisexual woman. Relax using deep breathing, yoga, meditation, and massage therapy. You can also take a few minutes to sit and listen to soft music or read a book. Talk to your friends or get help from a mental health professional if you need it.

Get help for domestic violence: Call the police or leave if you or your children are in danger. Call a crisis hotline or the National Domestic Violence Hotline at 800-799-SAFE or TDD 800-787-3224.

Chapter 5

Violence against Women and How to Get Help

What is domestic and intimate partner violence?

Domestic violence is when one person in a relationship purposely hurts another person physically or emotionally. Domestic violence is also called intimate partner violence because it often is caused by a husband, ex-husband, boyfriend, or ex-boyfriend. Women also can be abusers.

People of all races, education levels, and ages experience domestic abuse. In the United States, more than five million women are abused by an intimate partner each year.

Domestic violence includes the following:

- Physical abuse like hitting, shoving, kicking, biting, or throwing things

- Emotional abuse like yelling, controlling what you do, or threatening to cause serious problems for you

- Sexual abuse like forcing you to do something sexual you don't want to do

Here are some key points about domestic and intimate partner violence:

Excerpted from "Domestic and Intimate Partner Violence," U.S. Department of Health and Human Services Office on Women's Health (www.womenshealth.gov), May 18, 2011.

41

- If you are in immediate danger, you can call 911. It is possible for the police to arrest an abuser and to escort you and your children to a safe place.

- Often, abuse starts as emotional abuse and then becomes physical later. It's important to get help early.

- Your partner may try to make you feel like the abuse is your fault. Remember that you cannot make someone mistreat you. The abuser is responsible for his or her behavior.

- Violence can cause serious physical and emotional problems, including depression and posttraumatic stress disorder.

- There probably will be times when your partner is very kind. Unfortunately, abusers often begin the mistreatment again after these periods of calm. In fact, over time, abuse often gets worse, not better. Even if your partner promises to stop the abuse, make sure to learn about hotlines and other ways to get help for abuse.

- An abusive partner needs to get help from a mental health professional. But even if he or she gets help, the abuse may not stop.

How can you get help for domestic abuse?

If you are being abused, get help. The longer the abuse goes on, the more damage it can cause. You are not alone. There are people who will believe you and who want to help.

Consider these steps if you are in an abusive situation:

- If you are in immediate danger, call 911 or leave.

- If you are hurt, go to a local hospital emergency room.

- Call the National Domestic Violence Hotline at 800-799-SAFE (7233) or 800-787-3224 (TDD). The hotline offers help in many languages 24 hours a day, every day. Hotline staff can give you the phone numbers of local shelters and other resources.

- Plan ahead. Violence sometimes gets worse right after leaving, so think about a safe place to go.

- Look up state resources for a list of local places to get help.

- Review a full checklist of items to take if you leave, such as your marriage license, any children's birth certificates, and money. Put these things somewhere you can get them quickly. Of course, if you are in immediate danger, leave without them.

- Have a cell phone handy. Try not to call for help from your home phone or a shared cell phone since an abuser may be able to trace the numbers.

- Contact your state's family court for information about getting a court order of protection. If you need legal help but don't have much money, your local domestic violence agency may be able to help you find a lawyer who will work for free.

- Create a code word to use with friends and family to let them know you are in danger. If possible, agree on a secret location where they can pick you up.

- If you can, hide an extra set of car keys so you can leave if your partner takes away your keys.

- When you leave, try to bring any evidence of abuse, like threatening notes from your partner or copies of police reports.

- Reach out to someone you trust—a family member, friend, co-worker, or spiritual leader. Look into ways to get emotional help, like a support group or mental health professional.

Sometimes a woman may hit a man first, and then she ends up getting hurt badly because the man is stronger. Talk to your doctor or a mental health professional if you sometimes hit or use other kinds of violence.

What services are offered by domestic violence shelters?

Domestic violence shelters can give you and your children temporary housing, food and other basic items, and help finding other assistance. Usually you can stay at a shelter for free.

Transitional housing focuses on giving families a safe space and time to recover from domestic violence. Families live independently, in separate apartments, while they also receive needed services.

How does domestic abuse affect children?

Children living in a home where there is abuse may overhear adults fighting, see bruises after the abuse is over, or witness the actual abuse. These experience can have serious effects, including behavior problems, guilt, and mental and physical health problems.

In addition, children who see abuse at home are likely to think that abuse is a normal part of relationships. They are more likely than other children to abuse someone or be abused when they grow up.

If you are being abused and have children, you can take steps to help them:

- Get help for your children by getting help for yourself. Contact the National Domestic Violence Hotline for information about leaving an abusive situation or taking care of yourself and your children if you are not ready to leave.

- Talk to a health professional, like a pediatrician or a counselor.

- Be supportive and available to listen to your children.

- Make sure children know that the abuse is not their fault.

- Tell children to stay away if you are being hit.

- See if you can find ways to reduce your stress, like getting emotional support from a friend.

You also can get help from the court system. Your local domestic violence agency can help you understand your options and find a lawyer. Court options include the following:

- A court order of protection can keep an abuser away from you and your children. If you get an order that protects your children, give a copy to their school.

- A custody order can say that your children will live with you and not your partner. If your children are going to see their father, they may be able to see him at a visitation center, which is set up to be safe.

- An order can make the abuser pay child support.

Sometimes, abuse begins when you are pregnant. Abuse can cause serious health problems for a baby even before it is born. Also, some men try to stop their partners from using birth control. Talk to your doctor about protecting your health and about birth control that you can use without your partner knowing.

Is there a connection between violence against women and HIV risk?

Domestic violence and HIV are connected in a number of ways:

- If you are currently in an abusive relationship, you are more likely to get HIV. That's partly because abusive men are more likely to have sexual partners other than their wife. Also, if you are in an abusive relationship, your partner may force you to have sex, and forced sex can cause cuts that can let HIV enter your body.

- If you were physically or sexually abused as a child, you have an increased risk of getting HIV. That's because women who were abused as children are more likely to have a higher number of sex partners.

- Women with HIV may be at risk of violence when they tell a partner about their HIV status.

Why do some women choose to stay in an abusive relationship?

There are many reasons why a woman may stay in an abusive relationship. She may have little or no money and worry about supporting herself and her children. It may be hard for her to contact friends and family who could help her. Or she may feel too frightened, confused, or embarrassed to leave.

If you are in an abusive relationship and are not sure if you are ready to leave, keep these in mind:

- Abuse often gets worse. It may be possible for a partner to change, but it takes work and time.

- You deserve to be safe and happy.

- Even if you are not ready to leave, you can still contact a domestic violence hotline or a local shelter for support, safety planning, and services.

- People want to help. Many services are available at no cost, including childcare, temporary housing, job training, and legal aid.

- You need support. Reach out to people you trust.

If a friend or loved one is not leaving an abusive relationship, you may feel frustrated at times. Remember that your friend needs your support.

Part Two

Maintaining Women's Health and Wellness

Chapter 6

Nutrition and Exercise Recommendations

Chapter Contents

Section 6.1

Nutrition and Vitamins for Women

Excerpted from "The Healthy Woman: A Complete Guide for All Ages: Nutrition," U.S. Department of Health and Human Services Office on Women's Health (www.womenshealth.gov), November 1, 2008, and "Vitamins," U.S. Department of Health and Human Services Office on Women's Health (www.womenshealth.gov), June 17, 2008.

The Healthy Woman: Nutrition for Women

Life can be hectic, and sometimes it's hard to take the time to make healthy food choices. But making wise food choices—along with regular physical activity—can offer big benefits, now and in the future. Good nutrition may help you lower your risk of some chronic diseases, have healthy pregnancies and healthy babies, and reach and stay at a healthy body weight. Healthy eating habits can help you feel your best—today and every day.

Healthy Eating Plan

You might feel confused by all the conflicting information you hear about what to eat. But, in reality, a healthy eating plan can help you make wise food choices. A healthy eating plan includes the following:

- Fruits and vegetables
- Whole grains
- Fat-free or low-fat versions of milk, cheese, yogurt, and other milk products
- Lean meats, poultry, fish, dry beans and peas, eggs, and nuts

What should you limit? Your healthy eating plan should be low in the following:

- Saturated fat
- Trans fat
- Cholesterol

50

- Salt (sodium)

- Added sugars

- Alcohol

If you're a vegetarian, you can still have a healthy eating plan, even if you avoid some foods.

Healthy eating also means there's a balance between the number of calories you eat and the number of calories you burn. Your body burns calories two ways:

- Through daily routine activities and body functions, such as sitting, moving around, breathing, and digesting

- With physical activity, such as walking, biking, or other forms of exercise

Getting Personalized Recommendations about Eating

Where can you turn for reliable information, tailored to your needs? Here are two options.

- You can use the ChooseMyPlate food guidance system, a system developed by the U.S. Department of Agriculture (USDA) to help Americans make healthy food choices. At ChooseMyPlate.gov, you can get a food plan based on your age, weight, height, sex, and activity level.

- You can see a registered dietitian for a personalized nutrition plan. Your doctor can provide a referral. Or you can contact the American Dietetic Association for the name of a dietitian near you.

Tips for Making Wise Food Choices

A calorie is a measure of the energy used by the body and of the energy that food supplies to the body. Carbohydrates, proteins, fats, and alcohol all have calories. Your caloric needs are determined by your age, your size, how physically active you are, whether you are pregnant or breastfeeding, and other special conditions. Your caloric needs also depend on whether you want to lose or gain weight or keep your weight where it is.

Nutrients are substances found in food that nourish your body. Carbohydrates, proteins, and fats are all nutrients. Vitamins and minerals are also nutrients. It's best to get nutrients from foods instead of vitamin and mineral supplements because foods provide a number of other substances that keep you healthy. But sometimes you might need to take a supplement, such as when you're pregnant.

Grains: Make sure at least half of your grain choices are whole grain. Examples of grain foods are cereals, breads, crackers, and pasta. Check the list of ingredients for grain foods that list "whole" or "whole grain" as the first ingredient, such as whole wheat flour in bread. Whole grains haven't lost any fiber or nutrients from processing. They help meet your nutrient needs, as do foods made from enriched grains.

Vegetables: Choose a variety of vegetables, including the following:

- Dark green vegetables, such as broccoli, kale, and collard greens

- Orange vegetables, such as carrots, sweet potatoes, and pumpkin

- Dry beans and peas, such as pinto beans, kidney beans, black beans, garbanzo beans, split peas, and lentils

Fruits: For most of your fruit servings, choose a variety of fruits (without added sugars) in various forms, such as fresh, frozen, canned, or dried. For example, try fresh apples, frozen blueberries, canned peaches, or dried apricots. Look for canned fruit packed in water or 100% fruit juice, instead of syrup. Go easy on fruit juice because it lacks fiber. If you do have fruit juice, make sure it's 100% fruit juice.

Milk, cheese, and yogurt: Choose low-fat or fat-free milk, cheese, and yogurt. If you have lactose intolerance, you can still get calcium from reduced-lactose milk, other milk products, and non-dairy sources of calcium. Many people with lactose intolerance can eat small amounts of milk, cheese, yogurt, and other milk products without discomfort. If you can't or don't consume milk, cheese, or yogurt, choose other sources of calcium, such as calcium-fortified soy drinks, calcium-fortified tofu, collard greens, or fortified ready-to-eat cereals.

Meat, beans, and other foods high in protein: Choose low-fat or lean meats and poultry, such as chicken without the skin, or top round (a lean cut of beef). Prepare meat, fish, and poultry using low-fat cooking methods, such as baking, broiling, or grilling. Vary your protein choices. Try fish, beans, peas, nuts, and seeds. For example, try making a main dish without meat for dinner, such as pasta with beans, at least once a week.

Fats: Everyone needs some fat as part of a healthful diet. Fats should provide about 20% to 35% of your daily calories. Even though some fats are heart-healthy, they are still high in calories. Limit serving sizes of all fats.

- Choose heart-healthy fats (foods with monounsaturated fats and polyunsaturated fatty acids, such as salmon or corn oil). Most of the fat you eat should come from vegetable oils, nuts, and fish. For example, cook with canola oil. Snack on nuts. Have fish for dinner.

- Limit how often you have heart-harmful fats (foods with saturated fat, trans fat, and cholesterol, such as bacon, whole milk, and foods with hydrogenated or partially hydrogenated fats). Limit how often you have fats that are solid at room temperature and the foods that contain them, such as fatty cuts of meat.

Salt (sodium): Limit your sodium to less than 2,300 milligrams each day. Choose foods with little sodium. Fruits, vegetables, dry beans and peas, and fresh meat, poultry, and fish are naturally low in sodium. You can also check the Nutrition Facts label on food packages. Many processed foods are high in sodium. Try to cut back on how much salt you add while you cook and at the table.

Added sugars: Limit the amount of foods and drinks you consume with added sugars, such as cakes, cookies, regular soft drinks, and candy. Check the Nutrition Facts label to find added sugars. The Nutrition Facts label lists the total sugars content. However, the total includes naturally occurring sugar, such as the sugar in fruit, plus added sugar.

How to Start Changing the Way You Eat

Sometimes it's hard to change habits. But making a change step by step can help.

- Choose one small change you'd like to make.

- Make your idea as specific and realistic as possible. For example, instead of saying, "I will eat more high-fiber food," say, "I will have an orange three days a week for breakfast."

- Decide on when you will make this change, choosing a short period of time. For example, set a goal for this week.

- Write down your plan.

- When your idea has become a regular habit, choose something new to try.

Vitamins

Vitamins are substances found in foods that your body needs for growth and health. There are 13 vitamins your body needs. Each vitamin has specific jobs.

Vitamin A: Found in kale, broccoli, spinach, carrots, squash, sweet potatoes, liver, eggs, whole milk, cream, and cheese.

- Needed for vision
- Helps your body fight infections
- Helps keep your skin healthy

Vitamin B1: Found in yeasts, ham and other types of pork, liver, peanuts, whole-grain and fortified cereals and breads, and milk.

- Helps your body use carbohydrates for energy
- Good for your nervous system

Vitamin B2: Found in liver, eggs, cheese, milk, leafy green vegetables, peas, navy beans, lima beans, and whole-grain breads.

- Helps your body use proteins, carbohydrates, and fats
- Helps keep your skin healthy

Vitamin B3: Found in liver, yeast, bran, peanuts, lean red meats, fish, and poultry.

- Helps your body use proteins, carbohydrates, and fats
- Good for your nervous system and skin

Vitamin B5: Found in beef, chicken, lobster, milk, eggs, peanuts, peas, beans, lentils, broccoli, yeast, and whole grains.

- Helps your body use carbohydrates and fats
- Helps your body make red blood cells

Vitamin B6: Found in liver, whole grains, egg yolk, peanuts, bananas, carrots, and yeast.

- Helps your body use proteins and fats
- Good for your nervous system
- Helps your blood carry oxygen

Vitamin B9 (folic acid or folate): Found in green leafy vegetables, liver, yeast, beans, peas, oranges, and fortified cereals and grain products.

- Helps your body make and maintain new cells
- Prevents some birth defects

Vitamin B12: Found in milk, eggs, liver, poultry, clams, sardines, flounder, herring, eggs, blue cheese, cereals, nutritional yeast, and foods fortified with vitamin B12, including cereals, soy-based beverages, and veggie burgers.

- Helps your body make red blood cells
- Good for your nervous system

Vitamin C: Found in broccoli, green and red peppers, spinach, Brussels sprouts, oranges, grapefruits, tomatoes, potatoes, papayas, strawberries, and cabbage.

- Needed for healthy bones, blood vessels, and skin

Vitamin D: Found in fish liver oil and milk and cereals fortified with vitamin D. Your body may make enough vitamin D if you are exposed to sunlight for about 5 to 30 minutes at least twice a week.

- Needed for healthy bones

Vitamin E: Found in wheat germ oil, fortified cereals, egg yolk, beef liver, fish, milk, vegetable oils, nuts, fruits, peas, beans, broccoli, and spinach.

- Helps prevent cell damage
- Helps blood flow
- Helps repair body tissues

Vitamin H (biotin): Found in liver, egg yolk, soy flour, cereals, yeast, peas, beans, nuts, tomatoes, nuts, green leafy vegetables, and milk.

- Helps your body use carbohydrates and fats
- Needed for growth of many cells

Vitamin K: Found in alfalfa, spinach, cabbage, cheese, spinach, broccoli, Brussels sprouts, kale, cabbage, tomatoes, and plant oils. Your body usually makes all the vitamin K you need.

- Helps in blood clotting
- Helps form bones

Section 6.2

Folic Acid

Excerpted from "Folic Acid Fact Sheet," U.S. Department of Health and Human Services Office on Women's Health (www.womenshealth.gov), May 18, 2010.

What is folic acid?

Folic acid is a B vitamin. It helps the body make healthy new cells. "Folic acid" and "folate" mean the same thing. Folic acid is a man-made form of folate. Folate is found naturally in some foods. Most women do not get all the folic acid they need through food alone.

Who needs folic acid?

All people need folic acid. But folic acid is very important for women who are able to get pregnant. When a woman has enough folic acid in her body before and during pregnancy, it can prevent major birth defects, including the following:

- **Spina bifida** occurs when an unborn baby's spinal column does not close to protect the spinal cord. As a result, the nerves that control leg movements and other functions do not work. Children with spina bifida often have lifelong disabilities. They may also need many surgeries.

- **Anencephaly** is when most or all of the brain does not develop. Babies with this problem die before or shortly after birth.

The results of some studies suggest that folic acid might also help to prevent other types of birth defects.

Folic acid also helps keep your blood healthy. Not getting enough can cause anemia. Experts think that folic acid might also play a role in heart health and preventing cell changes that may lead to cancer. More research is needed to know this for certain.

How much folic acid do women need?

Women able to get pregnant need 400 to 800 mcg, or micrograms, of folic acid every day, even if they are not planning to get pregnant. (This is the same as 0.4 to 0.8 mg, or milligrams.) That way, if they do become pregnant, their babies will be less likely to have birth defects. Talk with your doctor about how much folic acid you need in the following situations:

- You are pregnant or are planning to become pregnant. Pregnant women need 400 to 800 mcg of folic acid in the very early stages of pregnancy often before they know they are pregnant. A pregnant woman should keep taking folic acid throughout pregnancy. Some doctors prescribe prenatal vitamins that contain higher amounts of folic acid.

- You are breastfeeding. Breastfeeding women need 500 mcg. Some doctors suggest that breastfeeding women keep taking their prenatal vitamins to be sure they are getting plenty of folic acid while they are breastfeeding and should they become pregnant again.

- You had a baby with a birth defect of the brain or spine and want to get pregnant again. Your doctor may give you a prescription for 4,000 mcg of folic acid. That is 10 times the normal dose. Taking this high dose of folic acid can lower the risk of having another baby with these birth defects.

- You have a family member with spina bifida. Your doctor may give you a prescription for 4,000 mcg folic acid.

- You have spina bifida and want to get pregnant.

Some people also need more folic acid. Talk to your doctor about how much folic acid you need in the following situations:

- If you are taking medicines used to treat any of the following conditions:

  - Epilepsy

  - Type 2 diabetes

  - Rheumatoid arthritis, lupus, psoriasis, asthma, or inflammatory bowel disease

57

- If you have kidney disease and are on dialysis
- If you have liver disease
- If you have sickle cell disease
- If you have celiac disease
- If you often consume more than one alcoholic drink a day

I don't plan on getting pregnant right now, and I am using birth control. Do I still need folic acid?

Yes. Birth defects of the brain and spine happen in the very early stages of pregnancy, often before a woman knows she is pregnant. By the time she finds out she is pregnant, it might be too late to prevent those birth defects. Also, half of all pregnancies in the United States are not planned. For these reasons, all women who are able to get pregnant need 400 to 800 mcg of folic acid every day.

How can I be sure I get enough folic acid each day?

Women can get enough folic acid by taking a vitamin pill every day. If you have a hard time swallowing pills, you might try a chewable or liquid product that has folic acid. Most U.S. multivitamins have at least 400 micrograms (mcg) of folic acid. Check the label on the bottle to be sure. Or you can take a pill that only contains folic acid. When choosing a brand of vitamins, look for "USP" or "NSF" on the label. These "seals of approval" mean that the pills have been made properly and contain the amounts of vitamins stated on the label. Please note, if you already are taking a daily prenatal vitamin, you probably are getting all the folic acid you need. Check the label to be sure.

What foods contain folic acid?

Folic acid is found naturally in some foods, including leafy vegetables, citrus fruits, beans (legumes), and whole grains. Folic acid is added to foods that are labeled "enriched," such as the following:

- Breakfast cereals (some have 100% of the Daily Value of folic acid in each serving)
- Breads
- Flours
- Pastas

- Cornmeal

- White rice

Check the label on the package to see if the food has folic acid. The label will tell you how much folic acid is in each serving. Sometimes, the label will say "folate" instead of folic acid.

Can I get enough folic acid through food alone?

The body does not use the natural form of folic acid (folate) as easily as the man-made form. We cannot be sure that eating foods that contain folate would have the same benefits as consuming folic acid. Also, even if you eat a healthy, well-balanced diet, you might not get all the nutrients you need every day from food alone. In the United States, most women who eat foods enriched with folic acid are still not getting all that they need. That's why it's important to take a vitamin with folic acid every day.

Can women get too much folic acid?

You can't get too much folic acid from foods that naturally contain it. But unless your doctor tells you otherwise, do not consume more than 1,000 mcg of folic acid a day. Consuming too much folic acid can hide signs that a person is lacking vitamin B12, which can cause nerve damage. Lacking vitamin B12 is rare among women of childbearing age. Plus, most prenatal vitamins also contain B12 to help women get all that they need. People at risk of not having enough vitamin B12 are mainly people 50 years and older and people who eat no animal products.

I am no longer of childbearing age. How much folic acid do I need?

Older adults need 400 mcg of folic acid every day for good health. But older adults need to be sure they also are getting enough vitamin B12. Too much folic acid can hide signs that a person is lacking vitamin B12. People older than 50 are at increased risk of not having enough vitamin B12. If you are 50 or older, ask your doctor what vitamins and supplements you might need.

Section 6.3

Physical Activity Guidelines for Women

Excerpted from "Physical Activity (Exercise) Fact Sheet,"
U.S. Department of Health and Human Services Office on Women's
Health (www.womenshealth.gov), February 26, 2009.

How can physical activity improve my health?

The 2008 *Physical Activity Guidelines for Americans* state that an active lifestyle can lower your risk of early death from a variety of causes. There is strong evidence that regular physical activity can also lower your risk of the following:

- Heart disease

- Stroke

- High blood pressure

- Unhealthy cholesterol levels

- Type 2 diabetes

- Metabolic syndrome

- Colon cancer

- Breast cancer

- Falls

- Depression

Regular activity can help prevent unhealthy weight gain and also help with weight loss, when combined with lower calorie intake. If you are overweight or obese, losing weight can lower your risk for many diseases. Being overweight or obese increases your risk of heart disease, high blood pressure, stroke, type 2 diabetes, breathing problems, osteoarthritis, gallbladder disease, sleep apnea (breathing problems while sleeping), and some cancers.

Regular physical activity can also improve your cardiorespiratory (heart, lungs, and blood vessels) and muscular fitness. For older adults, activity can improve mental function.

Physical activity may also provide these health benefits:

- Improve functional health for older adults
- Reduce waistline size
- Lower risk of hip fracture
- Lower risk of lung cancer
- Lower risk of endometrial cancer
- Maintain weight after weight loss
- Increase bone density
- Improve sleep quality

What is body mass index?

You can get an idea of whether you are obese, overweight, or of normal weight by figuring out your body mass index (BMI). BMI is a number calculated from your weight and height. Women with a BMI of 25 to 29.9 are considered overweight. Women with a BMI of 30 or more are considered obese. All adults (aged 18 years or older) with a BMI of 25 or higher are considered at risk for serious health problems. These health risks increase as your BMI rises. Your doctor or nurse can help you figure out your BMI, or you can use this online BMI calculator (nhlbisupport.com/bmi/bmicalc.htm).

How much physical activity should I do?

Health benefits are gained by doing the following each week:

- 2 hours and 30 minutes of moderate-intensity aerobic physical activity **or**
- 1 hour and 15 minutes of vigorous-intensity aerobic physical activity **or**
- A combination of moderate and vigorous-intensity aerobic physical activity **and**
- Muscle-strengthening activities on two or more days

This physical activity should be in addition to your routine activities of daily living, such as cleaning or spending a few minutes walking from the parking lot to your office.

Moderate activity: During moderate-intensity activities you should notice an increase in your heart rate, but you should still be able to talk comfortably. An example of a moderate-intensity activity is walking on a level surface at a brisk pace (about three to four miles per hour). Other examples include ballroom dancing, leisurely bicycling, moderate housework, and waiting tables.

Vigorous activity: If your heart rate increases a lot and you are breathing so hard that it is difficult to carry on a conversation, you are probably doing vigorous-intensity activity. Examples of vigorous-intensity activities include jogging, bicycling fast or uphill, singles tennis, and pushing a hand mower.

How much physical activity do I need to do to lose weight?

If you want to lose a substantial (more than 5% of body weight) amount of weight, you need a high amount of physical activity unless you also lower calorie intake. This is also the case if you are trying to keep the weight off. Many people need to do more than 300 minutes of moderate-intensity activity a week to meet weight-control goals.

Does the type of physical activity I choose matter?

Yes. Engaging in different types of physical activity is important to overall physical fitness. Your fitness routine should include aerobic and strength-training activities and may also include stretching activities.

Aerobic activities: These activities move large muscles in your arms, legs, and hips over and over again. Examples include walking, jogging, bicycling, swimming, and tennis.

Strength-training activities: These activities increase the strength and endurance of your muscles. Examples of strength-training activities include working out with weight machines, free weights, and resistance bands. Push-ups and sit-ups are examples of strength-training activities you can do without any equipment. You also can use soup cans to work out your arms.

Aim to do strength-training activities at least twice a week. In each strength-training session, you should do 8 to 10 different activities using the different muscle groups throughout your body, such as the muscles in your abdomen, chest, arms, and legs. Repeat each activity 8 to 12 times, using a weight or resistance that will make you feel tired. When you do strength-training activities, slowly increase the amount of weight or resistance that you use. Also, allow one day in between sessions to avoid excess strain on your muscles and joints.

Stretching: Stretching improves flexibility, allowing you to move more easily. This will make it easier for you to reach down to tie your shoes or look over your shoulder when you back the car out of your driveway. You should do stretching activities after your muscles are warmed up—for example, after strength training. Stretching your muscles before they are warmed up may cause injury.

How can I prevent injuries when I work out?

Being physically active is safe if you are careful. Take these steps to prevent injury:

- If you're not active at all or have a health problem, start your program with short sessions (5 to 10 minutes) of physical activity and build up to your goal. (Be sure to ask a doctor before you start if you have a health problem.)

- Use safety equipment such as a helmet for bike riding or supportive shoes for walking or jogging.

- Start every workout with a warm-up. If you plan to walk at a brisk pace, start by walking at an easy pace for 5 to 10 minutes. When you're done working out, do the same thing until your heart rate returns to normal.

- Drink plenty of fluids when you are physically active, even if you are not thirsty.

- Use sunscreen when you are outside.

- Always bend forward from the hips, not the waist. If you keep your back straight, you're probably bending the right way. If your back "humps," that's probably wrong.

- Stop your activity if you feel very out of breath, dizzy, nauseous, or have pain. If you feel tightness or pain in your chest, or you feel faint or have trouble breathing, stop the activity right away and talk to your doctor.

- Exercise should not hurt or make you feel really tired. You might feel some soreness, a little discomfort, or a bit weary. But you should not feel pain. In fact, in many ways, being active will probably make you feel better.

Can I stay active if I have a disability?

A disability may make it harder to stay active, but it shouldn't stop you. In most cases, people with disabilities can improve their flexibility, mobility, and coordination by becoming physically active. Getting regular physical activity can also help you stay independent by preventing illnesses, such as heart disease, that can make caring for yourself more difficult. Work with a doctor to develop a physical activity plan that works for you.

What are some tips to help me get moving?

Fit it into a busy schedule.

- If you can't set aside one block of time, do short activities throughout the day, such as three 10-minute walks.
- Create opportunities for activity. Try parking your car farther away from where you are headed. If you ride the bus or train, get off one or two stops early and walk.
- Walk or bike to work or to the store.
- Use stairs instead of the elevator or escalator.
- Take breaks at work to stretch or take quick walks, or do something active with co-workers at lunch.
- Walk while you talk, if you're using a cell phone or cordless phone.
- Doing yard work or household chores counts as physical activity. Turn on some upbeat music to help you do chores faster and speed up your heart rate.

Make it fun.

- Choose activities that you enjoy.
- Vary your activities, so you don't get bored. For instance, use different jogging, walking, or biking paths. Or bike one day, and jog the next.
- Reward yourself when you achieve your weekly goals. For instance, reward yourself by going to a movie.
- If you have children, make time to play with them outside. Set a good example.
- Plan active vacations that will keep you moving, such as taking tours and sightseeing on foot.

Make it social.

- Join a hiking or running club.

- Go dancing with your partner or friends.

- Turn activities into social occasions—for example, go to a movie after you and a friend work out.

Overcome challenges.

- Don't let cold weather keep you on the couch. You can find activities to do in the winter, such as indoor fitness classes or exercising to a workout video.

- If you live in a neighborhood where it is unsafe to be active outdoors, contact your local recreational center or church to see if they have indoor activity programs that you can join. You can also find ways to be active at home. For instance, you can do push-ups or lift hand weights. If you don't have hand weights, you can use canned foods or bottles filled with water or sand.

- Don't expect to notice body changes right away. It can take weeks or months before you notice some of the changes from being physically active, such as weight loss. And keep in mind, many benefits of physical activity are happening inside you and you cannot see them.

Do I need to talk to my doctor before I start?

You should talk to your doctor before you begin any physical activity program if the following apply to you:

- You have heart disease, had a stroke, or are at high risk for these diseases

- You have diabetes or are at high risk for diabetes

- You are obese (BMI of 30 or greater)

- You have an injury or disability

- You are pregnant

- You have a bleeding or detached retina, eye surgery, or laser treatment on your eye

- You have had recent hip surgery

Chapter 7

Obesity and Weight Loss

How many women in the United States are overweight or obese?

Over 60% of U.S. adult women are overweight, according to 2007 estimates from the National Center for Health Statistics of the Center for Disease Control and Prevention. Just over one-third of overweight adult women are obese.

How do I know if I'm overweight or obese?

Find out your body mass index (BMI). BMI is a measure of body fat based on height and weight. People with a BMI of 25 to 29.9 are considered overweight. People with a BMI of 30 or more are considered obese. You can find out your BMI by using this calculator (nhlbisupport.com/bmi/bmicalc.htm) or chart (www.nhlbi.nih.gov/guidelines/obesity/bmi_tbl.htm).

What causes someone to become overweight or obese?

You can become overweight or obese when you eat more calories than you use. A calorie is a unit of energy in the food you eat. Your body needs this energy to function and to be active. But if you take in more energy than your body uses, you will gain weight.

Excerpted from "Overweight, Obesity, and Weight Loss Fact Sheet," U.S. Department of Health and Human Services Office on Women's Health (www.womenshealth.gov), March 6, 2009.

Many factors can play a role in becoming overweight or obese. These factors include the following:

- Behaviors, such as eating too many calories or not getting enough physical activity
- Environment and culture
- Genes

Overweight and obesity problems keep getting worse in the United States. Some cultural reasons for this include the following:

- Bigger portion sizes
- Little time to exercise or cook healthy meals
- Using cars to get places instead of walking

What are the health effects of being overweight or obese?

Being overweight or obese can increase your risk of these conditions:

- Heart disease
- Stroke
- Type 2 diabetes
- High blood pressure
- Breathing problems
- Arthritis
- Gallbladder disease
- Some kinds of cancer

But excess body weight isn't the only health risk. The places where you store your body fat also affect your health. Women with a "pear" shape tend to store fat in their hips and buttocks. Women with an "apple" shape store fat around their waists. If your waist is more than 35 inches, you may have a higher risk of weight-related health problems.

What is the best way for me to lose weight?

The best way to lose weight is to use more calories than you take in. You can do this by following a healthy eating plan and being more active. Before you start a weight-loss program, talk to your doctor.

Safe weight-loss programs that work well have these characteristics:

- Set a goal of slow and steady weight loss—one to two pounds per week
- Offer low-calorie eating plans with a wide range of healthy foods
- Encourage you to be more physically active
- Teach you about healthy eating and physical activity
- Adapt to your likes and dislikes and cultural background
- Help you keep weight off after you lose it

How can I make healthier food choices?

The U.S. Department of Health and Human Services (HHS) and Department of Agriculture (USDA) offer tips for healthy eating in *Dietary Guidelines for All Americans.*

- **Focus on fruits.** Eat a variety of fruits—fresh, frozen, canned, or dried—rather than fruit juice for most of your fruit choices. For a 2,000-calorie diet, you will need two cups of fruit each day.

- **Vary your veggies.** Eat more of the following:
  - Dark green veggies, such as broccoli, kale, and other dark leafy greens
  - Orange veggies, such as carrots, sweet potatoes, pumpkin, and winter squash
  - Beans and peas, such as pinto beans, kidney beans, black beans, garbanzo beans, split peas, and lentils

- **Get your calcium-rich foods.** Each day, drink three cups of low-fat or fat-free milk. Or you can get an equivalent amount of low-fat yogurt and/or low-fat cheese. If you don't or can't consume milk, choose lactose-free milk products and/or calcium-fortified foods and drinks.

- **Make half your grains whole.** Eat at least three ounces of whole-grain cereals, breads, crackers, rice, or pasta each day. Look to see that grains such as wheat, rice, oats, or corn are referred to as "whole" in the list of ingredients.

- **Go lean with protein.** Choose lean meats and poultry. Bake it, broil it, or grill it. Vary your protein choices with more fish, beans, peas, nuts, and seeds.

- **Limit saturated fats.** Get less than 10% of your calories from saturated fatty acids. Most fats should come from sources of polyunsaturated and monounsaturated fatty acids, such as fish, nuts, and vegetable oils.

- **Limit salt.** Get less than 2,300 mg of sodium (about one teaspoon of salt) each day.

How can physical activity help?

The 2008 *Physical Activity Guidelines for Americans* state that an active lifestyle can lower your risk of early death from a variety of causes. Regular activity can help prevent unhealthy weight gain and also help with weight loss when combined with lower calorie intake. If you are overweight or obese, losing weight can lower your risk for many diseases. Regular physical activity can also improve your cardiorespiratory (heart, lungs, and blood vessels) and muscular fitness. For older adults, activity can improve mental function.

Health benefits are gained by doing the following each week:

- 2 hours and 30 minutes of moderate-intensity aerobic physical activity **or**

- 1 hour and 15 minutes of vigorous-intensity aerobic physical activity **or**

- A combination of moderate and vigorous-intensity aerobic physical activity **and**

- Muscle-strengthening activities on two or more days

This physical activity should be in addition to your routine activities of daily living, such as cleaning or spending a few minutes walking from the parking lot to your office.

Moderate activity: During moderate-intensity activities you should notice an increase in your heart rate, but you should still be able to talk comfortably. An example of a moderate-intensity activity is walking on a level surface at a brisk pace (about three to four miles per hour). Other examples include ballroom dancing, leisurely bicycling, moderate housework, and waiting tables.

Vigorous activity: If your heart rate increases a lot and you are breathing so hard that it is difficult to carry on a conversation, you are probably doing vigorous-intensity activity. Examples of vigorous-intensity activities include jogging, bicycling fast or uphill, singles tennis, and pushing a hand mower.

If you want to lose a substantial (more than 5% of body weight) amount of weight, you need a high amount of physical activity unless you also lower calorie intake. This is also the case if you are trying to keep the weight off. Many people need to do more than 300 minutes of moderate-intensity activity a week to meet weight-control goals.

What medicines are approved for long-term treatment of obesity?

The Food and Drug Administration has approved two medicines for long-term treatment of obesity:

- Sibutramine suppresses your appetite [see update on p. 73–74].

- Orlistat keeps your body from absorbing fat from the food you eat.

These medicines are for people who meet these criteria:

- Have a BMI of 30 or higher

- Have a BMI of 27 or higher and weight-related health problems or health risks

If you take these medicines, you will need to follow a healthy eating and physical activity plan at the same time. Before taking these medicines, talk with your doctor about the benefits and the side effects.

What surgical options are used to treat obesity?

Weight loss surgeries—also called bariatric surgeries—can help treat obesity. You should only consider surgical treatment for weight loss if you meet these criteria:

- Have a BMI of 40 or higher

- Have a BMI of 35 or higher and weight-related health problems

- Have not had success with other weight-loss methods

Common types of weight loss surgeries are the following:

- **Roux-en-Y gastric bypass:** The surgeon uses surgical staples to create a small stomach pouch. This limits the amount of food you can eat. Food bypasses the upper part of the small intestine and stomach, reducing the amount of calories and nutrients your body absorbs.

- **Laparoscopic gastric banding:** A band is placed around the upper stomach to create a small pouch and narrow passage into the rest of the stomach. This limits the amount of food you can eat. The size of the band can be adjusted. A surgeon can remove the band if needed.

- **Biliopancreatic diversion (BPD) or BPD with duodenal switch (BPD/DS):** In BPD, a large part of the stomach is removed, leaving a small pouch. The pouch is connected to the last part of the small intestine, bypassing other parts of the small intestine. In BPD/DS, less of the stomach and small intestine are removed. This surgery reduces the amount of food you can eat and the amount of calories and nutrients your body absorbs from food. This surgery is used less often than other types of surgery because of the high risk of malnutrition.

If you are thinking about weight-loss surgery, talk with your doctor about changes you will need to make after the surgery. You will need to do the following:

- Follow your doctor's directions as you heal
- Make lasting changes in the way you eat
- Follow a healthy eating plan and be physically active
- Take vitamins and minerals if needed

You should also talk to your doctor about risks and side effects of weight loss surgery. Side effects may include the following:

- Infection
- Leaking from staples
- Hernia
- Blood clots in the leg veins that travel to your lungs (pulmonary embolism)
- Dumping syndrome, in which food moves from your stomach to your intestines too quickly
- Not getting enough vitamins and minerals from food

Is liposuction a treatment for obesity?

Liposuction is not a treatment for obesity. In this procedure, a surgeon removes fat from under the skin. Liposuction can be used to reshape parts of your body. But this surgery does not promise lasting weight loss.

I'm concerned about my children's eating and physical activity levels. How can I help improve their habits?

The things children learn when they are young are hard to change as they get older. This is true for their eating and physical activity habits. Many children have a poor diet and are not very active. Kids who are overweight have a greater chance of becoming obese adults. Overweight children may develop weight-related health problems like high blood pressure and diabetes at a young age.

You can find out your child's BMI by using a calculator for children's BMI (at www.girlshealth.gov/nutrition/weight/bmi_calc.cfm).

You can help your child build healthy eating and activity habits.

- Limit time spent watching TV, playing video games, and using the computer.

- Make sure your child is physically active for one hour each day.

- Find out about activity programs in your community.

- Plan activities for the whole family—like hiking, walking, or playing ball.

- Help your children eat healthy foods.

- Have your children plan and cook healthy meals with you.

- Don't do other things while you eat, like watch TV.

- Give your kids healthy snacks, like fruits, whole-grain crackers, and vegetables.

- Limit your trips to fast-food restaurants.

- Involve the whole family in healthy eating. Don't single out your children by their weight.

We know children do what they see—not always what they are told. Set a good example for your children. Your kids will learn to eat right and be active by watching you. Setting a good example can mean a lifetime of good habits for you and your kids.

Sibutramine Update

On October 8, 2010, the U.S. Food and Drug Administration (FDA) asked Abbott Laboratories to voluntarily withdraw from the U.S. market, its weight loss drug Meridia (sibutramine) because of clinical trial data indicating an increased risk of cardiovascular adverse events, including heart attack and stroke, in the studied population. Abbott has agreed to voluntarily stop marketing of Meridia in the United States.

In January 2010, the European Medicines Agency's Committee for Medicinal Products for Human Use (CHMP) concluded that the risks of sibutramine-containing drugs is greater than the benefits and recommended the suspension of marketing authorizations for these medicines across the European Union.

Source: Excerpted from "Questions and Answers: FDA Recommends Against the Continued Use of Meridia (sibutramine)," U.S. Food and Drug Administration (www .fda.gov), October 8, 2010.

Chapter 8

Dealing with Sleep Disorders and Tips for Getting Better Sleep

Sleep Disorders

Most adults need at least eight hours of sleep every night to be well rested. Not everyone gets the sleep they need. About 40 million people in the United States suffer from sleep problems every year.

Not getting enough sleep for a long time can cause health problems. For example, it can make problems like diabetes and high blood pressure worse.

Insomnia

Insomnia includes the following symptoms:

- Trouble falling asleep

- Having trouble getting back to sleep

- Waking up too early

Most people will have trouble falling asleep from time to time. It is usually nothing to worry about. Stress or certain medicines can cause problems falling asleep. Drinking alcohol or eating too close to bedtime can keep you awake, too.

Excerpted from "Sleep Disorders," U.S. Food and Drug Administration (www .fda.gov), October 5, 2009, and "What Is Restless Legs Syndrome?" National Heart Lung and Blood Institute (www.nhlbi.gov), November 1, 2010.

Insomnia is called chronic (long-term) when it lasts most nights for a few weeks or more. You should see your doctor if this happens. Insomnia is more common in females, people with depression, and people older than 60.

Taking medicine together with some changes to your routine can help most people with insomnia (about 85%). Certain drugs work in the brain to help promote sleep.

The following are tips for better sleep:

- Go to bed and get up at the same times each day.
- Avoid caffeine, nicotine, beer, wine, and liquor in the four to six hours before bedtime.
- Don't exercise within two hours of bedtime.
- Don't eat large meals within two hours of bedtime.
- Don't nap later than 3 p.m.
- Sleep in a dark, quiet room that isn't too hot or cold for you.
- If you can't fall asleep within 20 minutes, get up and do something quiet.
- Wind down in the 30 minutes before bedtime by doing something relaxing.

Feeling Sleepy during the Day

Feeling tired every now and then is normal. It is not normal for sleepiness to interfere with your daily life. Watch for signs like the following:

- Slowed thinking
- Trouble paying attention
- Heavy eyelids
- Feeling cranky

Several sleep disorders can make you sleepy during the day. One of these is narcolepsy. People with narcolepsy feel very sleepy even after a full night's sleep. It is normal to take between 10 and 20 minutes to fall asleep. People who fall asleep in less than 5 minutes may have a serious sleep disorder.

Snoring

Snoring is noisy breathing during sleep. It is caused by vibrating in the throat. Some people can make changes that will stop snoring. These include the following:

- Losing weight
- Cutting down on smoking and alcohol
- Sleeping on your side instead of on your back

You can buy over-the-counter nasal strips to help prevent snoring. You place one over your nose before going to bed to make breathing easier.

Sleep Apnea

Snoring loud and often, together with too much daytime sleepiness, may be signs of sleep apnea. Sleep apnea is a very common sleep disorder. It is also very dangerous. The most common type of sleep apnea happens when your breathing stops during sleep. It can stop for about 10 seconds to as long as a minute. You wake up trying to breathe. This stop-and-start cycle of waking to breathe can repeat hundreds of times a night. The danger is that some time you may not wake up to breathe. If this happens, you can die.

You are likely to feel sleepy during the day if you have this problem. People with sleep apnea tend to be overweight. It is more common among men than women.

- The most common treatment is a device that pushes air through the airway. This device is called a CPAP.
- Avoid beer, wine, liquor, tobacco, and sleeping pills.
- Your doctor may also suggest you lose weight.
- In some cases, you may need surgery to make the airway bigger.

Restless Legs Syndrome

Restless legs syndrome (RLS) is a disorder that causes a strong urge to move your legs. This urge to move often occurs with strange and unpleasant feelings in your legs. Moving your legs relieves the urge and the unpleasant feelings.

People who have RLS describe the unpleasant feelings as creeping, crawling, pulling, itching, tingling, burning, aching, or electric shocks. Sometimes, these feelings also occur in the arms.

The urge to move and unpleasant feelings happen when you're resting and inactive. Thus, they tend to be worse in the evening and at night.

RLS can range from mild to severe based on the following:

- The strength of your symptoms and how often they occur
- How easily moving around relieves your symptoms
- How much your symptoms disturb your sleep

One type of RLS usually starts early in life (before 45 years of age) and tends to run in families. It may even start in childhood. Once this type of RLS starts, it usually lasts for the rest of your life. Over time, symptoms slowly get worse and occur more often. If you have a mild case, you may have long periods with no symptoms.

Another type of RLS usually starts later in life (after 45 years of age). It generally doesn't run in families. This type of RLS tends to have a more abrupt onset. The symptoms usually don't get worse over time.

Some diseases, conditions, and medicines may trigger RLS. For example, the disorder has been linked to kidney failure, Parkinson disease, diabetes, rheumatoid arthritis, pregnancy, and iron deficiency. When a disease, condition, or medicine causes RLS, the symptoms usually start suddenly.

Medical conditions or medicines often cause or worsen the type of RLS that starts later in life.

Outlook

RLS symptoms often get worse over time. However, some people's symptoms go away for weeks to months.

If a medical condition or medicine triggers RLS, the disorder may go away if the trigger is relieved or stopped. For example, RLS that occurs due to pregnancy tends to go away after giving birth. Kidney transplants (but not dialysis) relieve RLS linked to kidney failure.

Treatments for RLS include lifestyle changes and medicines. Some simple lifestyle changes often help relieve mild cases of RLS. Medicines often can relieve or prevent the symptoms of more severe RLS.

Chapter 9

Managing Stress

What is stress?

Stress is a feeling you get when faced with a challenge. In small doses, stress can be good for you because it makes you more alert and gives you a burst of energy. For instance, if you start to cross the street and see a car about to run you over, that jolt you feel helps you to jump out of the way before you get hit. But feeling stressed for a long time can take a toll on your mental and physical health. Even though it may seem hard to find ways to de-stress with all the things you have to do, it's important to find those ways. Your health depends on it.

What are the most common causes of stress?

Stress happens when people feel like they don't have the tools to manage all of the demands in their lives. Stress can be short-term or long-term. Missing the bus or arguing with your spouse or partner can cause short-term stress. Money problems or trouble at work can cause long-term stress. Even happy events, like having a baby or getting married, can cause stress. Some of the most common stressful life events include the following:

- Death of a spouse or close family member

Excerpted from "Stress and Your Health Fact Sheet," U.S. Department of Health and Human Services Office on Women's Health (www.womenshealth.gov), March 17, 2010.

- Divorce or marital separation
- Losing your job
- Major personal illness or injury
- Marriage
- Pregnancy
- Retirement
- Spending time in jail

What are some common signs of stress?

Everyone responds to stress a little differently. Your symptoms may be different from someone else's. Here are some of the signs to look for:

- Not eating or eating too much
- Feeling like you have no control
- Needing to have too much control
- Forgetfulness
- Headaches
- Lack of energy
- Lack of focus
- Trouble getting things done
- Poor self-esteem
- Short temper
- Trouble sleeping
- Upset stomach
- Back pain
- General aches and pains

These symptoms may also be signs of depression or anxiety, which can be caused by long-term stress.

Do women react to stress differently than men?

One recent survey found that women were more likely to experience physical symptoms of stress than men. But we don't have enough proof to say that this applies to all women. We do know that women often cope with stress in different ways than men. Women "tend and befriend," taking care of those closest to them but also drawing support from friends and family. Men are more likely to have the "fight or flight" response. They cope by "escaping" into a relaxing activity or other distraction.

Can stress affect my health?

The body responds to stress by releasing stress hormones. These hormones make blood pressure, heart rate, and blood sugar levels go up. Long-term stress can contribute to a variety of health problems, including the following:

- Mental health disorders, like depression and anxiety
- Obesity
- Heart disease
- High blood pressure
- Abnormal heart beats
- Menstrual problems
- Acne and other skin problems

Does stress cause ulcers?

No, stress doesn't cause ulcers, but it can make them worse. Most ulcers are caused by a germ called *H. pylori*. Researchers think people might get it through food or water. Most ulcers can be cured by taking a combination of antibiotics and other drugs.

What is posttraumatic stress disorder (PTSD)?

PTSD is a type of anxiety disorder that can occur after living through or seeing a dangerous event. It can also occur after a sudden traumatic event. You can start having PTSD symptoms right after the event. Or symptoms can develop months or even years later. Symptoms may include the following:

- Nightmares
- Flashbacks, or feeling like the event is happening again
- Staying away from places and things that remind you of what happened

- Being irritable, angry, or jumpy
- Feeling strong guilt, depression, or worry
- Trouble sleeping
- Feeling "numb"
- Having trouble remembering the event

Women are two to three times more likely to develop PTSD than men. Also, people with ongoing stress in their lives are more likely to develop PTSD after a dangerous event.

How can I help handle my stress?

Everyone has to deal with stress. There are steps you can take to help you handle stress in a positive way and keep it from making you sick. Try these tips to keep stress in check:

Develop a New Attitude

- Become a problem solver. Make a list of the things that cause you stress. From your list, figure out which problems you can solve now and which are beyond your control for the moment. From your list of problems that you can solve now, start with the little ones. Learn how to calmly look at a problem, think of possible solutions, and take action to solve the problem. Being able to solve small problems will give you confidence to tackle the big ones. And feeling confident that you can solve problems will go a long way to helping you feel less stressed.

- Be flexible. Sometimes, it's not worth the stress to argue. Give in once in awhile or meet people halfway.

- Get organized. Think ahead about how you're going to spend your time. Write a to-do list. Figure out what's most important to do and do those things first.

- Set limits. When it comes to things like work and family, figure out what you can really do. There are only so many hours in the day. Set limits for yourself and others. Don't be afraid to say NO to requests for your time and energy.

Relax

- Take deep breaths. If you're feeling stressed, taking a few deep breaths makes you breathe slower and helps your muscles relax.

- Stretch. Stretching can also help relax your muscles and make you feel less tense.

- Massage tense muscles. Having someone massage the muscles in the back of your neck and upper back can help you feel less tense.

- Take time to do something you want to do. We all have lots of things that we have to do. But often we don't take the time to do the things that we really want to do. It could be listening to music, reading a good book, or going to a movie. Think of this as an order from your doctor, so you won't feel guilty!

Take Care of Your Body

- Get enough sleep. Getting enough sleep helps you recover from the stresses of the day. Also, being well rested helps you think better so that you are prepared to handle problems as they come up. Most adults need seven to nine hours of sleep a night to feel rested.

- Eat right. Try to fuel up with fruits, vegetables, beans, and whole grains. Don't be fooled by the jolt you get from caffeine or high-sugar snack foods. Your energy will wear off, and you could wind up feeling more tired than you did before.

- Get moving. Getting physical activity can not only help relax your tense muscles but improve your mood. Research shows that physical activity can help relieve symptoms of depression and anxiety.

- Don't deal with stress in unhealthy ways. This includes drinking too much alcohol, using drugs, smoking, or overeating.

Connect with Others

- Share your stress. Talking about your problems with friends or family members can sometimes help you feel better. They might also help you see your problems in a new way and suggest solutions that you hadn't thought of.

- Get help from a professional if you need it. If you feel that you can no longer cope, talk to your doctor. She or he may suggest counseling to help you learn better ways to deal with stress. Your doctor may also prescribe medicines, such as antidepressants or sleep aids.

- Help others. Volunteering in your community can help you make new friends and feel better about yourself.

Chapter 10

Preventing Vision and Hearing Problems

Vision and hearing losses can happen as you age. Other problems with your eyes and ears can happen as you work and play. Prevention, early detection, and proper treatment for injury or disease to your eyes and ears will help you enjoy independence and a better quality of life.

Steps you can take include the following:

- Get your eyes examined according to this schedule:
  - If you are between the ages of 18 and 39, discuss with your doctor when you should have a comprehensive dilated eye exam.
  - Get a baseline exam at age 40, then every two to four years (or as your doctor advises) until age 49.
  - Have an exam every two to four years until age 55, then every one to three years until age 65, or as your doctor advises.
  - At ages 65 and older, get an exam every one to two years.

People at higher risk for eye diseases need to be examined more often. For example, adults with diabetes should have a dilated eye exam at least once a year. African Americans over age 40, people with a family history, and everyone over age 60 are at higher risk for glaucoma and should have a dilated eye exam every one to two years. Eye

Excerpted from "A Lifetime of Good Health: Your Guide to Staying Healthy," U.S. Department of Health and Human Services Office on Women's Health (www.womenshealth.gov), February 2011.

diseases often have no warning signs in their early stage and can only be detected by an eye care professional.

- Have regular dilated eye exams. This is the best thing you can do to make sure your eyes are healthy and you are seeing your best. Your eye care professional will tell you how often you need to have one.

- Wear sunglasses to protect your eyes from harmful ultraviolet (UV) rays when outdoors. Choose sunglasses with 99% to 100% UVA and UVB protection, to block both forms of ultraviolet rays.

- Wear protective eyewear, such as polycarbonate safety glasses, safety goggles, or face shields, when working outdoors or with materials that can harm eyes and when playing sports.

- Eating a diet rich in fruits and vegetables, particularly dark leafy greens such as spinach, kale, or collard greens, is important to keep your eyes healthy.

- Reduce eyestrain by adjusting your computer monitor appropriately, taking rest breaks when working on a computer, and sitting upright with your feet flat on the floor when working on a computer.

- Prevent hearing loss from noise. Pay attention to sounds around you that are at or above 85 decibels, such as concerts, fireworks, or lawn mowers. If you are around loud sounds for too long, wear earplugs or move away from the sound.

- Get a hearing exam every 10 years between the ages of 18 and 49 and every 3 years after that.

- Prevent ear infections. You can help prevent upper respiratory infections—and a resulting ear infection—by washing your hands often. Also, get a flu vaccine every year to help prevent flu-related ear infections.

- Ask your doctor if your medicines may hurt your ears. Some medicine (like certain antibiotics) can damage hearing.

- Be careful when listening to music through headphones. Many devices that people use today have noise levels much higher than 85 decibels. For example, an MP3 player at maximum level is roughly 105 decibels. Scientists recommend no more than 15 minutes of unprotected exposure to sounds that are 100 decibels. In addition, regular exposure to sounds at 110 decibels for more than one minute risks permanent hearing loss.

Chapter 11

Healthy Aging
Tips for Women

The average woman today has more than one-third of her life ahead of her after menopause. That means the menopausal transition is a good time for lifestyle changes that could help women make the most of the coming years.

Good Nutrition

A balanced diet will give you most of the nutrients and calories your body needs to stay healthy. Eat a variety of foods from the five major food groups. Look for foods that have lots of nutrients, like protein and vitamins, but not a lot of calories. These are called nutrient-dense foods. As you grow older, you need fewer calories for energy, but just as many nutrients.

The number of calories a woman over age 50 should eat daily depends on how physically active she is. Basically you need the following:

- 1,600 calories, if your physical activity level is low

- 1,800 calories, if you are moderately active

- 2,000–2,200 calories, if you have an active lifestyle

The more active you are, the more calories you can eat without gaining weight.

Excerpted from "Menopause: Time for a Change," National Institute on Aging (www.nia.gov), October 31, 2011.

Eating a variety of healthy foods will help you get needed nutrients. But people over 50 have trouble getting enough of some vitamins and minerals through diet alone, including calcium and vitamin D. Women past menopause who are still having a menstrual cycle because they are using menopausal hormone therapy might need some extra iron over the 8 mg (milligrams) recommended for women over age 50. Iron, important for healthy red blood cells, is found in meat, duck, peas, beans, and fortified bread and grain products.

Women over 50 also need more of two B vitamins. Getting 2.4 mcg (micrograms) of vitamin B12 per day will maintain the health of your blood and nerves. Some foods, such as cereals, are fortified with this vitamin. Vitamin B12 is also found in red meat and, to a lesser extent, fish and poultry. But, up to one-third of older people can no longer absorb natural vitamin B12 from their food. Furthermore, common medicines taken to control the symptoms of GERD (gastroesophageal reflux disease), also known as acid reflux, slow the release of certain stomach acids and, therefore, interfere with the body's absorption of vitamin B12. You might need a supplement if you have GERD.

Another B vitamin, B6, helps your body breakdown proteins and make hemoglobin, a part of red blood cells. Women should have 1.5 mg of vitamin B6 daily. This vitamin is found in fortified cereals, as well as meats, legumes, and eggs.

Don't forget to drink plenty of fluids, especially water. If you drink alcohol, do so in moderation—for a woman, only one drink a day according to the *Dietary Guidelines for Americans*. A drink could be one 12-ounce beer, 5 ounces of wine, or 1 1/2 ounces of 80-proof distilled spirits.

Health Care

Eating well, exercising, and not smoking are things you can do for yourself to stay healthy as you get older. It is also important to discuss your goals for healthy aging with your doctor. He or she may be able to help you prevent health problems or recognize problems early when they are probably easier to manage.

See your doctor: Continue to visit your doctor regularly. When you meet with any doctor, be prepared to discuss your family medical history. You might be at increased risk for certain diseases, like diabetes or heart disease, if other close family members had them. Knowing about this family history will help your doctor decide whether you need any screening tests, like cholesterol or blood sugar tests, more often or earlier than other people your age.

You should have routine screening tests, pelvic and breast exams, and a Pap test for cervical cancer. After age 50, you need to be checked for colon cancer, and don't forget your mammogram every one to two years, especially if you are still using menopausal hormone therapy. And remember to talk to your doctor about whether or not you are at risk for osteoporosis and what types of physical activity are best for you.

Skin: Check your skin every month for unusual blemishes, especially moles that seem to change size, shape, or color. Have your doctor look at your skin during checkups. Use sunscreen, SPF 15 or higher, when you are outside during the day. Try to stay out of the sun when it is strongest—from about 11 a.m. until 3 p.m.

Teeth and mouth: See your dentist once or twice a year. Not only will he or she clean your teeth, but the dentist will also check for cavities and gum disease. If you have dentures, you should still see a dentist periodically to check their fit and to look for gum problems.

Eyes: As you age, reading may become harder. You may need to hold things farther away in order to see them clearly. Reading glasses might help. Start regular visits to an eye care professional, who can check for glaucoma. This eye problem becomes more common after your forties. In glaucoma there is increased pressure on the optic nerve. The pressure can permanently damage your vision before you realize you have glaucoma. Special eye drops often control it.

Medications: Make sure all your doctors know which medications you are taking. This includes vitamins, minerals, other dictary supplements, and over-the-counter medicines like aspirin, antacids, or antihistamines. Some of these may change how your prescription medicines work; others might not be safe for you to use at all.

If your health care professional prescribes a medicine, take it as directed. Make sure you understand the possible side effects of the prescribed medicines.

Get vaccines: If you are over age 50, you should get a flu shot every fall, especially if you have other health problems. The Centers for Disease Control and Prevention (CDC) recommends that people over age 65 get the pneumococcal pneumonia vaccine—most need it only once. You should also have a tetanus shot every 10 years, or sooner if you have an injury that puts you at risk for getting tetanus.

A vaccine to prevent shingles is now available. Most adults 60 years and older should get one dose.

Listen to your body: Don't wait for your next checkup if you notice any suspicious changes in your body—swelling, unexpected weight loss or gain, persistent pain, unexplained fevers, a cough that won't go away, or recurring headaches, for example. Check with your doctor about any of these symptoms.

Know the warning signs of a heart attack, although the signs are sometimes less clear in a woman:

- Pain or an uncomfortable feeling in the center of your chest
- Pain or discomfort in other parts of the upper body, including the arms, back, neck, jaw, or stomach
- Other symptoms, such as shortness of breath, breaking out in a cold sweat, nausea, or light-headedness

Call 911 if you feel chest discomfort, especially with any of the other signs. If 911 emergency service is not available where you are, call the operator or get someone to drive you to the hospital.

You should also know the warning signs of a stroke. In the case of a stroke, one or more of these signs come on very suddenly:

- Numbness or weakness, usually in the face, arm, or leg, and often on just one side
- Strong headache for no reason
- Confusion or trouble speaking or understanding
- Problems seeing with one or both eyes
- Trouble walking, feeling dizzy, losing balance or coordination

There are drugs that can help if you get to an emergency room fast enough. Call the ambulance and get medical help as soon as possible, so you can get treatment that may lessen the damage.

Ovarian cancer (cancer of the ovaries) is rare and difficult to diagnose in its early stages, making it hard to treat. The early symptoms are often similar to signs of other illnesses:

- Pain in the abdomen or pelvis
- Urinating often or needing to urinate quickly
- Feeling full more quickly than usual when eating
- Frequent bloating in your abdomen

Normally these symptoms are nothing to worry about. But talk to your doctor if they happen frequently, perhaps more than twelve times a month, or if they continue for more than a few weeks.

Practice Safe Sex

After menopause, some women may think they needn't worry about sexually transmitted diseases. But, any woman, regardless of her age, who is not in a long-term relationship with a faithful partner and has unprotected sex, is at risk of sexually transmitted disease. If you have more than one sexual partner or have recently begun dating again, you need to be aware of the risk of these diseases and take necessary precautions to make sure you don't become infected.

The list of familiar and unfamiliar sexually transmitted diseases includes syphilis, gonorrhea, chlamydia, genital herpes, human papillomavirus/genital warts, and HIV/AIDS. Some can be cured—chlamydia, syphilis, and gonorrhea. But some—genital herpes, human papillomavirus/genital warts, and HIV/AIDS—can't. Being informed about HIV/AIDS is critical because an HIV infection that develops into AIDS is life-threatening. HIV/AIDS can be treated, although not cured, and new drugs enable people to live longer with HIV/AIDS.

HIV is found in body fluids such as blood, semen, and vaginal secretions. The virus can enter your body through any opening in the skin. Postmenopausal women are at special risk because of the fragile tissues of the vulva (the external female genital area around the opening of the vagina) and the lining of the vagina. These delicate tissues may be more susceptible to virus-infected fluids.

Other Lifestyle Changes

This new phase of your life can be as busy and fulfilling as you would like to make it. Stay active—not only physically, but also mentally. If you don't work outside of the home, you might consider getting a part-time job or volunteering with a nonprofit organization. You might find a hobby or learn to play a musical instrument. Maybe you would enjoy taking a class at a local community college or even working toward a degree. You could join a book group or learn to garden. This is the time to do something you always wanted to try, but never had the time before.

While exploring new things and keeping active, try to avoid adding stress to your life. Stress can make it harder to deal with the symptoms of menopause. Mid-life can be a complex time for many women. For example, if you have a family, there are probably changes at home— maybe you now have an "empty nest" because your children are leaving home for college, work, or marriage. Maybe you have young children who are still in need of attention, which can be extra challenging if you are tired because you aren't sleeping well at night.

91

Other possible stresses come from outside the home. If you work, you may be taking a different look at your career, starting to think about retirement, or feeling challenged by younger coworkers.

How do you know you are feeling stressed? Perhaps you feel overwhelmed by life, depressed, or anxious. Do your shoulder muscles feel tight? Do you sometimes realize your hands are clenched? Do you wake up with a sore jaw because you are grinding your teeth or tightening your jaw as you sleep? Do you have headaches, stomach problems, fatigue, trouble sleeping, or high blood pressure? These can be signs of stress.

Avoid stress as much as possible. That might be very hard to do if you are a caregiver—whether of a child or an adult. Try to identify the times when you feel overwhelmed so you can try to keep those situations to a minimum. Take time to relax, eat well, exercise regularly to release tension and feel better overall, and keep in touch with family and friends. Don't be reluctant to ask for help when you need it—from family or friends or even from a professional counselor.

Chapter 12

Complementary and Alternative Medicine Use by Women

Perhaps you have seen a bottle of an herbal medicine in the drugstore and wondered if it might help get rid of your cold. Or you have thought about going to a chiropractor to treat your back pain. Every year, millions of Americans try some form of complementary and alternative medicine—practices and products that are different from those normally used by your family doctor.

But you may wonder: Do these treatments work? Am I wasting my money? Most important, are they safe? Health experts are still trying to answer these questions. More research will hopefully shed light on the real benefits and risks of these alternative treatments.

What Is Complementary and Alternative Medicine?

The treatments used by most doctors are considered conventional medicine. Complementary and alternative medicine (CAM) consists of a group of health care practices and products that are considered out of the mainstream.

An "out-of-the-mainstream" treatment is considered complementary if you use it along with conventional medicine. An example would be using acupuncture along with painkilling drugs to reduce labor pains. A treatment is considered alternative if you use it instead of

Excerpted from "The Healthy Woman: A Complete Guide for All Ages," U.S. Department of Health and Human Services Office on Women's Health (www.womenshealth.gov), November 1, 2008.

conventional medicine. An example would be using acupuncture as your only treatment for headache.

Who Uses CAM?

Research shows that 40% of women in the United States use some form of CAM. If you include prayer for health reasons and taking large doses of vitamins as types of CAM, that number rises to 69%.

Why Do People Use CAM?

People try CAM for a variety of reasons, including the following:

- Conventional medicine has not helped solve their medical problem.

- They believe that products derived from nature are healthier and safer than prescription drugs, even though they may not be.

- They like the holistic approach taken by CAM therapists. A holistic approach involves paying attention to all of a client's needs to help her regain and maintain her health. These include not just physical but also emotional, social, and spiritual needs.

Although something can be said for all of these reasons, you should be aware of some of the downsides of using CAM treatments:

- No CAM treatment has been proven to work beyond a shadow of a doubt.

- Some CAM products, although derived from plants, can cause health problems. For instance, ephedra, a Chinese herbal product, was being sold in the United States to help people lose weight and to enhance athletic performance. Because ephedra increased the risk of heart problems and stroke, the U.S. Food and Drug Administration (FDA) banned the sale of ephedra.

- Some CAM products interfere with how prescription drugs work. For instance, St. John's wort, which some people take to treat depression, can interfere with the actions of drugs for treating HIV, cancer, and other diseases. It may also reduce the effectiveness of birth control pills.

- Some herbal products, such as black cohosh, are unsafe to use during pregnancy. The safety of many other herbal products, either during pregnancy or breastfeeding, has not been studied.

- Some people might use an unproven CAM treatment that may not work or may carry risks instead of a conventional treatment that is known to be effective.

If you choose to try a CAM treatment, be sure to discuss it first with your doctor. Your doctor should know whether the therapy may be helpful and is safe to try along with your current treatments. Some people don't mention their use of CAM treatments to their doctor because they think that their doctor will have negative feelings about CAM. If you are in this situation and would like to try a CAM treatment, perhaps you may want to find a doctor that you feel more comfortable talking to about this.

CAM Treatment Categories

CAM Treatments Found in Nature

Some CAM treatments use substances found in nature, such as herbs, vitamins, and minerals. The idea that natural substances might be used as medicines is not new. Practically since the beginning of time, people have used parts of plants and animals to treat diseases. In fact, some conventional drugs come from nature. For instance, aspirin is derived from a substance found in the bark of the willow tree.

Some CAM products are sold as dietary supplements. These are products taken by mouth that are intended to supplement, or add to, the diet. They come in many forms, including tablets, teas, and powders.

Examples include black cohosh and other plant products for treating menopausal symptoms, cranberry, echinacea, and ginger.

Energy Medicine

Some CAM therapies involve using different types of energy to treat illness. Some of these therapies use energies that everyone agrees exist, such as the energy field surrounding magnets. Other therapies claim to use a "life energy," which may or may not exist.

Therapies That Adjust the Body

Some CAM practices involve handling, pressing, or moving parts of the body. Examples include chiropractic, osteopathy, and massage.

Mind-Body Medicine

Perhaps you have noticed that your mood can affect whether or not you get sick. If you feel well, you are less likely to get sick. If you feel bad, you are more likely to get sick. In fact, research has shown that mood can affect your health. Mind-body medicine is a branch of CAM that seeks to understand how your mind and body affect each other. Mind-body therapies attempt to use this information to improve your health. Two examples of mind-body therapies are biofeedback and hypnosis.

Whole Medical Systems

Whole medical systems are health care methods that have evolved separately from conventional Western medicine. Each medical system involves several therapies that are often used in combination. Some examples are traditional Chinese medicine, Ayurveda, and homeopathy.

Tips on Selecting a CAM Therapist

- Talk with your primary care doctor about your interest in trying a CAM therapy. Discuss possible benefits and risks of the therapy. Ask if the therapy might interfere with your conventional treatments. Also, ask your doctor to recommend someone who practices the type of therapy that you are interested in.

- Some large medical centers have CAM therapists on staff. Check to see if there is such a center near you.

- Contact a national association for the therapy that you are interested in and ask for a list of certified therapists in your area. To find CAM associations, ask your local librarian for directories.

- Some states have agencies that regulate and license certain types of CAM therapists. The agency may be able to provide you with a list of therapists who meet their standards.

- Find out if your health insurance company will cover your visit to a CAM therapist. Most CAM therapies are not covered by insurance.

- After you choose a CAM therapist, go to your first visit with a list of questions that you want answered. Also, be prepared to discuss your health history and the other treatments that you are receiving.

Chapter 13

Avoiding Risk Factors for Common Health Concerns

Chapter Contents

Section 13.1

Women and High Cholesterol Prevention

"Women and Cholesterol" reprinted with permission from www.heart.org.
© 2012 American Heart Association, Inc.

The female sex hormone estrogen tends to raise HDL [high-density lipoprotein] cholesterol, and as a rule, women have higher HDL (good) cholesterol levels than men do. Estrogen production is highest during the childbearing years. This may help explain why premenopausal women are usually protected from developing heart disease.

Women also tend to have higher triglyceride levels. Triglyceride levels range from about 50 to 250 mg/dL [milligrams per deciliter], depending on age and sex. As people get older, more overweight, or both, their triglyceride and cholesterol levels tend to rise.

Postmenopausal hormone therapy (PHT) may benefit some women with osteoporosis or other medical conditions associated with menopause. However, the American Heart Association recommends that PHT not be used for cardiovascular prevention. The HERS trial of women who had previously had a heart attack showed that these women did not benefit from PHT. Recent clinical trials appear to confirm that PHT does not appear to reduce risk of cardiovascular disease and stroke in postmenopausal women. Women with a personal or family history of breast cancer or other endocrine-related cancers should not receive PHT either.

The American Heart Association recommends LDL[low-density lipoprotein] (bad) cholesterol-lowering drug therapy for most women with heart disease. Drug therapy should be combined with a diet low in saturated fat, *trans* fat, cholesterol, and sodium, and rich in fruits, vegetables, whole-grain and high-fiber foods, and fat-free and low-fat dairy. Fish (such as salmon, trout, or haddock) should be eaten twice a week. In addition, women should manage their weight, get regular physical activity, and not smoke.

Section 13.2

Preventing and Controlling High Blood Pressure

"What Is High Blood Pressure?" and "High Blood Pressure
and Women" reprinted with permission from www.heart.org.
© 2012 American Heart Association, Inc.

What Is High Blood Pressure?

What's so important about blood pressure?

High blood pressure, also known as HBP or hypertension, is a widely misunderstood medical condition. Some people think that those with hypertension are tense, nervous, or hyperactive, but hypertension has nothing to do with personality traits. The truth is, you can be a calm, relaxed person and still have HBP.

Let's look at the facts about blood pressure so you can better understand how your body works and why it is smart to start protecting yourself now, no matter what your blood pressure numbers are.

By keeping your blood pressure in the healthy range, you are:

- reducing your risk of the walls of your blood vessels walls becoming overstretched and injured;

- reducing your risk of having a heart attack or stroke and developing heart failure, kidney failure, and peripheral vascular disease;

- protecting your entire body so that your tissue receives regular supplies of blood that is rich in the oxygen it needs.

What happens in the body when blood pressure is high?

Blood pressure measures the force pushing outwards on your arterial walls.

The organs in your body need oxygen to survive. Oxygen is carried through the body by the blood. When the heart beats, it creates pressure that pushes blood through a network of tube-shaped arteries and

99

veins, also known as blood vessels and capillaries. The pressure—blood pressure—is the result of two forces. The first force occurs as blood pumps out of the heart and into the arteries that are part of the circulatory system. The second force is created as the heart rests between heart beats. (These two forces are each represented by numbers in a blood pressure reading.)

The problems from too much force: Healthy arteries are made of muscle and a semi-flexible tissue that stretches like elastic when the heart pumps blood through them. The more forcefully that blood pumps, the more the arteries stretch to allow blood to easily flow. Over time, if the force of the blood flow is often high, the tissue that makes up the walls of arteries gets stretched beyond its healthy limit. This creates problems in several ways.

- **Vascular weaknesses:** First, the overstretching creates weak places in the blood vessels, making them more prone to rupture. Problems such as strokes and aneurysms are caused by ruptures in the blood vessels.

- **Vascular scarring:** Second, the overstretching can cause tiny tears in the blood vessels that leave scar tissue on the walls of arteries and veins. These tears and the scar tissue are like nets and can catch debris such as cholesterol, plaque, or blood cells traveling in the bloodstream.

- **Increased risk of blood clots:** Trapped blood can form clots that can narrow (and sometimes block) the arteries. These clots sometimes break off and block vessels and the blood supply to different parts of the body. When this happens, heart attacks or strokes are often the result.

- **Increased plaque build-up:** The same principle applies to our blood flow. Cholesterol and plaque build-up in the arteries cause the blood flow to become limited or even cut off altogether. As this happens, pressure is increased on the rest of the system, forcing the heart to work harder to deliver blood to your body. Additionally, if pieces of plaque break off and travel to other parts of the body, or if the build-up completely blocks the vessel, then heart attacks and strokes occur.

- **Tissue and organ damage from narrowed and blocked arteries:** Ultimately, the arteries on the other side of the blockage do not receive enough freshly oxygenated blood, which results in tissue damage.

- **Increased workload on the circulatory system:** Think of it this way: In a home where several faucets are open and running, the water pressure flowing out of any one faucet is lower. But when pipes get clogged and therefore narrow, the pressure is much greater. And if all the household water is flowing through only one faucet, the pressure is higher still.

When the arteries are not as elastic because of the build-up of cholesterol or plaque or because of scarring, the heart pumps harder to get blood into the arteries. Over time, this increased work can result in damage to the heart itself. The muscles and valves in the heart can become damaged and heart failure can result.

Damage to the vessels that supply blood to your kidneys and brain may negatively affect these organs.

You may not feel that anything is wrong, but high blood pressure can permanently damage your heart, brain, eyes, and kidneys before you feel anything. High blood pressure can often lead to heart attack and heart failure, stroke, kidney failure, and other health consequences.

Take the time to learn about what the numbers in your blood pressure reading mean.

High Blood Pressure and Women

Many people mistakenly believe that high blood pressure, also called hypertension, is more common among men. The truth is nearly half of all adults with high blood pressure are women. Beginning at age 65, after the onset of menopause, women are actually more likely to have this disease than men.

While HBP isn't directly related to gender, certain woman's issues can increase your risk. Discover how high blood pressure relates to your stage in life.

Blood Pressure during Childbearing Years

Do birth control pills cause high blood pressure? Medical researchers have found that birth control pills increase blood pressure in some women. It's more likely to occur if you're overweight, have had high blood pressure during pregnancy, have a family history of HBP, or have mild kidney disease. The combination of birth control pills and cigarette use may be especially dangerous for some women.

Before you begin taking oral contraceptives:

- Talk to your doctor about the risks.

- Make sure your doctor measures and records your blood pressure before prescribing the pill.

- Have your blood pressure checked every six months or so.

Is it safe to get pregnant if my blood pressure is high? By following the recommendations of your doctor and carefully managing your blood pressure, you can help ensure a normal pregnancy and a healthy baby. However, high blood pressure can be dangerous for both mother and baby. If you are taking HBP medication and want to become pregnant, first consult your doctor. Also keep in mind that if you already have high blood pressure, pregnancy could make it more severe.

Is it safe to get pregnant if I am taking ACE inhibitors or ARBs for high blood pressure? If you're taking an ACE [angiotensin-converting enzyme] inhibitor or an ARB [angiotensin II receptor blocker] and think you might be pregnant, see your doctor immediately. These drugs have been shown to be dangerous to mother and baby alike during pregnancy. They can cause low blood pressure, severe kidney failure, dangerously high potassium levels, and even death of the newborn.

As a woman with high blood pressure, what precautions should I take if I want to become pregnant? Each pregnancy is different, and your doctor will give you recommendations for your situation. Most women with high blood pressure should follow these precautions before becoming pregnant.

- Get your blood pressure under control.

- Watch your diet and limit salt and sodium.

- Be active and exercise. Regular physical activity will help you control your blood pressure and increase your physical condition.

- If you're overweight, lose weight to help you have a safer pregnancy and a healthier baby.

- Stop using tobacco and alcohol.

- If you're on medication for high blood pressure (or any other condition), discuss all of your medications, including over-the-counter drugs and supplements, with all of your doctors. Never stop taking a prescription medication without first consulting the doctor who prescribed it.

Why is it so important to control my blood pressure during pregnancy? Failing to do so could result in:

- harm to the mother's kidneys and other organs,

- low birth weight and early delivery of the infant.

I'm pregnant, and I've never had high blood pressure before, but I do now. Will I always have it? Some women who have never had HBP develop it while they are pregnant. This condition is known as pregnancy induced hypertension (PIH). It usually disappears after delivery. According to the National Heart, Lung, and Blood Institute (NHLBI), high blood pressure affects 6%–8% of all pregnancies in the United States. Almost 70% of these cases are in first-time pregnancies. If the mother is not treated, HBP is dangerous to both the mother and baby. That's why doctors usually keep a close watch on a woman's blood pressure during pregnancy.

PIH is closely related to preeclampsia, or toxemia of pregnancy. This disorder can endanger the lives of both mother and child. Specifically, it can:

- harm the placenta;

- damage the mother's kidneys, liver, and brain;

- cause fetal complications such as low birth weight, premature birth, and stillbirth.

My prenatal clinic says I have preeclampsia because my urine has protein in it and my blood pressure is high. Are my baby and I in danger? Preeclampsia is a condition that typically begins after the 20th week of pregnancy and may continue six weeks after delivery. It's characterized by high blood pressure and elevated protein in the urine, which is caused by kidney problems. This kind of hypertension usually disappears after delivery. If it doesn't, it should be controlled with careful, long-term treatment as with all other types of HBP.

You are at a higher risk for developing preeclampsia if you:

- have high blood pressure before becoming pregnant;

- have developed high blood pressure or preeclampsia in a previous pregnancy;

- are obese prior to pregnancy;

- are under age 20 or over age 40;

- are pregnant with more than one baby;

- have diabetes, kidney disease, rheumatoid arthritis, lupus, or scleroderma.

The rate of preeclampsia has increased over the past decade by nearly one-third. This is due in part to a rise in numbers of older mothers and multiple births, where preeclampsia is more likely to develop.

Not all women have noticeable symptoms of preeclampsia. When symptoms do occur, they can include:

- swelling;
- sudden weight gain;
- headaches;
- changes in vision.

How can I be sure that I won't get pregnancy induced hypertension or preeclampsia? There is no proven way to prevent PIH or preeclampsia and no test that will predict or diagnose these conditions. Only regular visits to your doctor will ensure that you're having a safe pregnancy. Your doctor will track your blood pressure and check the level of protein in your urine. For a healthy pregnancy, you should:

- get early and regular care from your doctor (don't miss appointments);
- follow all of your doctor's recommendations;
- do what you can to help manage your blood pressure, including limiting sodium intake and getting regular physical activity.

Remember, even with HBP and preeclampsia, you can have a successful pregnancy if you follow this advice.

Am I At Greater Risk for High Blood Pressure after Menopause?

As a woman grows older, her chance of having high blood pressure becomes greater than a man's. You may have had normal blood pressure most of your life, but after menopause your chances of developing HBP increase considerably.

See your doctor regularly to have your blood pressure monitored. If you are diagnosed with HBP, follow the prescribed course of treatment.

Section 13.3

Health Risks of Smoking and How to Quit

Excerpted from "Why Should I Quit Now" and "How to Quit,"
U.S. Department of Health and Human Services Office on Women's
Health (www.womenshealth.gov), May 19, 2010.

Why Should I Quit Now?

Most women smokers say they want to quit. So how do you move
from wanting to quit to actually quitting? A first step is to find reasons
to quit that are important to you. Consider the many good reasons to
quit smoking.

Your Health

Your health begins to improve the minute you stop smoking, and you
begin to lower your long-term risk of many smoking-related diseases.
Smoking causes or can contribute to many serious health problems,
including the following:

- Cancers of the lung, throat, mouth, voice box, esophagus, pancreas, kidney, bladder, cervix, uterus, stomach, and blood
- Lung diseases
- Heart disease
- Stroke
- Atherosclerosis, or hardening and narrowing of the arteries
- Gum disease
- Eye diseases that can lead to blindness
- Osteoporosis and the risk of hip fracture

Smoking also does the following:

- Makes illnesses last longer
- Causes more wound infections after surgery
- Makes it harder to get pregnant

Smoking during pregnancy can hurt the mother and baby. It increases the risk of the following:

- Placenta previa, when placenta covers part of or the entire cervix inside of the uterus, which can lead to bed rest, early labor, and cesarean section

- Placental abruption, when the placenta separates too early from the wall of the uterus, which can lead to early labor or infant death

- Early rupture of membranes, or water breaking, before labor starts, so the baby is born too early

- A baby with a low birth weight; babies with low birth weight are more likely to die or have serious health problems or long-term disabilities, such as problems seeing or hearing

- Damage to an infant's lungs

- Sudden infant death syndrome (SIDS)

- Miscarriage

- Stillbirth

Your Quality of Life

When you quit, you will never again have to leave your workplace, your home, or other places to smoke. You won't need to worry about whether your smoke is bothering others. The money you would have spent on cigarettes can be saved or used to buy other things. Plus, you will be surprised by how good you feel overall. Over time, some of the ways you will look and feel better are as follows:

- You will breathe more easily.

- You will have more energy.

- Your lungs will be stronger, making it easier to be active.

- You will be able to smell and taste things better.

- Your hair, breath, and clothes will smell better.

- The stain marks on your fingers will fade.

- Your skin will look healthier.

- Your teeth and gums will be healthier.

- You will feel good about being able to quit!

Other People's Health

When you quit, you no longer create secondhand smoke, which is harmful to the people around you, and especially children. When you quit, you become a role model to children and other smokers who want to quit. When you quit, your own children are less likely to grow up to become smokers themselves.

How to Quit

If you have made the decision to quit smoking, congratulations! Not only will you improve your own health, you will also protect the health of your loved ones by no longer exposing them to secondhand smoke.

Did you know that many people try to quit two or three times before they give up smoking for good? Nicotine is a very addictive drug—as addictive as heroin and cocaine. The good news is that millions of people have given up smoking for good. It's hard work to quit, but you can do it! Freeing yourself of an expensive habit that threatens your health and the health of others will make you feel great!

Many women who smoke worry that they will gain weight if they quit. In fact, nearly 80% of people who quit smoking do gain weight, but the average weight gain is just five pounds. Keep in mind, however, that more than half of people who keep smoking will gain weight too. Plus, the health benefits of quitting far exceed any risks from the weight gain related to quitting.

Research has shown that these steps will help you to quit for good:

- **Pick a date to stop smoking:** Before that day, get rid of all cigarettes, ashtrays, and lighters everywhere you smoke. Do not allow anyone to smoke in your home. List the reasons why you want to quit and keep this list with you, so you can refer to it if you have an urge to light up. It will remind you why you want to stop.

- **Talk to your doctor or nurse about medicines to help you quit:** Many people have withdrawal symptoms when they quit smoking. These symptoms can include depression, trouble sleeping, feeling irritable or restless, and trouble thinking clearly. Medicines work well at relieving these symptoms and can boost your chances of quitting for good. Your chances of quitting are even better when medicine and counseling are used together. Most medicines help you quit smoking by giving you small, steady doses of nicotine, the drug in cigarettes that causes addiction. Also, for some people, certain combinations of medicine work better than using one medicine alone. Talk to your doctor or nurse to see if one of these medicines may be right for you:

- **Nicotine patch:** Worn on the skin and supplies a steady amount of nicotine to the body through the skin

- **Nicotine gum or lozenge:** Releases nicotine into the bloodstream through the lining in your mouth

- **Nicotine nasal spray:** Inhaled through your nose and passes into your bloodstream

- **Nicotine inhaler:** Inhaled through the mouth and absorbed in the mouth and throat

- **Bupropion (Zyban):** A medicine that reduces nicotine withdrawal symptoms and the urge to smoke

- **Varenicline (Chantix):** A medicine that reduces nicotine withdrawal symptoms and the pleasurable effects of smoking

- **Seek counseling:** You can improve your chances of quitting for good with professional help. Counseling can provide you with practical skills to overcome nicotine addiction, as well as support and encouragement. Many forms of counseling and support can help, whether alone, in a group, or through a telephone "quit line." Your chances of success are best with in-person, intense counseling and when all forms are used. Seeking frequent counseling, at least once a week, especially in the first months after quitting, also will boost your chances of success.

- **Get support from your family, friends, and co-workers:** You will be more likely to quit for good if you have help. Let the people important to you know the date you will be quitting and ask them for their support. Ask them not to smoke around you or leave cigarettes out.

- **Find substitutes for smoking and vary your routine:** When you get the urge to smoke, do something to take your mind off smoking. Talk to a friend, go for a walk, or go to the movies. Find ways other than smoking to reduce stress, such as exercise, meditation, hot baths, or reading. Try sugar-free gum or candy to help handle your cravings. Drink lots of water. You might want to try changing your daily routine as well. Try drinking tea instead of coffee, eating your breakfast in a different place, or taking a different route to work.

- **Be prepared for relapse:** Most people relapse, or start smoking again, within the first three months after quitting. Don't get discouraged if you relapse. Remember, many people try to quit several times before quitting for good. Think of what helped and didn't help the last time you tried to quit. Figuring these out before you try to quit again will increase your chances for success. Certain situations can increase your chances of smoking. These include drinking alcohol, being around other smokers, gaining weight, stress, or becoming depressed. Talk to your doctor or nurse to learn ways to cope with these situations.

Where to Get Help

Join a quit-smoking program or support group to help you quit. These programs can help you handle withdrawal and stress and teach you skills to resist the urge to smoke. Contact your local hospital, health center, or health department for information about quit-smoking programs and support groups in your area. Call the National Cancer Institute at 877-44U-QUIT to talk to a counselor. To get live, online assistance from the National Cancer Institute's LiveHelp service, go to www.smokefree.gov. LiveHelp for smoking cessation assistance is available Monday through Friday, 9:00 a.m. to 10:00 p.m. Eastern Standard Time.

Section 13.4

Women's Alcohol Consumption and How It Affects Health

"Excessive Alcohol Use and Risks to Women's Health," Centers for Disease Control and Prevention (www.cdc.gov), October 15, 2012.

Although men are more likely to drink alcohol and drink in larger amounts, gender differences in body structure and chemistry cause women to absorb more alcohol and take longer to break it down and remove it from their bodies (i.e., to metabolize it). In other words, upon drinking equal amounts, women have higher alcohol levels in their blood than men, and the immediate effects occur more quickly and last longer. These differences also make women more vulnerable to alcohol's long-term effects on their health.

Reproductive Health

- National surveys show that about one in two women of child-bearing age (i.e., aged 18–44 years) use alcohol, and 15% of women who drink alcohol in this age group binge drink.

- About 7.6% of pregnant women used alcohol.

- Excessive drinking may disrupt menstrual cycling and increase the risk of infertility, miscarriage, stillbirth, and premature delivery.

- Women who binge drink are more likely to have unprotected sex and multiple sex partners. These activities increase the risks of unintended pregnancy and sexually transmitted diseases.

Alcohol and Pregnancy

- Women who drink alcohol while pregnant increase their risk of having a baby with fetal alcohol spectrum disorders (FASD). The most severe form is fetal alcohol syndrome (FAS), which causes mental retardation and birth defects.

- FASD are completely preventable if a woman does not drink while pregnant or while she may become pregnant.

- Studies have shown that about 1 of 20 pregnant women drank excessively before finding out they were pregnant. No amount of alcohol is safe to drink during pregnancy. For women who drink during pregnancy, stopping as soon as possible may lower the risk of having a child with physical, mental, or emotional problems.

- Research suggests that women who drink alcohol while pregnant are more likely to have a baby die from sudden infant death syndrome (SIDS). This risk substantially increases if a woman binge drinks during her first trimester of pregnancy.

- The risk of miscarriage is also increased if a woman drinks excessively during her first trimester of pregnancy.

Other Health Concerns

- **Liver disease:** The risk of cirrhosis and other alcohol-related liver diseases is higher for women than for men.

- **Impact on the brain:** Excessive drinking may result in memory loss and shrinkage of the brain. Research suggests that women are more vulnerable than men to the brain damaging effects of excessive alcohol use, and the damage tends to appear with shorter periods of excessive drinking for women than for men.

- **Impact on the heart:** Studies have shown that women who drink excessively are at increased risk for damage to the heart muscle than men even for women drinking at lower levels.

- **Cancer:** Alcohol consumption increases the risk of cancer of the mouth, throat, esophagus, liver, colon, and breast among women. The risk of breast cancer increases as alcohol use increases.

- **Sexual assault:** Binge drinking is a risk factor for sexual assault, especially among young women in college settings. Each year, about 1 in 20 college women are sexually assaulted. Research suggests that there is an increase in the risk of rape or sexual assault when both the attacker and victim have used alcohol prior to the attack.

Section 13.5

Sunscreen Use and Avoiding Tanning Decrease Skin Cancer Risk

"Sunscreens and Tanning," U.S. Food and Drug Administration (www.fda.gov), April 22, 2010.

Many people like to spend time in the sun, but it can also cause harm. The sun can cause skin cancer, sunburn, wrinkles, and skin aging. Too much sun can even harm the body's immune system. You don't need to get a sunburn to have skin damage. Skin damage builds up over your lifetime.

What causes sunburn?

The sun's UV (ultraviolet) rays cause sunburn. The sun gives out two kinds of UV rays: UVA and UVB. You need to protect your skin from both kinds. Look for sunscreens and sunglasses that protect from both UVA and UVB rays.

A sunburn takes 6 to 48 hours to develop. You may not know your skin is burned until it is too late.

What does SPF mean?

SPF stands for "sun protection factor." Sunscreen labels have an SPF number. The higher the number, the better the protection.

What can I do to protect myself?

- Don't stay in the sun for a long time, especially in the middle of the day. The sun's rays are strongest from 10 a.m. to 4 p.m. in spring and summer.

- Use sunscreen with SPF 15 or more.

- Apply more sunscreen every two hours and after swimming, sweating, or towel drying.

- Use sunscreen even on a cloudy day. Glare from water and snow can expose you to UV.

- Wear clothing that covers your body and a hat with a wide brim to protect your head and face.

- Wear sunglasses that protect from UV. Not all tinted and dark glasses offer UV protection. Check the label before you buy them.

Are sunlamps and tanning beds hazardous to health?

Sunlamps and tanning beds give off UV rays just like the sun. Tanning beds can be as dangerous as tanning outdoors. They may be more dangerous than the sun because they can be used at any time. They can also be more dangerous because people can expose their entire bodies at each session, which would be difficult to do outdoors.

- All tanning beds put you at higher risk of skin cancer.

- The National Cancer Institute (NCI) reports that women who use tanning beds more than once a month are 55% more likely to develop melanoma, the deadliest form of skin cancer.

- The U.S. Food and Drug Administration (FDA) has standards for sunlamp products. All sunlamp products must have the following:

  - A warning label

  - An accurate timer

  - An emergency stop control

  - An exposure schedule

  - Protective goggles

Some people do things that make tanning beds even more dangerous:

- Not wearing goggles or wearing goggles that are loose or cracked

- Staying in the bed for the maximum time that is listed on the label

- Staying in the bed longer than recommended for your skin type (check the label for exposure times)

- Using medicines or cosmetics that make you more sensitive to UV rays (check with your doctor, nurse, or pharmacist)

What are "sunless" tanning products?

- Sunless tanning products are cosmetics that make the skin look tanned.

113

- Most of these products do not have sunscreen, so you still need to use sunscreen.

- If you go to a spray-on sunless tanning booth, ask for protection to keep from breathing in the spray. Keep it out of your mouth, eyes, and lips.

- FDA has not approved any tanning pills. These pills can have bad side effects including nausea, cramping, diarrhea, severe itching, and welts. Tanning pills also may cause yellow patches inside your eyes and affect your eyesight.

- Some lotions and pills claim to make you tan faster. There is no proof that these work. "Tanning accelerators" are not approved by the FDA.

Section 13.6

Safe Use of Cosmetics

Excerpted from "Cosmetics," October 5, 2009, and "Cosmetics Q&A,"
June 4, 2012, U.S. Food and Drug Administration (www.fda.gov).

Cosmetics

People use cosmetics to enhance their beauty. These products range from lipstick and foundation to deodorant, toothpaste, and hairspray. In 1938, Congress passed the U.S. Food, Drug, and Cosmetics Act. In the 70 years since the law was passed, the federal government has worked with industry to keep cosmetics safe.

How does the law protect you?

Cosmetics must follow these standards:

- Must be made and packaged in clean factories

- Cannot contain poisonous, rotten, or harmful ingredients

- May only use color additives that are FDA approved

- Must have a clear, truthful label

How does the label help you?

The law says a label must include the following:

- What the product is
- A list of what is in the product and how to use it safely
- How much of the product the package contains by weight
- The name of the company that makes or sells the product

Does FDA test cosmetics before they are sold?

FDA does not test cosmetics before they are sold in stores. Companies must make sure their products and ingredients are safe before they sell them. FDA can take action against companies who break the law.

What are safety tips for using cosmetics?

- Follow all directions on the label, including "Cautions" and "Warnings."
- Keep makeup containers clean and closed tight when not in use.
- Wash your hands before you put on makeup.
- Do not share makeup.
- Do not add saliva or water to makeup.
- Throw away makeup if the color or smell changes.
- Don't store your makeup above 85° F /29° C.
- Stop using a product if you get a rash or have a problem.
- Do not use spray cans while you are smoking or near an open flame. It could start a fire.
- Do not put on makeup while you are driving.

Will cosmetics expire?

- There is no law that cosmetics must have an expiration date.
- Expiration dates are just guidelines. A product may go bad sooner if you store it the wrong way.

Are "testers" at makeup counters safe?

- Testers can have lots of germs because so many people use them.

- When you test a product at the counter, use a new sponge or cotton swab.

Could I be allergic to something in a cosmetic?

- Some people may react to something in a product. For example, they may have itching, redness, rash, sneezing, or wheezing.

- Allergies may happen the first time you use a product or after you have used it more than once.

What should I do if I have a bad reaction to a cosmetic?

- Stop using the product.

- Call your doctor to find out how to take care of the problem.

- Call FDA's Center for Food Safety and Applied Nutrition (CFSAN) at 301-436-2405 or send an e-mail to CAERS@cfsan.fda.gov.

- Call the company that makes the product.

Cosmetics Q&A

How does FDA regulate cosmetics? Are they FDA approved?

FDA's legal authority over cosmetics is different from other products they regulate, such as drugs, biologics, and medical devices. FDA does not have the legal authority to approve cosmetics before they go on the market, although they do approve color additives used in them (except coal tar hair dyes). However, under the law, cosmetics must not be "adulterated" or "misbranded." For example, they must be safe for consumers when used as directed in their labeling or under customary conditions of use, and they must be properly labeled. Companies and individuals who market cosmetics have a legal responsibility for the safety and labeling of their products.

FDA can take action against a cosmetic on the market if they have reliable information showing that it is adulterated or misbranded.

What ingredients are prohibited from use in cosmetics?

With the exception of color additives and a few prohibited ingredients, a cosmetic manufacturer may use almost any raw material as a cosmetic ingredient and market the product without an approval from FDA. The Federal Food, Drug, and Cosmetic Act requires that color additives used in cosmetics must be tested for safety and be listed by the FDA for their intended uses.

Regulations restrict or prohibit the use of the following ingredients in cosmetics: bithionol, mercury compounds, vinyl chloride, halogenated salicylanilides, zirconium complexes in aerosol cosmetics, chloroform, methylene chloride, chlorofluorocarbon propellants, methyl methacrylate monomer, and hexachlorophene.

In addition to the ingredients that are controlled by regulation or were the subject of a court ruling, cosmetic and fragrance trade associations have recommended eliminating or limiting the use of certain ingredients associated with health risks.

What is the shelf life of cosmetics?

The shelf life for eye-area cosmetics is more limited than for other products. Because of repeated microbial exposure during use by the consumer and the risk of eye infections, some industry experts recommend replacing mascara three months after purchase. If mascara becomes dry, discard it.

Among other cosmetics that are likely to have an unusually short shelf life are certain "all natural" products that may contain plant-derived substances conducive to microbial growth. It also is important for consumers and manufacturers to consider the increased risk of contamination in products that contain nontraditional preservatives, or no preservatives at all.

Consumers should be aware that expiration dates are simply "rules of thumb" and that a product's safety may expire long before the expiration date if the product has not been properly stored. Cosmetics that have been improperly stored—for example, exposed to high temperatures or sunlight, or opened and examined by consumers prior to final sale—may deteriorate substantially before the expiration date. On the other hand, products stored under ideal conditions may be acceptable long after the expiration date has been reached.

What are "hypoallergenic" cosmetics?

Hypoallergenic cosmetics are products that manufacturers claim produce fewer allergic reactions than other cosmetic products. Consumers with hypersensitive skin, and even those with "normal" skin, may be led to believe that these products will be gentler to their skin than non-hypoallergenic cosmetics.

There are no federal standards or definitions that govern the use of the term "hypoallergenic." The term means whatever a particular company wants it to mean. Manufacturers of cosmetics labeled as hypoallergenic are not required to submit substantiation of their hypoallergenicity claims to FDA.

Are tattoos and permanent makeup safe? How about henna and other temporary tattoos?

FDA is looking into the safety of tattoos and permanent makeup because of their growing popularity. For example, they are looking at tattoo removal, adverse reactions to tattoo colors, and infections that result from the use of these products.

Consumers should be aware of some of the risks presented by tattoos and permanent makeup:

- No color additives are approved for tattoos, including those used in permanent makeup. Some people have had bad reactions to pigments used in tattoo and permanent makeup inks. Some have suffered permanent disfigurement.

- Unsterile tattooing equipment and needles can transmit infectious disease, such as hepatitis; it is extremely important to confirm that all equipment is clean and sanitary before use.

- Tattoos and permanent makeup are not easily removed and in some cases may cause permanent discoloration. Think carefully before getting a tattoo and consider the possibility of an allergic reaction.

- If you get a tattoo at a facility not regulated by your state or at facilities that use unsterile equipment, or re-use ink, you may not be accepted as a blood or plasma donor for 12 months.

Temporary tattoos, such as those applied to the skin with a moistened wad of cotton, fade several days after application. Many contain color additives approved for cosmetic use on the skin. However, FDA has received reports of allergic reactions to some temporary tattoos.

Henna, a coloring made from a plant, is approved only for use as a hair dye, not for direct application to the skin. FDA has received reports of injuries to the skin from products marketed as henna.

Do cosmetics contain harmful contaminants, such as lead? What does FDA do to guard against them?

Under the Federal Food, Drug, and Cosmetic Act, cosmetics must be safe for consumers when used as intended. If a cosmetic is harmful to consumers, it is adulterated under the law, and it is against the law to market adulterated cosmetics in interstate commerce. It doesn't matter whether the safety problem is caused by ingredients or contaminants. Companies and individuals who market cosmetics have a legal responsibility for the safety of their products.

FDA monitors cosmetics on the market to watch for potential safety problems, including potential contaminants. They take action against products that do not comply with the law.

These are some of the ways FDA watches out for cosmetics that may contain harmful contaminants:

Inspecting imports: One way that FDA guards against contaminated cosmetics is by working with U.S. Customs and Border Protection staff to inspect imported products. FDA issues Import Alerts to help inspection staff look out for products that are most likely to pose a safety hazard. A number of Import Alerts for cosmetics warn about products that may contain harmful contaminants. Cosmetics that are found to be unsafe are refused entry into this country.

Inspecting manufacturers: FDA has issued guidance to manufacturers on how to keep two kinds of contaminants, nitrosamines and 1,4-dioxane, from forming during the manufacturing process. FDA inspectors check to make sure manufacturers are following the proper procedures.

Color additives: Except for those intended as coal tar hair dyes, each color additive used in cosmetics must be approved by FDA and listed in a regulation that states its permitted use, as well as all specifications and restrictions. These regulations set strict limits on contaminants. FDA sets these limits based on how much of the color additive a person is likely to be exposed to and the routes of exposure under the intended conditions of use.

What precautions should you take if you dye your hair?

People who dye their hair should follow these safety precautions:

- Follow the directions in the package. Pay attention to all "Caution" and "Warning" statements.

- Do a patch test before using dye on your hair. Rub a tiny bit of the dye on the inside of your elbow or behind your ear. Leave it there for two days. If you get a rash, don't use the dye on your hair. You should do the test each time you dye your hair. (Salons should also do the patch test before dyeing your hair.)

- Never dye your eyebrows or eyelashes. This can hurt your eyes. You might even go blind. FDA does not allow using hair dyes on eyelashes and eyebrows.

- Keep hair dyes out of the reach of children.

- Don't leave the dye on longer than the directions say you should.

- Rinse your scalp well with water after dyeing.

- Wear gloves when you apply the hair dye.

- Never mix different hair dye products. This can hurt your hair and scalp.

What precautions should you take when using eye cosmetics?

If you use eye cosmetics, FDA urges you to follow these safety tips:

- If any eye cosmetic causes irritation, stop using it immediately. If irritation persists, see a doctor.

- Avoid using eye cosmetics if you have an eye infection or the skin around the eye is inflamed. Wait until the area is healed. Discard any eye cosmetics you were using when you got the infection.

- Be aware that there are bacteria on your hands that, if placed in the eye, could cause infections. Wash your hands before applying eye cosmetics.

- Make sure that any instrument you place in the eye area is clean.

- Don't share your cosmetics. Another person's bacteria may be hazardous to you.

- Don't allow cosmetics to become covered with dust or contaminated with dirt or soil. Keep containers clean.

- Don't use old containers of eye cosmetics. Discard mascara three months after purchase.

- Discard dried-up mascara. Don't add saliva or water to moisten it. The bacteria from your mouth may grow in the mascara and cause infection. Adding water may introduce bacteria and will dilute the preservative that is intended to protect against microbial growth.

- Don't store cosmetics at temperatures above 85° F. Cosmetics held for long periods in hot cars, for example, are more susceptible to deterioration of the preservative.

- When applying or removing eye cosmetics, be careful not to scratch the eyeball or other sensitive area. Never apply or remove eye cosmetics in a moving vehicle.

- Don't use any cosmetics near your eyes unless they are intended specifically for that use. For instance, don't use a lip liner as an eye liner. You may be exposing your eyes to contamination from your mouth or to color additives that are not approved for use in the area of the eye.

- Avoid color additives that are not approved for use in the area of the eye, such as "permanent" eyelash tints and kohl. Be especially careful to keep kohl away from children, since reports have linked it to lead poisoning.

Chapter 14

Recommended Screenings for Women

Chapter Contents

Section 14.1

Preventive Health Care Screenings for Women

Excerpted from "A Lifetime of Good Health: Your Guide to Staying Healthy," U.S. Department of Health and Human Services Office on Women's Health (www.womenshealth.gov), February 2011.

Prevention is important to living long and living well. Getting preventive screenings and immunizations are among the most important things you can do for yourself. Take time to review these guidelines for screening tests and immunizations. These are guidelines only. Your doctor or nurse will personalize the timing of each test and immunization to meet your health care needs.

General Health

Full checkup, including weight and height: Ask your doctor or nurse about health topics such as the following:

• Overweight and obesity

• Tobacco use

• Alcohol use

• Depression

• Thyroid (TSH) testing

• Skin and mole exam

HIV test: Get tested at least once to find out your HIV status. Ask your doctor or nurse if and when you need the test again.

Heart Health

Blood pressure test: For adult women, this should be checked at least every two years.

Cholesterol test: Start at age 20; discuss frequency with your doctor or nurse.

Bone Health

Bone mineral density test: Starting at age 50, discuss with your doctor or nurse. You should be tested at least once by age 65. Talk to your doctor or nurse about repeat testing.

Diabetes

Blood glucose or A1C test: Start at age 45, then retest every three years.

Breast Health

Mammogram (X-ray of the breast): Starting at age 40, have a mammogram every one to two years.

Clinical breast exam: Discuss with your doctor or nurse.

Reproductive Health

Pap test: Every two years starting at age 21. Women 30 and older should be tested every three years. Age 65 and older, discuss with your doctor or nurse.

Pelvic exam: Test yearly beginning at age 21. If younger than 21 and sexually active, discuss with your doctor or nurse.

Chlamydia test: Test yearly until age 24 if sexually active. Age 25 and older, get this test if you have new or multiple partners.

Sexually transmitted infection (STI) tests: Discuss with your doctor or nurse.

Colorectal Health

Screening tests for colorectal cancer: Beginning around age 50, discuss with your doctor or nurse which test is best for you and how often you need it.

Eye and Ear Health

Comprehensive eye exam: If younger than 40, discuss with your doctor. Get a baseline exam at age 40, then every two to four years or as your doctor advises. After age 55, every one to three years is appropriate.

Hearing screening: Every 10 years until age 50. After 50, receive a hearing screening every 3 years.

Oral Health

Dental and oral cancer exam: This exam should be performed routinely; discuss with your dentist.

Section 14.2

What Are Mammograms (Breast Cancer Screening)?

Excerpted from "Mammograms Fact Sheet," U.S. Department of Health and Human Services Office on Women's Health (www.womenshealth.gov), November 17, 2010.

What is a mammogram?

A mammogram is a low-dose X-ray exam of the breasts to look for changes that are not normal. The results are recorded on X-ray film or directly into a computer for a doctor called a radiologist to examine.

A mammogram allows the doctor to have a closer look for changes in breast tissue that cannot be felt during a breast exam. It is used for women who have no breast complaints and for women who have breast symptoms, such as a change in the shape or size of a breast, a lump, nipple discharge, or pain. Breast changes occur in almost all women. In fact, most of these changes are not cancer and are called "benign," but only a doctor can know for sure. Breast changes can also happen monthly, due to your menstrual period.

What is the best method of detecting breast cancer as early as possible?

A high-quality mammogram plus a clinical breast exam, an exam done by your doctor, is the most effective way to detect breast cancer early. Finding breast cancer early greatly improves a woman's chances for successful treatment.

Like any test, mammograms have both benefits and limitations. For example, some cancers can't be found by a mammogram, but they may be found in a clinical breast exam.

Checking your own breasts for lumps or other changes is called a breast self-exam (BSE). Studies so far have not shown that BSE alone helps reduce the number of deaths from breast cancer. BSE should not take the place of routine clinical breast exams and mammograms.

If you choose to do BSE, remember that breast changes can occur because of pregnancy, aging, menopause, menstrual cycles, or from taking birth control pills or other hormones. It is normal for breasts to feel a little lumpy and uneven. Also, it is common for breasts to be swollen and tender right before or during a menstrual period. If you notice any unusual changes in your breasts, contact your doctor.

How is a mammogram done?

You stand in front of a special X-ray machine. The person who takes the X-rays, called a radiologic technician, places your breasts, one at a time, between an X-ray plate and a plastic plate. These plates are attached to the X-ray machine and compress the breasts to flatten them. This spreads the breast tissue out to obtain a clearer picture. You will feel pressure on your breast for a few seconds. It may cause you some discomfort; you might feel squeezed or pinched. This feeling only lasts for a few seconds, and the flatter your breast, the better the picture. Most often, two pictures are taken of each breast—one from the side and one from above. A screening mammogram takes about 20 minutes from start to finish.

Are there different types of mammograms?

Screening mammograms are done for women who have no symptoms of breast cancer. It usually involves two X-rays of each breast. Screening mammograms can detect lumps or tumors that cannot be felt. They can also find microcalcifications, or tiny deposits of calcium in the breast, which sometimes mean that breast cancer is present.

Diagnostic mammograms are used to check for breast cancer after a lump or other symptom or sign of breast cancer has been found. Signs of breast cancer may include pain, thickened skin on the breast, nipple discharge, or a change in breast size or shape. This type of mammogram also can be used to find out more about breast changes found on a screening mammogram or to view breast tissue that is hard to see on a screening mammogram. A diagnostic mammogram takes longer than a screening mammogram because it involves more X-rays in order to obtain views of the breast from several angles. The technician can magnify a problem area to make a more detailed picture, which helps the doctor make a correct diagnosis.

A digital mammogram also uses X-rays to produce an image of the breast, but instead of storing the image directly on film, the image is stored directly on a computer. This allows the recorded image to be magnified for the doctor to take a closer look. Current research has not shown that digital images are better at showing cancer than x-ray film images in general.

How often should I get a mammogram?

The National Cancer Institute recommends the following:

• Women 40 years and older should get a mammogram every one to two years.

• Women who have had breast cancer or other breast problems or who have a family history of breast cancer might need to start getting mammograms before age 40, or they might need to get them more often. Talk to your doctor about when to start and how often you should have a mammogram.

What can mammograms show?

The radiologist will look at your X-rays for breast changes that do not look normal and for differences in each breast. He or she will compare your past mammograms with your most recent one to check for changes.

• **Lump or mass:** The size, shape, and edges of a lump sometimes can give doctors information about whether or not it may be cancer. On a mammogram, a growth that is benign often looks smooth and round with a clear, defined edge. Breast cancer often has a jagged outline and an irregular shape.

• **Calcification:** A calcification is a deposit of the mineral calcium in the breast tissue. Calcifications appear as small white spots on a mammogram. There are two types:

  • Macrocalcifications are large calcium deposits often caused by aging. These usually are not a sign of cancer.

  • Microcalcifications are tiny specks of calcium that may be found in an area of rapidly dividing cells.

If calcifications are grouped together in a certain way, it may be a sign of cancer. Depending on how many calcium specks you have, how big they are, and what they look like, your doctor may suggest that you have other tests.

What if my screening mammogram shows a problem?

If you have a screening test result that suggests cancer, your doctor must find out whether it is due to cancer or to some other cause. Your doctor may ask about your personal and family medical history. You may have a physical exam. Your doctor also may order some of these tests:

- **Diagnostic mammogram:** This test can focus on a specific area of the breast.

- **Ultrasound:** This imaging test uses sound waves to create a picture of your breast. The pictures may show whether a lump is solid or filled with fluid. A cyst is a fluid-filled sac. Cysts are not cancer. But a solid mass may be cancer.

- **Magnetic resonance imaging (MRI):** This test uses a powerful magnet linked to a computer. MRI makes detailed pictures of breast tissue.

- **Biopsy:** In this test, fluid or tissue is removed from your breast to help find out if there is cancer. Your doctor may refer you to a surgeon or to a doctor who is an expert in breast disease for a biopsy.

Where can I get a high-quality mammogram?

Women can get high-quality mammograms in breast clinics, hospital radiology departments, mobile vans, private radiology offices, and doctors' offices. The Food and Drug Administration (FDA) certifies mammography facilities that meet strict quality standards for their X-ray machines and staff and are inspected every year. You can ask your doctor or the staff at the mammography center about FDA certification before making your appointment. A list of FDA-certified facilities can be found on the internet (at www.fda.gov/cdrh/mammography/certified.html).

Your doctor, medical clinic, or health department can tell you where to get no-cost or low-cost mammograms. You can also call the National Cancer Institute's Cancer Information Service toll free at 800-422-6237.

What if I have breast implants?

Women with breast implants should also have mammograms. A woman who had an implant after breast cancer surgery in which the entire breast was removed (mastectomy) should ask her doctor whether she needs a mammogram of the reconstructed breast.

If you have breast implants, be sure to tell your mammography facility that you have them when you make your appointment. The technician and radiologist must be experienced in X-raying patients with breast implants. Implants can hide some breast tissue, making it harder for the radiologist to see a problem when looking at your mammogram.

How do I get ready for my mammogram?

First, check with the place you are having the mammogram for any special instructions you may need to follow before you go. Here are some general guidelines to follow:

- If you are still having menstrual periods, try to avoid making your mammogram appointment during the week before your period. Your breasts will be less tender and swollen. The mammogram will hurt less and the picture will be better.

- If you have breast implants, be sure to tell your mammography facility that you have them when you make your appointment.

- Wear a shirt with shorts, pants, or a skirt. This way, you can undress from the waist up when you get your mammogram.

- Don't wear any deodorant, perfume, lotion, or powder under your arms or on your breasts on the day of your mammogram appointment. These things can make shadows show up on your mammogram.

- If you have had mammograms at another facility, have those X-ray films sent to the new facility so that they can be compared to the new films.

Are there any problems with mammograms?

Although they are not perfect, mammograms are the best method to find breast changes that cannot be felt. As with any medical test, mammograms have limits. These limits include the following:

- They are only part of a complete breast exam. Your doctor also should do a clinical breast exam. If your mammogram finds something abnormal, your doctor will order other tests.

- Finding cancer does not always mean saving lives. Even though mammography can detect tumors that cannot be felt, finding a small tumor does not always mean that a woman's life will be saved. Mammography may not help a woman with a fast-growing cancer that has already spread to other parts of her body.

- False negatives can happen. This means everything may look normal, but cancer is actually present. False negatives don't happen often. Younger women are more likely to have a false negative mammogram than are older women.

- False positives can happen. This is when the mammogram results look like cancer is present, even though it is not. False positives are more common in younger women, women who have had breast biopsies, women with a family history of breast cancer, and women who are taking estrogen, such as menopausal hormone therapy.

- Mammograms use very small doses of radiation. The risk of any harm is very slight, but repeated X-rays could cause cancer. The benefits nearly always outweigh the risk. Talk to your doctor about the need for each X-ray. Ask about shielding to protect parts of the body that are not in the picture. You should always let your doctor and the technician know if there is any chance that you are pregnant.

Section 14.3

Mammogram and Breast Self-Examination Recommendations

Excerpted from "Screening for Breast Cancer:
Recommendation Statement," U.S. Preventive Services Task Force
(www.uspreventiveservicestaskforce.org), December 2009.

Summary of Recommendation and Evidence

- The U.S. Preventive Services Task Force (USPSTF) recommends biennial screening mammography for women aged 50 to 74 years.

- The decision to start regular, biennial screening mammography before the age of 50 years should be an individual one and take patient context into account, including the patient's values regarding specific benefits and harms.

- The USPSTF concludes that the current evidence is insufficient to assess the additional benefits and harms of screening mammography in women 75 years or older.

- The USPSTF recommends against teaching breast self-examination (BSE).

- The USPSTF concludes that the current evidence is insufficient to assess the additional benefits and harms of clinical breast examination (CBE) beyond screening mammography in women 40 years or older.

- The USPSTF concludes that the current evidence is insufficient to assess the additional benefits and harms of either digital mammography or MRI instead of film mammography as screening modalities for breast cancer.

Rationale

Importance

Breast cancer is the second-leading cause of cancer death among women in the United States. Widespread use of screening, along with treatment advances in recent years, have been credited with significant reductions in breast cancer mortality.

Detection

Mammography, as well as physical examination of the breasts (CBE and BSE), can detect presymptomatic breast cancer. Because of its demonstrated effectiveness in randomized, controlled trials of screening, film mammography is the standard for detecting breast cancer.

Benefits of Detection and Early Intervention

There is convincing evidence that screening with film mammography reduces breast cancer mortality, with a greater absolute reduction for women aged 50 to 74 years than for women aged 40 to 49 years. The strongest evidence for the greatest benefit is among women aged 60 to 69 years.

Among women 75 years or older, evidence of benefits of mammography is lacking.

Adequate evidence suggests that teaching BSE does not reduce breast cancer mortality. The evidence for additional effects of CBE beyond mammography on breast cancer mortality is inadequate.

The evidence for benefits of digital mammography and MRI of the breast, as a substitute for film mammography, is also lacking.

Harms of Detection and Early Intervention

The harms resulting from screening for breast cancer include psychological harms, unnecessary imaging tests and biopsies in women without cancer, and inconvenience due to false positive screening results. Furthermore, one must also consider the harms associated with treatment of cancer that would not become clinically apparent during a woman's lifetime (overdiagnosis), as well as the harms of unnecessary earlier treatment of breast cancer that would have become clinically apparent but would not have shortened a woman's life. Radiation exposure (from radiologic tests), although a minor concern, is also a consideration.

Adequate evidence suggests that the overall harms associated with mammography are moderate for every age group considered, although the main components of the harms shift over time. Although false positive test results, overdiagnosis, and unnecessary earlier treatment are problems for all age groups, false positive results are more common for women aged 40 to 49 years, whereas overdiagnosis is a greater concern for women in the older age groups.

There is adequate evidence that teaching BSE is associated with harms that are at least small. There is inadequate evidence concerning harms of CBE.

Section 14.4

Pap Tests
(Cervical Cancer Screening)

Excerpted from "Pap Test Fact Sheet," U.S. Department of Health and Human Services Office on Women's Health (www.womenshealth.gov), January 14, 2009.

What is a Pap test?

The Pap test, also called a Pap smear, checks for changes in the cells of your cervix. The cervix is the lower part of the uterus (womb) that opens into the vagina (birth canal). The Pap test can tell if you have an infection, abnormal (unhealthy) cervical cells, or cervical cancer.

Why do I need a Pap test?

A Pap test can save your life. It can find the earliest signs of cervical cancer. If caught early, the chance of curing cervical cancer is very high. Pap tests also can find infections and abnormal cervical cells that can turn into cancer cells. Treatment can prevent most cases of cervical cancer from developing.

Getting regular Pap tests is the best thing you can do to prevent cervical cancer. In fact, regular Pap tests have led to a major decline in the number of cervical cancer cases and deaths.

Do all women need Pap tests?

It is important for all women to have Pap tests, along with pelvic exams, as part of their routine health care. You need a Pap test if you are 21 years or older.

Women who have gone through menopause (when a woman's periods stop) still need regular Pap tests. Women ages 65 and older can talk to their doctor about stopping after at least three normal Pap tests and no abnormal results in the last 10 years.

How often do I need to get a Pap test?

It depends on your age and health history. Talk with your doctor about what is best for you. Most women can follow these guidelines:

- Starting at age 21, have a Pap test every two years.
- If you are 30 years old and older and have had three normal Pap tests for three years in a row, talk to your doctor about spacing out Pap tests to every three years.
- If you are over 65 years old, ask your doctor if you can stop having Pap tests.

Ask your doctor about more frequent testing in these situations:

- You have a weakened immune system because of organ transplant, chemotherapy, or steroid use
- Your mother was exposed to diethylstilbestrol (DES) while pregnant
- You are HIV positive

Women who are living with HIV, the virus that causes AIDS, are at a higher risk of cervical cancer and other cervical diseases. The U.S. Centers for Disease Control and Prevention recommends that all HIV-positive women get an initial Pap test and get retested six months later. If both Pap tests are normal, then these women can get yearly Pap tests in the future.

Who does not need regular Pap tests?

The only women who do not need regular Pap tests are the following:

- Women over age 65 who have had three normal Pap tests and in a row and no abnormal test results in the last 10 years and have been told by their doctors that they don't need to be tested anymore.

- Women who do not have a cervix and are at low risk for cervical cancer. These women should speak to their doctor before stopping regular Pap tests.

I had a hysterectomy. Do I still need Pap tests?

It depends on the type of hysterectomy (surgery to remove the uterus) you had and your health history. Women who have had a hysterectomy should talk with their doctor about whether they need routine Pap tests.

Usually during a hysterectomy, the cervix is removed with the uterus. This is called a total hysterectomy. Women who have had a total hysterectomy for reasons other than cancer may not need regular Pap tests. Women who have had a total hysterectomy because of abnormal cells or cancer should be tested yearly for vaginal cancer until they have three normal test results. Women who have had only their uterus removed but still have a cervix need regular Pap tests. Even women who have had hysterectomies should see their doctors yearly for pelvic exams.

How can I reduce my chances of getting cervical cancer?

Aside from getting Pap tests, the best way to avoid cervical cancer is by steering clear of the human papillomavirus (HPV). HPV is a major cause of cervical cancer. HPV infection is also one of the most common sexually transmitted infections (STI). So, a woman boosts her chances of getting cervical cancer if she engages in these behaviors:

- Starts having sex before age 18

- Has many sex partners

- Has sex partners who have other sex partners

- Has or has had a STI

What should I know about HPV?

Human papillomaviruses are a group of more than 100 different viruses.

- About 40 types of HPV are spread during sex.

- Some types of HPVs can cause cervical cancer when not treated.

- HPV infection is one of the most common STIs.
- About 75% of sexually active people will get HPV sometime in their life.
- Most women with untreated HPV do not get cervical cancer.
- Some HPVs cause genital warts, but these HPVs do not cause cervical cancer.
- Since HPV rarely causes symptoms, most people don't know they have the infection.

How would I know if I had HPV?

Most women never know they have HPV. It usually stays hidden and doesn't cause symptoms like warts. When HPV doesn't go away on its own, it can cause changes in the cells of the cervix. Pap tests usually find these changes.

How do I prepare for a Pap test?

Many things can cause wrong test results by washing away or hiding abnormal cells of the cervix. So doctors suggest that for two days before the test you avoid the following:

- Douching
- Using tampons
- Using vaginal creams, suppositories, and medicines
- Using vaginal deodorant sprays or powders
- Having sex

Doctors suggest you schedule a Pap test when you do not have your period. The best time to be tested is 10 to 20 days after the first day of your last period.

How is a Pap test done?

Your doctor can do a Pap test during a pelvic exam. It is a simple and quick test. While you lie on an exam table, the doctor puts an instrument called a speculum into your vagina, opening it to see the cervix. She will then use a special stick or brush to take a few cells from inside and around the cervix. The cells are placed on a glass slide and sent to a lab for examination. While usually painless, a Pap test is uncomfortable for some women.

When will I get the results of my Pap test?

Usually it takes three weeks to get Pap test results. Most of the time, test results are normal. If the test shows that something might be wrong, your doctor will contact you to schedule more tests. There are many reasons for abnormal Pap test results. It usually does not mean you have cancer.

What do abnormal Pap test results mean?

It is scary to hear that your Pap test results are "abnormal." But abnormal Pap test results usually do not mean you have cancer. Most often there is a small problem with the cervix.

Some abnormal cells will turn into cancer. But most of the time, these unhealthy cells will go away on their own. By treating these unhealthy cells, almost all cases of cervical cancer can be prevented. If you have abnormal results, talk with your doctor about what they mean.

My Pap test was "abnormal," what happens now?

There are many reasons for "abnormal" Pap test results. If results of the Pap test are unclear or show a small change in the cells of the cervix, your doctor will probably repeat the Pap test.

If the test finds more serious changes in the cells of the cervix, the doctor will suggest more powerful tests that will help your doctor decide on the best treatment:

- **Colposcopy:** The doctor uses a tool called a colposcope to see the cells of the vagina and cervix in detail.

- **Endocervical curettage:** The doctor takes a sample of cells from the endocervical canal with a small spoon-shaped tool called a curette.

- **Biopsy:** The doctor removes a small sample of cervical tissue. The sample is sent to a lab to be studied under a microscope.

The FDA recently approved the LUMA Cervical Imaging System. The doctor uses this device right after a colposcopy. This system can help doctors see areas on the cervix that are likely to contain precancerous cells.

My Pap test result was a "false positive." What does this mean?

Pap tests are not always 100% correct. False positive and false negative results can happen. This can be upsetting and confusing.

A false positive Pap test is when a woman is told she has abnormal cervical cells, but the cells are really normal. If your doctor says your Pap results were a false positive, there is no problem.

A false negative Pap test is when a woman is told her cells are normal, but in fact there is a problem with the cervical cells that was missed. False negatives delay the discovery and treatment of unhealthy cells of the cervix. But having regular Pap tests boosts your chances of finding any problems. If abnormal cells are missed at one time, they will probably be found on your next Pap test.

If I don't have health insurance, how can I get a free or low-cost Pap test?

Programs funded by the National Breast and Cervical Cancer Early Detection Program (NBCCEDP) offer free or low-cost Pap tests to women in need. To find contact information for a program near you, visit the NBCCEDP website (www.cdc.gov/cancer/nbccedp) or call 800-232-4636. Also, your state or local health department can direct you to places that offer free or low-cost Pap tests.

Planned Parenthood offers low-cost Pap tests as well. To find the Planned Parenthood office in your area, call 800-230-7526 or visit their website (www.plannedparenthood.org).

Section 14.5

Colorectal Cancer Screening

"Colorectal Cancer Screening," Centers for Disease Control
and Prevention (www.cdc.gov), March 8, 2012.

Colorectal cancer almost always develops from precancerous polyps (abnormal growths) in the colon or rectum. Screening tests can find precancerous polyps, so that they can be removed before they turn into cancer. Screening tests can also find colorectal cancer early, when treatment works best.

When should I begin to get screened?

You should begin screening for colorectal cancer soon after turning 50, then continue getting screened at regular intervals. However, you may need to be tested earlier than 50 or more often than other people if the following apply to you:

- You or a close relative have had colorectal polyps or colorectal cancer.

- You have inflammatory bowel disease.

- You have genetic syndromes such as familial adenomatous polyposis (FAP) or hereditary non-polyposis colorectal cancer.

Speak with your doctor about when you should begin screening and how often you should be tested.

What is colorectal cancer screening?

A screening test is used to look for a disease when a person is not experiencing any symptoms. Cancer screening tests, including those for colorectal cancer, are effective when they can detect disease early. Detecting disease early can lead to more effective treatment. In some cases, screening tests can detect something that shouldn't be there, such as a polyp in the colon or rectum, before it has a chance to turn into cancer. Removing polyps in the colon and rectum prevents colorectal cancer from developing. (A diagnostic test differs from a screening test because it is used when a person has symptoms. A diagnostic test is used to find the cause of the symptoms.)

How can I find free or low-cost screening options?

CDC's Colorectal Cancer Control Program (CRCCP) provides funding to 25 states and four tribes across the United States. The program supports population-based screening efforts and provides colorectal cancer screening services to low-income men and women aged 50–64 years who are underinsured or uninsured for screening, when no other insurance is available. In addition to colorectal cancer screening, the program sites also provide diagnostic follow-up.

If you live in one of the CRCCP-funded states, you may be eligible for free or low-cost colorectal cancer screening. If you are not eligible for the program, or live outside the areas in which the CRCCP operates, please call 800-4-CANCER or 800-ACS-2345 to learn more about screening options in your community. You also may be able to find information about free or low-cost screening by calling your local department of health.

Section 14.6

Osteoporosis Screening (Bone Density Testing)

"Bone Mass Measurement: What the Numbers Mean,"
National Institute of Arthritis and Musculoskeletal and Skin Diseases
(www.niams.nih.gov), January 2012.

A bone mineral density (BMD) test is the best way to determine your bone health. The test can identify osteoporosis, determine your risk for fractures (broken bones), and measure your response to osteoporosis treatment. The most widely recognized BMD test is called a dual-energy X-ray absorptiometry, or DXA test. It is painless—a bit like having an X-ray. The test can measure bone density at your hip and spine.

A DXA test measures your bone mineral density and compares it to that of an established norm or standard to give you a score. Although no bone density test is 100% accurate, the DXA test is the single most important predictor of whether a person will have a fracture in the future.

T-Score

Most commonly, your DXA test results are compared to the ideal or peak bone mineral density of a healthy 30-year-old adult, and you are given a T-score. A score of 0 means your BMD is equal to the norm for a healthy young adult. Differences between your BMD and that of the healthy young adult norm are measured in units called standard deviations (SDs). The more standard deviations below 0, indicated as negative numbers, the lower your BMD and the higher your risk of fracture.

As shown in Table 14.1, a T-score between +1 and −1 is considered normal or healthy. A T-score between −1 and −2.5 indicates that you have low bone mass, although not low enough to be diagnosed with osteoporosis. A T-score of −2.5 or lower indicates that you have osteoporosis. The greater the negative number, the more severe the osteoporosis.

142

Table 14.1. World Health Organization Definitions Based on Bone Density Levels

Level	Definition
Normal	Bone density is within 1 SD (+1 or –1) of the young adult mean.
Low bone mass	Bone density is between 1 and 2.5 SD below the young adult mean (–1 to –2.5 SD).
Osteoporosis	Bone density is 2.5 SD or more below the young adult mean (–2.5 SD or lower).
Severe (established) osteoporosis	Bone density is more than 2.5 SD below the young adult mean, and there have been one or more osteoporotic fractures.

Z-Score

Sometimes your bone mineral density is compared to that of a typical individual whose age is matched to yours. This comparison gives you a Z-score. Because a low BMD level is common among older adults, comparisons with the BMD of a typical individual whose age is matched to yours can be misleading. Therefore, the diagnosis of osteoporosis or low bone mass is based on your T-score. However, a Z-score can be useful for determining whether an underlying disease or condition is causing bone loss.

Low Bone Mass versus Osteoporosis

The information provided by a BMD test can help your doctor decide which prevention or treatment options are right for you.

If you have low bone mass that is not low enough to be diagnosed as osteoporosis, this is sometimes referred to as osteopenia. Low bone mass can be caused by many factors:

- Heredity

- The development of less-than-optimal peak bone mass in your youth

- A medical condition or medication to treat such a condition that negatively affects bone

- Abnormally accelerated bone loss

Although not everyone who has low bone mass will develop osteoporosis, everyone with low bone mass is at higher risk for the disease and the resulting fractures.

People with low bone mass can take steps to help slow down bone loss and prevent osteoporosis in the future. Your doctor will want you to develop—or keep—healthy habits such as eating foods rich in calcium and vitamin D and doing weight-bearing exercise such as walking, jogging, or dancing. In some cases, your doctor may recommend medication to prevent osteoporosis.

If you are diagnosed with osteoporosis, these healthy habits will help, but your doctor will probably also recommend that you take medication. Several effective medications are available to slow—or even reverse—bone loss. If you do take medication to treat osteoporosis, your doctor can advise you concerning the need for future BMD tests to check your progress.

Who Should Get a Bone Density Test?

The U.S. Preventive Services Task Force recommends that all women over age 65 should have a bone density test. Women who are younger than age 65 and at high risk for fractures should also have a bone density test.

In addition, a panel convened by the National Institutes of Health in 2000 recommended that bone density testing be considered in people taking glucocorticoid medications for two months or more and in those with conditions that place them at high risk for an osteoporosis-related fracture.

However, the panel did not find enough scientific evidence upon which to base universal recommendations about when all women and men should obtain a BMD test. Instead, an individualized approach is recommended.

Section 14.7

How to Spot Skin Cancer

Why Self Exams Are So Important

Skin cancer is the most common of all cancers, afflicting more than two million Americans each year, a number that is rising rapidly. It is also the easiest to cure, if diagnosed and treated early. When allowed to progress, however, skin cancer can result in disfigurement and even death.

Who Should Do It

You should! And if you have children, begin teaching them how to at an early age so they can do it themselves by the time they are teens. Coupled with yearly skin exams by a doctor, self-exams are the best way to ensure that you don't become a statistic in the battle against skin cancer.

When to Do It

Performed regularly, self-examination can alert you to changes in your skin and aid in the early detection of skin cancer. It should be done often enough to become a habit, but not so often as to feel like a bother. For most people, once a month is ideal, but ask your doctor if you should do more frequent checks.

You may find it helpful to have a doctor do a full-body exam first, to assure you that any existing spots, freckles, or moles are normal or treat any that may not be. After the first few times, self-examination should take no more than 10 minutes—a small investment in what could be a life-saving procedure.

What to Look For

There are three main types of skin cancer: basal cell carcinoma, squamous cell carcinoma, and melanoma. Because each has many different appearances, it is important to know the early warning signs.

Look especially for change of any kind. Do not ignore a suspicious spot simply because it does not hurt. Skin cancers may be painless, but dangerous all the same. If you notice one or more of the warning signs, see a doctor right away, preferably one who specializes in diseases of the skin.

The Warning Signs

- A skin growth that increases in size and appears pearly, translucent, tan, brown, black, or multicolored
- A mole, birthmark, beauty mark, or any brown spot that:
  - changes color;
  - increases in size or thickness;
  - changes in texture;
  - is irregular in outline;
  - is bigger than six millimeters or one-quarter inch, the size of a pencil eraser;
  - appears after age 21.
- A spot or sore that continues to itch, hurt, crust, scab, erode, or bleed
- An open sore that does not heal within three weeks

If You Spot It...

Don't overlook it. Don't delay. See a physician, preferably one who specializes in diseases of the skin, if you note any change in an existing mole, freckle, or spot or if you find a new one with any of the warning signs of skin cancer.

Protection Stops It, Too

About 90% of non-melanoma skin cancers are associated with exposure to ultraviolet (UV) radiation from the sun. Since its inception in 1979, the Skin Cancer Foundation has always recommended using a sunscreen with an SPF 15 or higher as one important part of a complete sun protection regimen. Sunscreen alone is not enough, however. Read our full list of skin cancer prevention tips.

- Seek the shade, especially between 10 a.m. and 4 p.m.
- Do not burn.

- Avoid tanning and UV tanning booths.

- Cover up with clothing, including a broad-brimmed hat and UV-blocking sunglasses.

- Use a broad spectrum (UVA/UVB) sunscreen with an SPF of 15 or higher every day.

- For extended outdoor activity, use a water-resistant, broad-spectrum (UVA/UVB) sunscreen with an SPF of 30 or higher.

- Apply one ounce (two tablespoons) of sunscreen to your entire body 30 minutes before going outside.

- Reapply every two hours or immediately after swimming or excessive sweating.

- Keep newborns out of the sun. Sunscreens should be used on babies over the age of six months.

- Examine your skin head to toe every month.

- See your physician every year for a professional skin exam.

Chapter 15

Immunizations for Women

Chapter Contents

Section 15.1

Recommended Immunizations for Adults

"Vaccinations for Adults," August 2012. Reprinted with permission from the Immunization Action Coalition, www.immunize.org.

You're never too old to get immunized! Getting immunized is a lifelong, life-protecting job. Don't leave your health care provider's office without making sure you've had all the vaccinations you need. Consult your health care provider about your level of risk for various infections.

Hepatitis A (HepA)

Do you need it? Maybe. You need this vaccine if you have a specific risk factor for hepatitis A virus infection or simply want to be protected from this disease. The vaccine is usually given in two doses, 6–18 months apart.

Hepatitis B (HepB)

Do you need it? Maybe. You need this vaccine if you have a specific risk factor for hepatitis B virus infection or simply want to be protected from this disease. The vaccine is given in three doses, usually over six months.

Human Papillomavirus (HPV)

Do you need it? Maybe. You need this vaccine if you are a woman age 26 years or younger or a man age 21 years or younger. Men age 22 through 26 years with a risk condition also need vaccination. Any other man age 22 through 26 who wants to be protected from HPV may receive it, too. The vaccine is given in three doses over six months.

Influenza

Do you need it? Yes! You need a dose every fall (or winter) for your protection and for the protection of others around you.

Measles, Mumps, Rubella (MMR)

Do you need it? Maybe. You need at least one dose of MMR if you were born in 1957 or later. You may also need a second dose.

Meningococcal (MCV4, MPSV4)

Do you need it? Maybe. You need this vaccine if you have one of several health conditions, or if you are 19–21 and a first-year college student living in a residence hall and you either have never been vaccinated or were vaccinated before age 16.

Pneumococcal (PPSV23, PCV13)

Do you need it? Maybe. You need one dose of PPSV23 at age 65 years (or older) if you've never been vaccinated or you were previously vaccinated at least five years ago when you were younger than age 65 years. You also need one to two doses if you smoke cigarettes or have certain chronic health conditions. Some adults with certain high risk conditions also need vaccination with PCV13. Talk to your health care provider to find out if you need this vaccine.

Tetanus, Diphtheria, Whooping Cough (Pertussis) (Tdap, Td)

Do you need it? Yes! All adults need to get a one-time dose of Tdap vaccine (the adult whooping cough vaccine). After that, you need a Td booster dose every 10 years. Consult your health care provider if you haven't had at least three tetanus- and diphtheria-containing shots sometime in your life or have a deep or dirty wound.

Varicella (Chickenpox)

Do you need it? Maybe. If you've never had chickenpox or were vaccinated but received only one dose, talk to your health care provider to find out if you need this vaccine.

Zoster (Shingles)

Do you need it? Maybe. If you are age 60 years or older, you should get a one-time dose of this vaccine now.

Are you planning to travel outside the United States? If so, you may need additional vaccines. The Centers for Disease Control and Prevention (CDC) provides information to assist travelers and their health care providers in deciding which vaccines, medications, and other measures are necessary to prevent illness and injury during international travel. Visit CDC's website at www.cdc.gov/travel or call 800-CDC-INFO (800-232-4636). You may also consult a travel clinic or your health care provider.

Section 15.2

Human Papillomavirus (HPV) Vaccine

Excerpted from "Human Papillomavirus (HPV) and Genital Warts
Fact Sheet," U.S. Department of Health and Human Services Office on
Women's Health (www.womenshealth.gov), January 1, 2009.

What is human papillomavirus (HPV)?

Human papillomavirus, or HPV, is the name for a group of viruses that includes more than 100 types. More than 40 types of HPV can be passed through sexual contact.

The types of HPV that infect the genital area are called genital HPV. Over half of sexually active people will have HPV at some point in their lives. But most people never know it. This is because HPV most often has no symptoms and goes away on its own.

Genital HPV is the most common sexually transmitted infection (STI) in the United States. About 20 million Americans ages 15 to 49 currently have HPV.

What is the difference between the high-risk and low-risk types of HPV?

Some types of HPV can cause cervical cancer. These types of HPV are called high risk. High-risk HPV can lead to cancer. Most often, high-risk HPV causes no health problems and goes away on its own. High-risk HPV cases that don't go away are the biggest risk factor for cervical cancer. If you have high-risk HPV, your doctor can look for changes on your cervix during Pap tests. Changes can be treated to try to prevent cervical cancer. Be sure to have regular Pap tests so changes can be found early.

Low-risk HPV can cause genital warts. Warts can form weeks, months, or years after sexual contact with an infected person. The size of genital warts varies. Some are so small you can't see them. They can be flat and flesh-colored or look bumpy like cauliflower. They often form in clusters or groups. They may itch, burn, or cause discomfort.

Low-risk HPV doesn't always cause warts. In fact, most people with low-risk HPV never know they are infected. This is because they don't get warts or any other symptoms.

How do women get HPV?

Genital HPV is passed by skin-to-skin and genital contact. It is most often passed during vaginal and anal sex. Although much less common, it is possible to pass HPV during oral sex or hand-to-genital contact.

Should I get the HPV vaccine?

It depends on your age and whether or not you already have had sex. Two vaccines (Cervarix and Gardasil) can protect girls and young women against the types of HPV that cause most cervical cancers. The vaccines work best when given before a person's first sexual contact, when she could be exposed to HPV. Both vaccines are recommended for 11- and 12-year-old girls. But the vaccines also can be used in girls as young as 9 and in women through age 26 who did not get any or all of the shots when they were younger. These vaccines are given in a series of three shots. It is best to use the same vaccine brand for all three doses. The vaccine does not replace the need to wear condoms to lower your risk of getting other types of HPV and other sexually transmitted infections. Women who have had the HPV vaccine still need to have regular Pap tests.

How do I know if I have an HPV infection?

A Pap test is when a cell sample is taken from your cervix and looked at with a microscope. A Pap test can find changes on the cervix caused by HPV. To do a Pap test, your doctor will use a small brush to take cells from your cervix. It's simple, fast, and the best way to find out if your cervix is healthy.

If you are age 30 or older, your doctor may also do an HPV test with your Pap test. This is a DNA test that detects most of the high-risk types of HPV. It helps with cervical cancer screening. If you're younger than 30 years old and have had an abnormal Pap test result, your doctor may give you an HPV test. This test will show if HPV caused the abnormal cells on your cervix.

Do I still need a Pap test if I got the HPV vaccine?

Yes. There are three reasons why:

- The vaccine does not protect against all HPV types that cause cancer.
- Women who don't get all the vaccine doses (or at the right time) might not be fully protected.
- Women may not fully benefit from the vaccine if they got it after getting one or more of the four HPV types.

What happens if I have an abnormal Pap test?

An abnormal result does not mean you have HPV or cervical cancer. Other reasons for an abnormal Pap test result include the following:

- Yeast infections
- Irritation
- Hormone changes

If your Pap test is abnormal, your doctor may do the test again. You may also have an HPV test or these tests:

- **Colposcopy:** A device is used to look closely at your cervix. It lets the doctor look at any abnormal areas.
- **Schiller test:** The test involves coating the cervix with an iodine solution. Healthy cells turn brown and abnormal cells turn white or yellow.
- **Biopsy:** A small amount of cervical tissue is taken out and looked at under a microscope.

Could I have HPV even if my Pap test was normal?

Yes. You can have HPV but still have a normal Pap test. Changes on your cervix may not show up right away; or they may never appear. For women older than 30 who get an HPV test and a Pap test, a negative result on both the Pap and HPV tests means no cervical changes or HPV were found on the cervix. This means you have a very low chance of getting cervical cancer in the next few years.

Can HPV be cured?

There is no cure for the virus HPV. But there are treatments for the changes HPV can cause on the cervix. Genital warts can also be treated. Sometimes, the virus goes away on its own.

What treatments are used to get rid of abnormal cells on the cervix?

If you have abnormal cells on the cervix, follow up with your doctor. If the problem is mild, your doctor may wait to see if the cells heal on their own. Or your doctor may suggest taking out the abnormal tissue. Treatment options include the following:

- Cryosurgery, when abnormal tissue is frozen off

- Loop electrosurgical excision procedure (LEEP), where tissue is removed using a hot wire loop

- Laser treatment, which uses a beam of light to destroy abnormal tissue

- Cone biopsy, where a cone-shaped sample of abnormal tissue is removed from the cervix and looked at under the microscope for signs of cancer

How are genital warts treated?

Genital warts can be treated or not treated. Some people may want warts taken off if they cause itching, burning, and discomfort. Others may want to clear up warts you can see with the eye.

If you decide to have warts removed, do not use over-the-counter medicines meant for other kinds of warts. There are special treatments for genital warts. Surgery is also an option.

Even when warts are treated, the HPV virus may remain. This is why warts can come back after treatment. The warts will not turn into cancer.

How do I protect myself from HPV?

Using condoms may reduce the risk of getting genital warts and cervical cancer. But condoms don't always protect you from HPV. The best ways to protect yourself from HPV are to not have sex or be faithful, meaning you and your partner only have sex with each other and no one else.

155

How does HPV affect a pregnancy?

Most women who had genital warts, but no longer have them, do not have problems during pregnancy or birth. For women who have genital warts during pregnancy, the warts may grow or become larger and bleed. In rare cases, a pregnant woman can pass HPV to her baby during vaginal delivery. Rarely, a baby who is exposed to HPV gets warts in the throat or voice box.

If the warts block the birth canal, a woman may need to have a cesarean section (C-section) delivery. But HPV infection or genital warts are not sole reasons for a C-section.

Part Three

Breast and Gynecological Concerns

Chapter 16

Nonmalignant
Breast Conditions

Chapter Contents

Section 16.1

Breast Changes

Excerpted from "Understanding Breast Changes: A Health Guide
for Women NIH Publication No. 12-3536," National Cancer Institute
(www.cancer.gov), November 2, 2012.

Check with Your Health Care Provider about Breast Changes

Check with your health care provider if you notice that your breast looks or feels different. No change is too small to ask about. In fact, the best time to call is when you first notice a breast change.

Breast changes to see your health care provider about include the following:

A Lump (Mass) or a Firm Feeling

- A lump in or near your breast or under your arm

- Thick or firm tissue in or near your breast or under your arm

- A change in the size or shape of your breast

Lumps come in different shapes and sizes. Most lumps are not cancer.

If you notice a lump in one breast, check your other breast. If both breasts feel the same, it may be normal. Normal breast tissue can sometimes feel lumpy.

Some women do regular breast self-exams. Doing breast self-exams can help you learn how your breasts normally feel and make it easier to notice and find any changes. Breast self-exams are not a substitute for mammograms.

Always get a lump checked. Don't wait until your next mammogram. You may need to have tests to be sure that the lump is not cancer.

Nipple Discharge or Changes

- Nipple discharge (fluid that is not breast milk)

- Nipple changes, such as a nipple that points or faces inward (inverted) into the breast

Nipple discharge may be different colors or textures. Nipple discharge is not usually a sign of cancer. It can be caused by birth control pills, some medicines, and infections.

Get nipple discharge checked, especially fluid that comes out by itself or fluid that is bloody.

Skin Changes

- Itching, redness, scaling, dimples, or puckers on your breast

If the skin on your breast changes, get it checked as soon as possible.

Talk with Your Health Care Provider

It can help to prepare before you meet with your health care provider. Write down the breast changes you notice, as well as your personal medical history and your family medical history before your visit.

Tell your health care provider about the following:

- What the breast change looks or feels like
- Where the breast change is
- When you first noticed the breast change and what happened since then

Share your personal medical history:

- The breast problems you've had in the past
- The breast exams and tests you have had
- Your last mammogram date
- Your last menstrual period date
- The medicines or herbs you take
- If you have breast implants, are pregnant, or are breastfeeding
- If you've had cancer before

Share your family medical history:

- Breast problems or diseases your family members have had
- Family members who have had breast cancer
- Age of family members when they had breast cancer

Breast Changes during Your Lifetime That Are Not Cancer

Most women have changes in their breasts during their lifetime. Many of these changes are caused by hormones. For example, your breasts may feel more lumpy or tender at different times in your menstrual cycle.

Other breast changes can be caused by the normal aging process. As you near menopause, your breasts may lose tissue and fat. They may become smaller and feel lumpy. Most of these changes are not cancer; they are called benign changes. However, if you notice a breast change, don't wait until your next mammogram. Make an appointment to get it checked.

Young women who have not gone through menopause often have more dense tissue in their breasts. Dense tissue has more glandular and connective tissue and less fat tissue. This kind of tissue makes mammograms harder to interpret—because both dense tissue and tumors show up as solid white areas on X-ray images. Breast tissue gets less dense as women get older.

Before or during your menstrual periods, your breasts may feel swollen, tender, or painful. You may also feel one or more lumps during this time because of extra fluid in your breasts. These changes usually go away by the end of your menstrual cycle. Because some lumps are caused by normal hormone changes, your health care provider may have you come back for a return visit at a different time in your menstrual cycle.

During pregnancy, your breasts may feel lumpy. This is usually because the glands that produce milk are increasing in number and getting larger.

While breastfeeding, you may get a condition called mastitis. This happens when a milk duct becomes blocked. Mastitis causes the breast to look red and feel lumpy, warm, and tender. It may be caused by an infection and is often treated with antibiotics. Sometimes the duct may need to be drained. If the redness or mastitis does not go away with treatment, call your health care provider.

As you approach menopause, your menstrual periods may come less often. Your hormone levels also change. This can make your breasts feel tender, even when you are not having your menstrual period. Your breasts may also feel more lumpy than they did before.

If you are taking hormones (such as menopausal hormone therapy, birth control pills, or injections) your breasts may become more dense. This can make a mammogram harder to interpret. Be sure to let your health care provider know if you are taking hormones.

When you stop having menstrual periods (menopause), your hormone levels drop, and your breast tissue becomes less dense and more fatty. You may stop having any lumps, pain, or nipple discharge that you used to have. And because your breast tissue is less dense, mammograms may be easier to interpret.

Section 16.2

Breast Infection

© 2013 A.D.A.M. Inc.
Reprinted with permission.

A breast infection is an infection in the tissue of the breast.

Causes

Breast infections are usually caused by a common bacteria (*Staphylococcus aureus*) found on normal skin. The bacteria enter through a break or crack in the skin, usually on the nipple.

The infection takes place in the fatty tissue of the breast and causes swelling. This swelling pushes on the milk ducts. The result is pain and lumps in the infected breast.

Breast infections usually occur in women who are breastfeeding. Breast infections that are not related to breastfeeding might be a rare form of breast cancer.

Symptoms

- Breast enlargement on one side only
- Breast lump
- Breast pain
- Fever and flu-like symptoms including nausea and vomiting
- Itching
- Nipple discharge (may contain pus)

163

- Nipple sensation changes
- Swelling, tenderness, redness, and warmth in breast tissue
- Tender or enlarged lymph nodes in armpit on the same side

Exams and Tests

Breastfeeding women are usually not tested. However, an exam is often helpful to confirm the diagnosis and rule out complications such as an abscess.

Sometimes for infections that keep returning, milk from the nipple will be cultured. In women who are not breastfeeding, testing may include mammography or breast biopsy.

Treatment

Self-care may include applying moist heat to the infected breast tissue for 15 to 20 minutes four times a day.

Antibiotic medications are usually very effective in treating a breast infection. You are encouraged to continue to breastfeed or to pump to relieve breast engorgement from milk production while receiving treatment.

Outlook (Prognosis)

The condition usually clears quickly with antibiotic therapy.

Possible Complications

In severe infections, an abscess may develop. Abscesses need to be drained, either as an office procedure or with surgery. Women with abscesses may be told to temporarily stop breastfeeding.

When to Contact a Medical Professional

Call your health care provider if:

- any portion of the breast tissue becomes reddened, tender, swollen, or hot;
- you are breastfeeding and develop a high fever;
- the lymph nodes in the armpit become tender or swollen.

Prevention

The following may help reduce the risk of breast infections:

- Careful nipple care to prevent irritation and cracking

- Feeding often and pumping milk to prevent engorgement of the breast

- Proper breastfeeding technique with good latching by the baby

- Weaning slowly, over several weeks, rather than abruptly stopping breastfeeding

Section 16.3

Fibrocystic Breast Disease

© 2013 A.D.A.M. Inc. Reprinted with permission.

Fibrocystic breast disease is a commonly used phrase to describe painful, lumpy breasts.

The word "disease" may make you worry that the breasts are abnormal. However, doctors say this is not really a disease. Some doctors or nurses say "fibrocystic change" instead.

Causes

Hormones made in the ovaries can make a woman's breasts feel swollen, lumpy, or painful before or during menstruation each month.

Some women feel that eating chocolate, drinking caffeine, or eating a high-fat diet cause their symptoms, but there is no clear proof of this.

Fibrocystic changes in the breast with the menstrual cycle affect over half of women. It most commonly starts during the thirties. Women who take birth control pills have fewer symptoms. Women who take hormone replacement therapy may have more symptoms. Symptoms usually get better after menopause.

Symptoms

Symptoms are usually worse right before the menstrual period and then improve after the period starts.

Symptoms can include:

- pain or discomfort in both breasts;
- the pain commonly comes and goes with the period, but can last through the whole month;
- breasts that feel full, swollen, and heavy;
- pain or discomfort under the arms;
- thick or lumpy breasts.

You may notice a lump in the same area that becomes larger before your menstrual cycle and then shrinks afterward. These type of lumps will move if you push on them. They do not feel stuck or fixed to anything.

Some women will have discharge from the nipple. If the discharge is clear, red, or bloody, talk to your health care provider right away.

Exams and Tests

Tell your doctor or nurse if you notice any breast changes.

Your health care provider will examine you. This will include a breast exam.

Ask your doctor or nurse how often you should have a mammogram to screen for breast cancer. Usually women should have a mammogram every year, beginning at age 40.

You may need further tests if you have:

- a lump found during a breast exam,
- abnormal screening mammogram.

Another mammogram and breast ultrasound may be done.

Treatment

If you have painful breasts, the following may help:

- Take medication such as acetaminophen or ibuprofen.
- Use heat or ice on the breast.
- Wear a well-fitting bra.

Although some women believe that eating less fat, caffeine, or chocolate helps with their symptoms, there is no good evidence that this helps.

Vitamin E, thiamine, magnesium, and evening primrose oil are not harmful in most cases, but they have not shown any benefit in most studies. Before taking any medication or supplement, be sure to talk with your health care provider.

Most women are not as worried about their symptoms if their breast exam and imaging tests are normal. Remember that most of these symptoms will go away over time.

Outlook (Prognosis)

Fibrocystic breast changes do not increase your risk of breast cancer. Symptoms usually improve after menopause.

Possible Complications

Women who have very lumpy breasts may be more difficult to examine. Mammograms may be harder to interpret. Therefore, early cancer might be more difficult to detect.

When to Contact a Medical Professional

Call your health care provider if:

- you find any new or different lumps on your breast self exam;
- you have a new discharge from the nipple or any discharge becomes bloody or clear;
- you have any redness or puckering of the skin, or flattening or indentation of the nipple.

Prevention

There is no proof that anything you do or don't do will prevent symptoms.

Chapter 17

Premenstrual Syndrome and Premenstrual Dysphoric Disorder

What is premenstrual syndrome (PMS)?

Premenstrual syndrome (PMS) is a group of symptoms linked to the menstrual cycle. PMS symptoms occur one to two weeks before your period (menstruation or monthly bleeding) starts. The symptoms usually go away after you start bleeding. PMS can affect menstruating women of any age, and the effect is different for each woman. For some people, PMS is just a monthly bother. For others, it may be so severe that it makes it hard to even get through the day. PMS goes away when your monthly periods stop, such as when you get pregnant or go through menopause.

What causes PMS?

The causes of PMS are not clear, but several factors may be involved. Changes in hormones during the menstrual cycle seem to be an important cause. These changing hormone levels may affect some women more than others. Chemical changes in the brain may also be involved. Stress and emotional problems, such as depression, do not seem to cause PMS, but they may make it worse. Some other possible causes include the following:

Excerpted from "Premenstrual Syndrome (PMS) Fact Sheet," U.S. Department of Health and Human Services Office on Women's Health (www.womens health.gov), May 18, 2010.

- Low levels of vitamins and minerals

- Eating a lot of salty foods, which may cause you to retain (keep) fluid

- Drinking alcohol and caffeine, which may alter your mood and energy level

What are the symptoms of PMS?

PMS often includes both physical and emotional symptoms, such as the following:

- Acne

- Swollen or tender breasts

- Feeling tired

- Trouble sleeping

- Upset stomach, bloating, constipation, or diarrhea

- Headache or backache

- Appetite changes or food cravings

- Joint or muscle pain

- Trouble with concentration or memory

- Tension, irritability, mood swings, or crying spells

- Anxiety or depression

Symptoms vary from woman to woman.

How do I know if I have PMS?

Your doctor may diagnose PMS based on which symptoms you have, when they occur, and how much they affect your life. If you think you have PMS, keep track of which symptoms you have and how severe they are for a few months. Record your symptoms each day on a calendar or PMS symptom tracker (at womenshealth.gov/publications/our-publications/PMS-symptom-tracker.pdf). Take this form with you when you see your doctor about your PMS.

Your doctor will also want to make sure you don't have one of the following conditions that shares symptoms with PMS:

- Depression

- Anxiety

- Menopause

- Chronic fatigue syndrome (CFS)

- Irritable bowel syndrome (IBS)

- Problems with the endocrine system, which makes hormones

How common is PMS?

There's a wide range of estimates of how many women suffer from PMS. The American College of Obstetricians and Gynecologists estimates that at least 85% of menstruating women have at least one PMS symptom as part of their monthly cycle. Most of these women have fairly mild symptoms that don't need treatment. Others (about 3% to 8%) have a more severe form of PMS, called premenstrual dysphoric disorder (PMDD).

PMS occurs more often in women who fit these criteria:

- Are between their late twenties and early forties

- Have at least one child

- Have a family history of depression

- Have a past medical history of either postpartum depression or a mood disorder

What is the treatment for PMS?

Many things have been tried to ease the symptoms of PMS. No treatment works for every woman. You may need to try different ones to see what works for you.

Lifestyle changes: If your PMS isn't so bad that you need to see a doctor, some lifestyle changes may help you feel better. The following are some steps you can take that may help ease your symptoms.

- Exercise regularly. Each week, you should get the following:

  - 2 hours and 30 minutes of moderate-intensity physical activity **or**

  - 1 hour and 15 minutes of vigorous-intensity aerobic physical activity **or**

  - A combination of moderate and vigorous-intensity activity **and**

  - Muscle-strengthening activities on two or more days

- Eat healthy foods, such as fruits, vegetables, and whole grains.

- Avoid salt, sugary foods, caffeine, and alcohol, especially when you're having PMS symptoms.

- Get enough sleep. Try to get about eight hours of sleep each night.

- Find healthy ways to cope with stress. Talk to your friends, exercise, or write in a journal. Some women also find yoga, massage, or relaxation therapy helpful.

- Don't smoke.

Medications: Over-the-counter pain relievers may help ease physical symptoms, such as cramps, headaches, backaches, and breast tenderness.

In more severe cases of PMS, prescription medicines may be used to ease symptoms. One approach has been to use drugs that stop ovulation, such as birth control pills. Women on the pill report fewer PMS symptoms, such as cramps and headaches, as well as lighter periods.

Alternative therapies: Certain vitamins and minerals have been found to help relieve some PMS symptoms. These include the following:

- Folic acid (400 micrograms)

- Calcium with vitamin D

- Magnesium (400 milligrams)

- Vitamin B-6 (50 to 100 mg)

- Vitamin E (400 international units)

Some women find their PMS symptoms relieved by taking supplements such as the following:

- Black cohosh

- Chasteberry

- Evening primrose oil

Talk with your doctor before taking any of these products. Many have not been proven to work and may interact with other medicines you are taking.

What is premenstrual dysphoric disorder (PMDD)?

A brain chemical called serotonin may play a role in PMDD, a severe form of PMS. The main symptoms, which can be disabling, include the following:

- Feelings of sadness or despair, or even thoughts of suicide
- Feelings of tension or anxiety
- Panic attacks
- Mood swings or frequent crying
- Lasting irritability or anger that affects other people
- Lack of interest in daily activities and relationships
- Trouble thinking or focusing
- Tiredness or low energy
- Food cravings or binge eating
- Trouble sleeping
- Feeling out of control
- Physical symptoms, such as bloating, breast tenderness, headaches, and joint or muscle pain

You must have five or more of these symptoms to be diagnosed with PMDD. Symptoms occur during the week before your period and go away after bleeding starts. Making some lifestyle changes may help ease PMDD symptoms.

Antidepressants called selective serotonin reuptake inhibitors (SSRIs) have also been shown to help some women with PMDD. These drugs change serotonin levels in the brain.

Yaz (drospirenone and ethinyl estradiol) is the only birth control pill approved by the U.S. Food and Drug Administration (FDA) to treat PMDD. Individual counseling, group counseling, and stress management may also help relieve symptoms.

Chapter 18

Menstrual Irregularities

Chapter Contents

Section 18.1

Dysfunctional Uterine Bleeding

Dysfunctional uterine bleeding (DUB) is abnormal bleeding from the vagina that is due to changes in hormone levels.

Causes

Every woman's menstrual cycle, or period, is different. On average, a woman's period occurs every 28 days. Most women have cycles between 24 and 34 days apart. It usually lasts 4–7 days.

Young girls may get their periods anywhere from 21 to 45 days or more apart. Women in their forties will often notice their period occurring less often.

About every month, the levels of female hormones in a woman's body rise and fall. Estrogen and progesterone are two very important hormones. These hormones play an important role in ovulation, the time when the ovaries release an egg.

Dysfunctional uterine bleeding (DUB) most commonly occurs when the ovaries do not release an egg. Changes in hormone levels cause your period to be later or earlier and sometimes heavier than normal.

Symptoms

Symptoms of dysfunctional uterine bleeding may include:

- bleeding or spotting from the vagina between periods;

- periods that occur less than 28 days apart (more common) or more than 35 days apart;

- time between periods changes each month;

- heavier bleeding (such as passing large clots, needing to change protection during the night, soaking through a sanitary pad or tampon every hour for two to three hours in a row);

- bleeding lasts for more days than normal or for more than seven days.

Other symptoms caused by changes in hormone levels may include:

- excessive growth of body hair in a male pattern (hirsutism);
- hot flashes;
- mood swings;
- tenderness and dryness of the vagina.

A woman may feel tired or have fatigue if she is loses too much blood over time. This is a symptom of anemia.

Exams and Tests

The health care provider will do a pelvic examination and may perform a Pap smear. Tests that may be done include:

- complete blood count (CBC);
- blood clotting profile;
- hormone tests;
- pregnancy test;
- thyroid function tests;
- pap smear and culture to look for infection.

Your health care provider may recommend the following:

- Biopsy to look for infection, precancer, or cancer, or to help decide on hormone treatment
- Hysteroscopy, performed in the doctor's office, to look into the uterus through the vagina
- Transvaginal ultrasound to look for problems in the uterus or pelvis

Treatment

Young women within a few years of their first period are often not treated unless symptoms are very severe, such as heavy blood loss causing anemia.

In other women, the goal of treatment is to control the menstrual cycle. Treatment may include:

- birth control pills or progesterone only pills;

- intrauterine device (IUD) that releases the hormone progestin;

- ibuprofen or naproxen taken just before the period starts.

The health care provider may recommend iron supplements for women with anemia.

If you want to get pregnant, you may be given medication to stimulate ovulation.

Women with severe symptoms that do not get better with other treatments may consider the following procedures if they no longer want to have children:

- Endometrial ablation or resection to destroy or remove the lining of the uterus

- Hysterectomy to remove the uterus

- D and C to remove polyps and diagnose certain conditions

Outlook (Prognosis)

Hormone therapy usually relieves symptoms. Treatment may not be needed if you do not develop anemia due to blood loss.

Possible Complications

- Infertility (inability to get pregnant)

- Severe anemia due to a lot of blood loss over time

- Increased risk for endometrial cancer

When to Contact a Medical Professional

Call your health care provider if you have unusual vaginal bleeding.

Section 18.2

Amenorrhea
(Absent Menstrual Periods)

Amenorrhea is the absence of menstruation. Menstruation is a woman's monthly period.

Primary amenorrhea is when a girl has not yet started her monthly periods, and she:

- has gone through other normal changes that occur during puberty,
- is older than 15.

Causes

Most girls begin menstruating between ages 9 and 18, with an average of around 12 years old. Primary amenorrhea typically occurs when a girl is older than 15, if she has gone through other normal changes that occur during puberty. Primary amenorrhea may occur with or without other signs of puberty.

Being born with poorly formed genital or pelvic organs can lead to primary amenorrhea. Some of these defects include:

- blockages or narrowing of the cervix;
- imperforate hymen;
- missing uterus or vagina;
- vaginal septum.

Hormones play a big role in a woman's menstrual cycle. Hormone problems can occur when:

- changes occur to the parts of the brain where hormones that help manage the menstrual cycle are produced, or
- the ovaries are not working correctly.

Either of these problems may be due to:

- anorexia;
- chronic or long-term illnesses, such as cystic fibrosis or heart disease;
- genetic defects or disorders;
- infections that occur in the womb or after birth;
- other birth defects;
- poor nutrition;
- tumors.

In many cases, the cause of primary amenorrhea is not known.

Symptoms

A female with amenorrhea will have no menstrual flow with or without other signs of puberty.

Exams and Tests

The doctor will perform a physical exam and ask questions about your medical history. A pregnancy test will be done.

Blood tests and other tests may be done.

Treatment

Treatment depends on the cause of the missing period. Primary amenorrhea caused by birth defects may require medications (hormones), surgery, or both.

If the amenorrhea is caused by a tumor in the brain (pituitary tumor):

- medications may shrink certain types of tumors;
- surgery to remove the tumor may also be needed;
- radiation therapy is usually only performed when other treatments have not worked.

If the condition is caused by a body-wide (systemic) disease, treatment of the disease may allow menstruation to begin.

If the amenorrhea is due to anorexia or too much exercise, periods will often begin when the weight returns to normal or the exercise level is decreased.

If the amenorrhea cannot be corrected, medicines can sometimes create a menstrual-like situation (pseudomenstruation). Medicines can help the woman feel more like her friends and family and protect the bones from becoming too thin (osteoporosis).

Outlook (Prognosis)

The outlook depends on the cause of the amenorrhea and whether it can be corrected with treatment or lifestyle changes.

Periods are unlikely to start on their own if the amenorrhea was caused by one of the following conditions:

- Congenital defects of the upper genital system

- Craniopharyngioma

- Cystic fibrosis

- Genetic disorders

You may have emotional distress because you feel different from friends or family or worry that you might not be able to have children.

When to Contact a Medical Professional

Call your health care provider if your daughter is older than 15 and has not yet begun menstruating or if she is 14 and shows no other signs of puberty.

Section 18.3

Dysmenorrhea
(Painful Menstrual Periods)

Painful menstrual periods are periods in which a woman has crampy lower abdominal pain, sharp or aching pain that comes and goes, or possibly back pain.

Although some pain during your period is normal, excessive pain is not. The medical term for painful menstrual periods is dysmenorrhea.

Considerations

Many women have painful periods. Sometimes, the pain makes it difficult to perform normal household, job, or school-related activities for a few days during each menstrual cycle. Painful menstruation is the leading cause of lost time from school and work among women in their teens and twenties.

Causes

Painful menstrual periods fall into two groups, depending on the cause:

- Primary dysmenorrhea
- Secondary dysmenorrhea

Primary dysmenorrhea is menstrual pain that occurs around the time that menstrual periods first begin in otherwise healthy young women. This pain is usually not related to a specific problem with the uterus or other pelvic organs. Increased activity of the hormone prostaglandin, which is produced in the uterus, is thought to play a role in this condition.

Secondary dysmenorrhea is menstrual pain that develops later in women who have had normal periods and is often related to problems in the uterus or other pelvic organs, such as:

- endometriosis;
- fibroids;
- intrauterine device (IUD) made of copper;
- pelvic inflammatory disease;
- premenstrual syndrome (PMS);
- sexually transmitted infection;
- stress and anxiety.

Home Care

The following steps may allow you to avoid prescription medications:

- Apply a heating pad to your lower belly area, below your belly button. Never fall asleep with the heating pad on.
- Do light circular massage with your fingertips around your lower belly area.
- Drink warm beverages.
- Eat light but frequent meals.
- Follow a diet rich in complex carbohydrates such as whole grains, fruits, and vegetables, but low in salt, sugar, alcohol, and caffeine.
- Keep your legs raised while lying down, or lie on your side with your knees bent.
- Practice relaxation techniques such as meditation or yoga.
- Try over-the-counter anti-inflammatory medicine, such as ibuprofen. Start taking it the day before your period is expected to start, and continue taking it regularly for the first few days of your period.
- Try vitamin B6, calcium, and magnesium supplements, especially if your pain is from PMS.
- Take warm showers or baths.
- Walk or exercise regularly, including pelvic rocking exercises.
- Lose weight if you are overweight. Get regular, aerobic exercise.

If these self-care measures do not work, your doctor may prescribe medications such as:

- antibiotics;

- antidepressants;

- birth control pills;

- prescription anti-inflammatory medicines;

- prescription pain relievers (including narcotics, for brief periods).

When to Contact a Medical Professional

Call your doctor right away if you have:

- increased or foul-smelling vaginal discharge;

- fever and pelvic pain;

- sudden or severe pain, especially if your period is more than one week late and you have been sexually active.

Also call your doctor if:

- treatments do not relieve your pain after three months;

- you have pain and had an IUD placed more than three months ago;

- you pass blood clots or have other symptoms with the pain;

- your pain occurs at times other than menstruation, begins more than five days before your period, or continues after your period is over.

What to Expect at Your Office Visit

Your doctor will examine you and ask questions about your medical history and symptoms. Tests and procedures that may be done include:

- complete blood count (CBC);

- cultures to rule out sexually transmitted infections;

- laparoscopy;

- ultrasound.

Treatment depends on what is causing your pain.

Your health care provider may prescribe birth control pills to relieve menstrual pain. If you don't need them for birth control, you can stop using the pills after 6 to 12 months. Many women continue to have symptom relief even after stopping the medication.

Your doctor may prescribe prescription pain medications. For pain caused by an IUD, your doctor may recommend:

- waiting one year after it was placed (painful periods go away in many women during this time);

- removing the IUD and using other types of birth control;

- changing to a different type of IUD that contains progesterone, which usually makes the periods lighter and less painful.

Surgery may be needed if other treatments do not relieve your pain. Surgery may be done to remove endometriosis, cysts, fibroids, scar tissue, or your uterus (hysterectomy).

Section 18.4

Menorrhagia
(Heavy Menstrual Bleeding)

"Heavy Menstrual Bleeding,"
Centers for Disease Control and Prevention (www.cdc.gov),
December 12, 2011.

Menorrhagia is menstrual bleeding that lasts more than seven days. It can also be bleeding that is very heavy. How do you know if you have heavy bleeding? If you need to change your tampon or pad after less than two hours or you pass clots the size of a quarter or larger, that is heavy bleeding. If you have this type of bleeding, you should see a doctor.

Untreated heavy or prolonged bleeding can stop you from living your life to the fullest. It also can cause anemia. Anemia is a common blood problem that can leave you feeling tired or weak. If you have a bleeding problem, it could lead to other health problems. Sometimes treatments, such as dilation and curettage (D&C) or a hysterectomy, might be done when these procedures could have been avoided.

185

Causes

Possible causes fall into the following three areas:

- Uterine-related problems:
  - growths or tumors of the uterus that are *not* cancer; these can be called uterine fibroids or polyps;
  - cancer of the uterus or cervix;
  - certain types of birth control—for example, an IUD;
  - problems related to pregnancy, such as a miscarriage or ectopic pregnancy
- Hormone-related problems
- Other illnesses or disorders:
  - bleeding-related disorders, such as von Willebrand disease (VWD) or platelet function disorder;
  - nonbleeding-related disorders such as liver, kidney, or thyroid disease; pelvic inflammatory disease; and cancer.

In addition, certain drugs, such as aspirin, can cause increased bleeding. Doctors have not been able to find the cause in half of all women who have this problem. If you have bleeding such as this, and your gynecologist has not found any problems during your routine visit, you should be tested for a bleeding disorder.

Signs

You might have menorrhagia if you have the following:

- Have a menstrual flow that soaks through one or more pads or tampons every hour for several hours in a row
- Need to double up on pads to control your menstrual flow
- Need to change pads or tampons during the night
- Have menstrual periods lasting more than seven days
- Have a menstrual flow with blood clots the size of a quarter or larger
- Have a heavy menstrual flow that keeps you from doing the things you would do normally
- Have constant pain in the lower part of the stomach during your periods

- Are tired, lack energy, or are short of breath

Diagnosis

Finding out if a woman has heavy menstrual bleeding often is not easy because each person might think of "heavy bleeding" in a different way. Usually, menstrual bleeding lasts about four to five days and the amount of blood lost is small (two to three tablespoons). However, women who have menorrhagia usually bleed for more than seven days and lose twice as much blood. If you have bleeding that lasts longer than seven days per period, or is so heavy that you have to change your pad or tampon nearly every hour, you need to talk with your doctor.

To find out if you have menorrhagia, your doctor will ask you about your medical history and menstrual cycles. Your doctor may also ask if any of your family members have had heavy menstrual bleeding.

You might want to track your periods by writing down the dates of your periods and how heavy you think your flow is (maybe by counting how many pads or tampons you use). Do this before you visit the doctor so that you can give the doctor as much information as possible. Your doctor also will do a pelvic exam and might tell you about other tests that can be done to help find out if you have menorrhagia.

Tests

Your doctor might tell you that one or more of the following tests will help find out if you have a bleeding problem:

Blood test: In this test, your blood will be taken using a needle. It will then be looked at to check for anemia, problems with the thyroid, or problems with the way the blood clots.

Pap test: For this test, cells from your cervix are removed and then looked at to find out if you have an infection, inflammation, or changes in your cells that might be cancer or might cause cancer.

Endometrial biopsy: Tissue samples are taken from the inside lining of your uterus or "endometrium" to find out if you have cancer or other abnormal cells. You might feel as if you were having a bad menstrual cramp while this test is being done. But it does not take long, and the pain usually goes away when the test ends.

Ultrasound: This is a painless test using sound waves and a computer to show what your blood vessels, tissues, and organs look like. Your doctor then can see how they are working and check your blood flow.

Using the results of these first tests, the doctor might recommend more tests, including the following:

Sonohysterogram: This ultrasound scan is done after fluid is injected through a tube into the uterus by way of your vagina and cervix. This lets your doctor look for problems in the lining of your uterus. Mild to moderate cramping or pressure can be felt during this procedure.

Hysteroscopy: This is a procedure to look at the inside of the uterus using a tiny tool to see if you have fibroids, polyps, or other problems that might be causing bleeding. You might be given drugs to put you to sleep or drugs simply to numb the area being looked at.

Dilation and curettage (D&C): This is a procedure that can be used to find and treat the cause of bleeding. During a D&C, the inside lining of your uterus is scraped and looked at to see what might be causing the bleeding. A D&C is a simple procedure. Most often it is done in an operating room, but you will not have to stay in the hospital afterwards. You might be given drugs to make you sleep during the procedure, or you might be given something that will numb only the area to be worked on.

Treatment

The type of treatment you get will depend on the cause of your bleeding and how serious it is. Your doctor also will look at things such as your age, general health, and medical history; how well you respond to certain medicines, procedures, or therapies; and your wants and needs. For example, some women do not want to have a period, some want to know when they can usually expect to have their period, and some want just to reduce the amount of bleeding. Some women want to make sure they can still have children in the future. Others want to lessen the pain more than they want to reduce the amount of bleeding. Some treatments are ongoing and others are done one time. You should discuss all of your options with your doctor to decide which is best for you. Following is a list of the more common treatments.

Drug Therapy

Iron supplements: To get more iron into your blood to help it carry oxygen if you show signs of anemia

Ibuprofen: To help reduce pain, menstrual cramps, and the amount of bleeding; in some women, these drugs can increase the risk of bleeding

Birth control pills: To help make periods more regular and reduce the amount of bleeding

Intrauterine contraception (IUC): To help make periods more regular and reduce the amount of bleeding through drug-releasing devices placed into the uterus

Hormone therapy (drugs that contain estrogen and/or progesterone): To reduce the amount of bleeding

Desmopressin nasal spray: To stop bleeding in people who have certain bleeding disorders, such as von Willebrand disease and mild hemophilia, by releasing a clotting protein or "factor" that helps the blood to clot and temporarily increases the level of these proteins in the blood

Antifibrinolytic medicines (tranexamic acid, aminocaproic acid): To reduce the amount of bleeding by stopping a clot from breaking down once it has formed

Surgical Treatment

D&C: D&C is a procedure in which the top layer of the uterus lining is removed to reduce menstrual bleeding.

Operative hysteroscopy: This surgical procedure, using a special tool to view the inside of the uterus, can be used to help remove polyps and fibroids, correct abnormalities of the uterus, and remove the lining of the uterus to manage heavy menstrual flow.

Endometrial ablation or resection: This includes two types of surgical procedures using different techniques in which all or part of the lining of the uterus is removed to control menstrual bleeding. While some patients will stop having menstrual periods altogether, others may continue to have periods but the menstrual flow will be lighter than before. Although the procedures do not remove the uterus, they will prevent women from having children in the future.

Hysterectomy: This is a major operation requiring hospitalization that involves surgically removing the entire uterus. After having this procedure, a woman can no longer become pregnant and will stop having her period.

Menorrhagia is common among women. But many women do not know that they can get help for it. Others do not get help because they are too embarrassed to talk with a doctor about their problem. Talking openly with your doctor is very important in making sure you are diagnosed properly and get the right treatment.

Heavy bleeding is one of the most common problems women report to their doctors. It affects more than 10 million American women each year. This means that about one out of every five women has it.

Chapter 19

Menopausal Concerns

Chapter Contents

Section 19.1

Premature Menopause (Premature Ovarian Failure)

Excerpted from "Early Menopause (Premature Menopause)," U.S. Department of Health and Human Services Office on Women's Health (www.womenshealth.gov), September 29, 2010.

What is early menopause?

When menopause happens before age 40, it is considered early. Early menopause can be caused by certain medical treatments, or it can just happen on its own.

Medical treatments that may cause early menopause include the following:

- **Chemotherapy or pelvic radiation treatments for cancer:** These treatments can damage the ovaries and cause your periods to stop. Effects like having trouble getting pregnant can happen right away or several months later. The chances of going into menopause depend on the type and amount of chemotherapy that was used. Also, the younger a woman is, the lower the chances that she will experience menopause.

- **Surgery to remove the ovaries:** Surgical removal of both ovaries, also called a bilateral oophorectomy, causes menopause right away. A woman's periods will stop after this surgery, and her hormones drop quickly. She may immediately have strong menopausal symptoms.

- **Surgery to remove the uterus:** Some women who have a hysterectomy, which removes the uterus, are able to keep their ovaries. They will not enter menopause right away because their ovaries will continue to make hormones. But they no longer have their periods and cannot get pregnant. They might have hot flashes because the surgery can sometimes affect the blood supply to the ovaries. Later on, they might have natural menopause a year or two earlier than expected.

192

Sometimes menopause happens early on its own. Some possible causes include the following:

- **Chromosome defects:** Problems in the chromosomes can cause premature menopause. For example, women with Turner syndrome are born without all or part of one X chromosome. The ovaries don't form normally, and early menopause results.

- **Genetics:** Women with a family history of early menopause are more likely to have early menopause themselves.

- **Autoimmune diseases:** The body's immune system, which normally fights off diseases, may mistakenly attack the ovaries and prevent them from making hormones. Thyroid disease and rheumatoid arthritis are two diseases that can cause this to happen.

When menopause comes early on its own, it sometimes has been called "premature menopause" or "premature ovarian failure." But a better term is "primary ovarian insufficiency," which describes the decreased activity in the ovaries. In some cases, women have ovaries that still make hormones from time to time, and their menstrual periods return. Some women can even become pregnant after the diagnosis.

How can you know if you have early menopause?

Usually, menopause is confirmed when a woman hasn't had her period for 12 months in a row. To help determine if you may be reaching menopause, your doctor will ask if you've had signs like hot flashes, irregular periods, sleep problems, and vaginal dryness. But these signs are not enough to determine that you are reaching menopause.

Blood tests that can measure estrogen and related hormones, like follicle-stimulating hormone (FSH), can help determine if you have reached early menopause. You may choose to get tested if you want to know whether you can still get pregnant. Your hormone levels change daily, though, so you may need to have a test more than once to know for sure.

What are the effects of early menopause?

Women who enter menopause early can have symptoms similar to those of regular menopause. These can include hot flashes, mood changes, vaginal dryness, and decreased sex drive. For some women with early menopause, these symptoms are quite severe. In addition, women who go through menopause early may have a higher risk of certain health problems, such as heart disease and osteoporosis. Talk to your doctor about treatments like menopausal hormone therapy that can help with symptoms. Discuss ways to protect your health.

Women who want to have children and go through early menopause may feel extremely upset. If you want to be a parent, talk to your doctor about other options, like donor egg programs or adoption. Your doctor may suggest that you see an infertility specialist. You also can talk to your doctor or a therapist about painful feelings from the loss of fertility and other effects of reaching menopause early.

Section 19.2

Treating the Symptoms of Menopause

Excerpted from "Menopause Symptom Relief and Treatments," U.S. Department of Health and Human Services Office on Women's Health (www.womenshealth.gov), September 29, 2010.

Learning about Menopause Treatment Options

Most women do not need treatment of menopausal symptoms. Some women find that their symptoms go away by themselves, and some women just don't find the symptoms very uncomfortable. But if you are bothered by symptoms, there are many ways to deal with them, including medications and lifestyle changes. You may find it hard to decide about treatment options like menopausal hormone therapy because of the possible side effects. Talk to your doctor about the possible risks and benefits so you can choose what's best for you. No one treatment is right for all women.

When you talk about treatment options with your doctor, discuss the following issues:

- Your symptoms and how much they bother you

- Your personal risks based on your age, your overall health, and your risk for diseases such as heart disease or cancer

- Whether you have used a treatment like menopausal hormone therapy (MHT) before

- Whether you have already gone through menopause and, if so, how long ago

Dealing with Specific Menopause Symptoms

Hot Flashes

- Try to notice what triggers your hot flashes and avoid those things. Possible triggers to consider include spicy foods, alcohol, caffeine, stress, or being in a hot place.

- Dress in layers and remove some when you feel a flash starting.

- Use a fan in your home or workplace.

- If you still have menstrual periods, ask your doctor if you might take low-dose oral contraceptives (birth control pills). These may help symptoms and prevent pregnancy.

- Menopausal hormone therapy is the most effective treatment for hot flashes and night sweats. Ask your doctor if the benefits of MHT outweigh the risks for you.

- If MHT is not an option for you, ask your doctor about prescription medicines that are usually used for other conditions. These include antidepressants, epilepsy medicine, and blood pressure medicine.

- Try taking slow, deep breaths when a flash starts.

- If you're overweight, losing weight might help with hot flashes, according to one recent study.

Vaginal Dryness

- A water-based, over-the-counter vaginal lubricant like K-Y Jelly or Astroglide can help make sex more comfortable.

- An over-the-counter vaginal moisturizer like Replens can help keep needed moisture in your vagina if used every few days and can make sex more comfortable.

Problems Sleeping

- One of the best ways to get a good night's sleep is to be physically active. You might want to avoid exercise close to bedtime, though, since it might make you more awake.

- Avoid large meals, smoking, and working right before bedtime, avoid caffeine after noon, and avoid alcohol close to bedtime.

- Try drinking something warm before bedtime, such as caffeine-free tea or warm milk.

- Keep your bedroom dark, quiet, and cool. Use your bedroom only for sleep and sex.

- Avoid napping during the day, and try to go to bed and get up at the same times every day.

- If you wake during the night and can't get back to sleep, get up and do something relaxing until you're sleepy.

- Talk to your doctor about your sleep problems.

- If hot flashes are the cause of sleep problems, treating the hot flashes will usually improve sleep.

Mood Swings

- Getting enough sleep and staying physically active will help you feel your best.

- Avoid taking on too many duties. Look for positive ways to ease your stress.

- Talk to your doctor. He or she can look for signs of depression, which is a serious illness that needs treatment. You also could consider seeing a therapist to talk about your problems.

- Try a support group for women who are going through the same things as you.

- If you are using MHT for hot flashes or another menopause symptom, your mood swings may get better too.

Memory Problems

- Some women complain of memory problems or trouble focusing in midlife. But studies suggest that natural menopause has little effect on these functions. Women should not use MHT to protect against memory loss or brain diseases, including dementia and Alzheimer disease.

- Getting enough sleep and keeping physically active might help improve symptoms. Mental exercises may help too, so ask your doctor about them.

- If forgetfulness or other mental problems are affecting your daily life, see your doctor.

Other symptoms that might bother you around this time are having less interest in sex and having trouble holding in your urine.

Medications and Menopause

A number of medications can help with symptoms during the years around menopause.

- **Low-dose oral contraceptives (birth control pills)** are an option if you are in perimenopause (the years leading up to your final period). Low-dose contraceptives may stop or reduce hot flashes, vaginal dryness, and moodiness. They can also help with very heavy, frequent, or unpredictable periods. Your doctor may advise you not to take the pill, though, if you smoke or have a history of blood clots or certain types of cancer.

- **Prescription medications** that are usually used for other conditions may help with hot flashes and moodiness. These include medications for epilepsy, depression, and high blood pressure.

- **Menopausal hormone therapy** can be very good at helping with moderate to severe symptoms of menopause. It has certain possible risks, though.

- **Over-the-counter medicines (OTC)** can treat vaginal discomfort. A water-based vaginal lubricant can help make sex more comfortable. A vaginal moisturizer can provide lubrication and help keep needed moisture in vaginal tissues.

- **Prescription medicines for vaginal discomfort** may be an option if OTC treatments don't work. These include estrogen creams, tablets, or rings that you put in your vagina. If you have severe vaginal dryness, the most effective treatment may be an MHT pill or patch.

Section 19.3

Menopause and Sexuality

Excerpted from "Menopause and Sexuality,"
U.S. Department of Health and Human Services Office on Women's
Health (www.womenshealth.gov), September 29, 2010.

Sexual Issues and Menopause

In the years around menopause, you may experience changes in your sexual life. Some women say they enjoy sex more after they don't have to worry about getting pregnant. Other women find that they think about sex less often or don't enjoy it as much.

Changes in sexuality at this time of life have several possible causes, including the following:

- Decreased hormones can make vaginal tissues drier and thinner, which can make sex uncomfortable.

- Decreased hormones may reduce sex drive.

- Night sweats can disturb a woman's sleep and make her too tired for sex.

- Emotional changes can make a woman feel too stressed for sex.

Keep in mind that being less interested in sex as you get older is not a medical condition that needs treatment. But if you are upset about sexual changes, you can get help. Don't be shy about talking with your doctor or nurse. They certainly have talked with many women about these issues before.

Lifestyle Changes

Some simple steps may help with sexual issues you face at this time:

- **Get treated for any medical problems:** Your overall health can affect your sexual health. For example, you need healthy arteries to supply blood to your vagina.

- **Try to exercise:** Physical activity can increase your energy, lift your mood, and improve your body image—all of which can help with sexual interest.

- **Don't smoke:** Cigarette smoking can reduce both the blood flow to the vagina and the effects of estrogen, which are important to sexual health.

- **Avoid drugs and alcohol:** They can slow down how your body responds.

- **Try to have sex more often:** Sex can increase blood flow to your vagina and help keep tissues healthy.

- **Allow time to become aroused during sex:** Moisture from being aroused protects tissues. Also, avoid sex if you have any vaginal irritation.

- **Practice pelvic floor exercises:** These can increase blood flow to the vagina and strengthen the muscles involved in orgasm.

- **Avoid products that irritate your vagina:** Bubble bath and strong soaps might cause irritation. Don't douche. If you're experiencing vaginal dryness, allergy and cold medicines may add to the problem.

Treatment Options

Discuss your symptoms and personal health issues with your doctor to decide whether one or more treatment options are right for you. If vaginal dryness is an issue, take these precautions:

- Using an over-the-counter, water-based vaginal lubricant when you have sex can lessen discomfort.

- An over-the-counter vaginal moisturizer can help put moisture back in vaginal tissues. You may need to use it every few days.

- Prescription medicines that are put into a woman's vagina may increase moisture and sensation. These include estrogen creams, tablets, or rings. If you have severe vaginal dryness, the most effective treatment may be menopausal hormone therapy.

If sexual interest is an issue:

- Treating vaginal dryness may help. Talking with your partner or making lifestyle changes also may help.

199

- You may wonder about Viagra. This medication has helped men with erection problems, but it has not proven effective in increasing women's sexual interest.

- Some women try products like pills or creams that contain the male hormone testosterone or similar products. The U.S. Food and Drug Administration (FDA) has not approved these products for treating reduced female sex drive because there is not enough research proving them safe and effective.

- The FDA has approved menopausal hormone therapy for symptoms like hot flashes, but research has not proven that MHT increases sex drive.

Talking with Your Partner

Talking with your partner about your sexual changes can be very helpful. Some possible topics to discuss include the following:

- What feels good and what doesn't

- Times that you may feel more relaxed

- Which positions are more comfortable

- Whether you need more time to get aroused than you used to

- Concerns you have about the way your appearance may be changing

- Ways to enjoy physical connection other than intercourse, like massage

Talking with your partner can strengthen your sexual relationship and your overall connection. If you need help, consider meeting with a therapist or sex counselor for individual or couples therapy.

Section 19.4

Menopausal Hormone Therapy

Excerpted from "Menopause and Menopause Treatments Fact Sheet,"
U.S. Department of Health and Human Services Office on Women's
Health (www.womenshealth.gov), September 28, 2010.

Can menopausal hormone therapy help treat my symptoms?

MHT, which used to be called hormone replacement therapy (HRT),
involves taking the hormones estrogen and progesterone. (Women
who don't have a uterus anymore take just estrogen.) MHT can be
very good at relieving moderate to severe menopausal symptoms and
preventing bone loss. But MHT also has some risks, especially if used
for a long time.

MHT can help with menopause in the following ways:

- Reducing hot flashes and night sweats and related problems
  such as poor sleep and irritability

- Treating vaginal symptoms, such as dryness and discomfort, and
  related problems, such as pain during sex

- Slowing bone loss

- Possibly easing mood swings and mild depressive mood

For some women, MHT may increase their chance of these symptoms:

- Blood clots

- Heart attack

- Stroke

- Breast cancer

- Gall bladder disease

Research into the risks and benefits of MHT continues. For example,
a recent study suggests that the low-dose patch form of MHT may
not have the possible risk of stroke that other forms can have. Talk

with your doctor about the positives and negatives of MHT based on your medical history and age. Keep in mind, too, that you may have symptoms when you stop MHT. You can also ask about other treatment options. Lower-dose estrogen products (vaginal creams, rings, and tablets) are a good choice if you are bothered only by vaginal symptoms, for example. And other drugs may help with bone loss.

If you choose MHT, experts recommend that you do the following:

- Use it at the lowest dose that helps

- Use it for the shortest time needed

If you take MHT, call your doctor if you develop any of the following side effects:

- Vaginal bleeding

- Bloating

- Breast tenderness or swelling

- Headaches

- Mood changes

- Nausea

Who should not take MHT for menopause?

Women who fit these criteria should not take MHT:

- Think they are pregnant

- Have problems with undiagnosed vaginal bleeding

- Have had certain kinds of cancers (such as breast or uterine cancer)

- Have had a stroke or heart attack

- Have had blood clots

- Have liver disease

- Have heart disease

Can MHT prevent heart disease or Alzheimer disease?

A major study called the Women's Health Initiative (WHI) has looked at the effects of MHT on heart disease and other health concerns. It has explored many questions relating to MHT, including whether MHT's effects are different depending on when a woman starts it.

Future research may tell experts even more about MHT. For now, MHT should not be used to prevent heart disease, memory loss, dementia, or Alzheimer disease. MHT sometimes is used to treat bone loss and menopausal symptoms.

What is "bioidentical" hormone therapy?

Bioidentical hormone therapy (BHT) means man-made hormones that are the same as the hormones the body makes. There are several prescription BHT products that are well tested and approved by the FDA.

Often, people use the term "BHT" to mean medications that are custom-made by a pharmacist for a specific patient based on a doctor's order. These custom-made products are also sometimes called bioidentical hormone replacement therapy (BHRT). Despite claims, there is no proof that these products are better or safer than drugs approved by the FDA. Also, many insurance and prescription programs do not pay for these drugs because they are viewed as experimental.

Section 19.5

Hormone Replacement Therapy Use and Health Risks for Women

Excerpted from "Menopausal Hormonal Therapy and Cancer," National Cancer Institute (www.cancer.gov), December 5, 2011, and "Menopausal Hormone Therapy and Heart Disease," National Heart, Lung, and Blood Institute (www.nhlbi.nih.gov), February 29, 2012.

Menopausal Hormonal Therapy and Cancer

What is menopausal hormone therapy?

Menopausal hormone therapy (MHT) is a treatment that doctors may recommend to relieve common symptoms of menopause and to address long-term biological changes, such as bone loss, that result from declining levels of the natural hormones estrogen and progesterone in a woman's body during and after the completion of menopause.

How do the hormones used in MHT differ from the hormones produced by a woman's body?

The hormones used in MHT come from a variety of plants and animals, or they can be made in a laboratory. The chemical structure of these hormones is similar, although usually not identical, to those of hormones produced by women's bodies.

The FDA has approved many hormone products for use in MHT. FDA-approved products have undergone extensive testing and are produced under standardized conditions to ensure that every dose—whether in a pill, a skin patch, or a cream—contains the proper amount of the appropriate hormones. These FDA-approved products are available only with a doctor's prescription.

Where does evidence about risks and benefits of MHT come from?

The most comprehensive evidence about risks and benefits of MHT comes from two randomized clinical trials that were sponsored by the National Institutes of Health as part of the Women's Health Initiative.

More than 27,000 healthy women who were 50 to 79 years of age at the time of enrollment took part in the two trials, either the WHI Estrogen-plus-Progestin Study or WHI Estrogen-Alone Study. Although both trials were stopped early (in 2002 and 2004, respectively) when it was determined that both types of therapy were associated with specific health risks, longer-term follow-up of the participants continues to provide new information about the health effects of MHT.

What are the benefits of menopausal hormone therapy?

Research from the WHI Estrogen-plus-Progestin study has shown that women taking combined hormone therapy had the following benefits:

- One-third fewer hip and vertebral fractures than women taking the placebo

- One-third lower risk of colorectal cancer than women taking the placebo

However, a follow-up study found that neither benefit persisted after the study participants stopped taking combined hormone therapy medication.

Women taking estrogen alone experienced the following benefits:

- One-third lower risk for hip and vertebral fractures than women taking the placebo

- A 23% reduced risk of breast cancer than women taking the placebo

After 10.7 years of follow-up, however, the risk of hip fractures was slightly higher in the estrogen-alone group, but the risk of breast cancer remained lower than that among women who took the placebo.

What are the health risks of MHT?

Before the WHI studies began, it was known that MHT with estrogen alone increased the risk of endometrial cancer in women with an intact uterus. It was for this reason that, in the WHI trials, women randomly assigned to receive hormone therapy took estrogen plus progestin if they had a uterus and estrogen alone if they didn't have one.

Research from the WHI studies has shown that MHT is associated with the following harms:

- **Urinary incontinence:** Use of estrogen plus progestin increased the risk of urinary incontinence.

- **Dementia:** Use of estrogen plus progestin doubled the risk of developing dementia among postmenopausal women age 65 and older.

- **Stroke, blood clots, and heart attack:** Women who took either combined hormone therapy or estrogen alone had an increased risk of stroke, blood clots, and heart attack. For women in both groups, however, this risk returned to normal levels after they stopped taking the medication.

- **Breast cancer:** Women who took estrogen plus progestin were more likely to be diagnosed with breast cancer. The breast cancers in these women were larger and more likely to have spread to the lymph nodes by the time they were diagnosed. The number of breast cancers in this group of women increased with the length of time that they took the hormones and decreased after they stopped taking the hormones.

These studies also showed that both combination and estrogen-alone hormone use made mammography less effective for the early detection of breast cancer. Women taking hormones had more repeat mammograms to check on abnormalities found in a screening mammogram and more breast biopsies to determine whether abnormalities detected in mammograms were cancer.

The rate of death from breast cancer among those taking estrogen plus progestin was 2.6 per 10,000 women per year, compared with 1.3 per 10,000 women per year among those taking the placebo. The rate of death from any cause after a diagnosis of breast cancer was 5.3 per 10,000 women per year among women taking combined hormone therapy, compared with 3.4 per 10,000 women per year among those taking the placebo.

- **Lung cancer:** Women who took combined hormone therapy had the same risk of lung cancer as women who took the placebo. However, among those who were diagnosed with lung cancer, women who took estrogen plus progestin were more likely to die of the disease than those who took the placebo.

  There were no differences in the number of cases or the number of deaths from lung cancer among women who took estrogen alone compared with those among women who took the placebo.

- **Colorectal cancer:** In the initial study report, women taking combined hormone therapy had a lower risk of colorectal cancer than women who took the placebo. However, the colorectal tumors that arose in the combined hormone therapy group were more advanced at detection than those in the placebo group. There was no difference in either the risk of colorectal cancer or the stage of disease at diagnosis between women who took estrogen alone and those who took the placebo.

  However, a subsequent analysis of the WHI trials found no strong evidence that either estrogen alone or estrogen plus progestin had any effect on the risk of colorectal cancer, tumor stage at diagnosis, or death from colorectal cancer.

Does hysterectomy affect the cancer risks associated with MHT?

Women who had a hysterectomy and who are prescribed MHT generally take estrogen alone.

In 2004, when the WHI Estrogen-Alone Study was stopped early, women taking estrogen alone had a 23% reduced risk of breast cancer compared with those who took the placebo. An analysis conducted after study participants had been followed for an average of 10.7 years found that women who had taken estrogen alone still had a lower risk of breast cancer than women who had taken the placebo.

Do the cancer risks from MHT change over time?

Women who have had a hysterectomy and who use estrogen-alone MHT have a reduced risk of breast cancer that continues for at least five years after they stop taking MHT.

Women who take combined hormone therapy have an increased risk of breast cancer that continues after they stop taking the medication. In the WHI study, where women took the combined hormone therapy for an average of 5.6 years, this increased risk persisted after an average follow-up period of 11 years. Breast cancers diagnosed in this group of women were larger and more likely to have spread to the lymph nodes (a sign of more advanced disease).

Studies have documented a decline in breast cancer diagnoses in the United States after the sharp reduction in the use of MHT that followed publication of the initial results of the Estrogen-plus-Progestin Study in July 2002. Additional factors, such as a reduction in the use of mammography, may also have contributed to this decline.

Is it safe for women who have had a cancer diagnosis to take MHT?

One of the roles of naturally occurring estrogen is to promote the normal growth of cells in the breast and uterus. For this reason, it is generally believed that MHT may promote further tumor growth in women who have already been diagnosed with breast cancer. However, studies of hormone use to treat menopausal symptoms in breast cancer survivors have produced conflicting results.

What should women do if they have menopausal symptoms but are concerned about taking MHT?

Although MHT provides short-term benefits such as relief from hot flashes and vaginal dryness, several health concerns are associated with its use. Women should discuss whether to take MHT and what alternatives may be appropriate for them with their health care provider. The FDA currently advises women to use MHT for the shortest time and at the lowest dose possible to control menopausal symptoms.

Women who are concerned about the health effects that occur naturally with the decline in hormone production that occurs during menopause can make changes in their lifestyle and diet to reduce certain risks. For example, eating foods that are rich in calcium and vitamin D or taking dietary supplements containing these nutrients may help to prevent osteoporosis. FDA-approved drugs have been shown in randomized trials to prevent bone loss.

Medications approved by the FDA for treating depression and seizures may help to relieve menopausal symptoms such as hot flashes.

Some women seek relief from menopausal symptoms with over-the-counter complementary and alternative therapies. Some of these remedies contain estrogen-like compounds derived from sources such as soy products, whole-grain cereals, oilseeds (primarily flaxseed), legumes, or the plant black cohosh. To date, however, randomized clinical trials have not shown that any of these remedies is superior to a placebo in relieving hot flashes. Trials of other herbal remedies, such as evening primrose oil, ginseng, and wild yam, have also not shown that they effectively reduce menopausal symptoms.

What questions remain in this area of research?

The WHI trials were landmark studies that have transformed our understanding of the health effects of MHT. Follow-up studies have expanded and refined the original findings of these two trials. Many questions, however, remain to be answered, such as the following:

- Are different forms of hormones, lower doses, different hormones, or different methods of administration safer or more effective than those tested in the WHI trials?

- Does hormone use present different risks and benefits for women younger than those studied in the WHI trials?

- Is there an optimal age at which to initiate MHT or an optimal duration of therapy that maximizes benefits and minimizes risks?

It's important to note that women who were enrolled in the WHI trials were, on average, 63 years old, although about 5,000 of them were under age 60, so the results of the study may also apply to younger women. However, women in the study were not using MHT to relieve menopausal symptoms. In addition, the WHI trials tested single-dose strengths of one estrogen-only medication (Premarin) and one estrogen-plus-progestin medication (Prempro).

NIA is sponsoring the Early Versus Late Intervention Trial With Estradiol (ELITE) to try to answer some of these remaining questions. This clinical trial is comparing the effects of estrogen in a group of women who are within 6 years of menopause and another group of women who are at least 10 years past menopause. Women are randomly assigned to take either estradiol (Estrace) or a placebo for 5 years. Women with a uterus will also use a progesterone gel or a placebo gel for the last 10 days of each month. This trial has enrolled 643 women and is expected to be completed in the summer of 2013.

Menopausal Hormone Therapy and Heart Disease

Menopausal hormone therapy once seemed the answer for many of the conditions women face as they age. It was thought that hormone therapy could ward off heart disease, osteoporosis, and cancer, while improving women's quality of life. But beginning in July 2002, findings emerged from clinical trials that showed this was not so. In fact, long-term use of hormone therapy poses serious risks and may increase the risk of heart attack and stroke. The findings come from the Women's Health Initiative (WHI), launched in 1991 to test ways to prevent a number of medical disorders in postmenopausal women. It consists of a set of clinical studies on hormone therapy, diet modification, and calcium and vitamin D supplements; an observational study; and a community prevention study.

The two hormone therapy clinical studies were both stopped early because of serious risks and the failure to prevent heart disease. Briefly, the estrogen-plus-progestin therapy increased women's risk for heart attacks, stroke, blood clots, and breast cancer. These risks diminished after stopping estrogen plus progestin. Estrogen plus progestin also doubled the risk of dementia and did not protect women against memory loss. However, the therapy had some benefits: it reduced the risk for colorectal cancer and bone fractures. Estrogen-alone therapy increased the risk for stroke and venous thrombosis (blood clot, usually in one of the deep veins of the legs). It had no effect on heart disease and colorectal cancer and an uncertain effect on breast cancer. Estrogen alone gave no protection against memory loss, and there were more cases of dementia in those who took the therapy than those on the placebo, although the increase was not statistically significant. Estrogen alone reduced the risk for bone fractures.

While questions remain, the findings make possible some advice about using hormone therapy: Estrogen alone or with progestin should not be used to prevent heart disease. Talk with your doctor about other ways of preventing heart attack and stroke, including lifestyle changes and medicines such as cholesterol-lowering statins and blood pressure drugs.

- If you are considering using menopausal hormone therapy to prevent osteoporosis, talk with your doctor about the possible benefits weighed against your personal risks for heart attack, stroke, blood clots, and breast cancer. Ask your doctor about alternative treatments that are safe and effective in preventing osteoporosis and bone fractures.

209

- Do not take menopausal hormone therapy to prevent dementia or memory loss.

- If you are considering menopausal hormone therapy to provide relief from menopausal symptoms such as hot flashes, talk with your doctor about whether this treatment is right for you. WHI findings confirm that menopausal hormone therapy relieves menopausal symptoms. At the average age of menopause the absolute risks (numbers) of heart attack, stroke, and blood clots are low and little affected by short-term menopausal hormone therapy. The current U.S. Food and Drug Administration recommendation for menopausal hormone therapy is that it should be used at the lowest dose for the shortest period of time to reach treatment goals.

- And remember: Your risk for heart disease, stroke, osteoporosis, and other conditions may change as you age. So review your health regularly with your doctor. New treatments that are safe and effective may become available. Stay informed.

If you have heart disease: Menopausal hormone therapy was once thought to lower the risk of heart attack and stroke for women with heart disease. But research now shows that women with heart disease should not take it. Menopausal hormone therapy can involve the use of estrogen alone or estrogen plus progestin. For women with heart disease, estrogen alone will not prevent heart attacks, and estrogen plus progestin increases the risk for heart attack during the first few years of use. Estrogen plus progestin also increases the risk for blood clots, stroke, and breast cancer.

Chapter 20

Ovarian Pain and Disorders of the Ovaries

Chapter Contents

Section 20.1

Ovarian Cysts

Excerpted from "Ovarian Cysts Fact Sheet,"
U.S. Department of Health and Human Services Office on Women's
Health (www.womenshealth.gov), September 23, 2008.

What are ovaries?

The ovaries are a pair of organs in the female reproductive system. They are located in the pelvis, one on each side of the uterus. The uterus is the hollow, pear-shaped organ where a baby grows. Each ovary is about the size and shape of an almond. The ovaries produce eggs and female hormones. Hormones are chemicals that control the way certain cells or organs function.

Every month, during a woman's menstrual cycle, an egg grows inside an ovary. It grows in a tiny sac called a follicle. When an egg matures, the sac breaks open to release the egg. The egg travels through the fallopian tube to the uterus for fertilization. Then the sac dissolves. The empty sac becomes corpus luteum. Corpus luteum makes hormones that help prepare for the next egg.

The ovaries are the main source of the female hormones estrogen and progesterone. These hormones affect the following:

- The way breasts and body hair grow

- Body shape

- The menstrual cycle

- Pregnancy

What are ovarian cysts?

A cyst is a fluid-filled sac. They can form anywhere in the body. Ovarian cysts form in or on the ovaries. The most common type of ovarian cyst is a functional cyst.

Functional cysts often form during the menstrual cycle. The two types are as follows:

- **Follicle cysts:** These cysts form when the sac doesn't break open to release the egg. Then the sac keeps growing. This type of cyst most often goes away in one to three months.

- **Corpus luteum cysts:** These cysts form if the sac doesn't dissolve. Instead, the sac seals off after the egg is released. Then fluid builds up inside. Most of these cysts go away after a few weeks. They can grow to almost four inches. They may bleed or twist the ovary and cause pain. They are rarely cancerous. Some drugs used to cause ovulation can raise the risk of getting these cysts.

Other types of ovarian cysts are the following:

- **Endometriomas:** These cysts form in women who have endometriosis. This problem occurs when tissue that looks and acts like the lining of the uterus grows outside the uterus. The tissue may attach to the ovary and form a growth. These cysts can be painful during sex and during your period.

- **Cystadenomas:** These cysts form from cells on the outer surface of the ovary. They are often filled with a watery fluid or thick, sticky gel. They can become large and cause pain.

- **Dermoid cysts:** These cysts contain many types of cells. They may be filled with hair, teeth, and other tissues that become part of the cyst. They can become large and cause pain.

- **Polycystic ovaries:** These cysts are caused when eggs mature within the sacs but are not released. The cycle then repeats. The sacs continue to grow and many cysts form.

What are the symptoms of ovarian cysts?

Many ovarian cysts don't cause symptoms. Others can cause the following:

- Pressure, swelling, or pain in the abdomen
- Pelvic pain
- Dull ache in the lower back and thighs
- Problems passing urine completely
- Pain during sex
- Weight gain
- Pain during your period

- Abnormal bleeding
- Nausea or vomiting
- Breast tenderness

If you have these symptoms, get help right away:

- Pain with fever and vomiting
- Sudden, severe abdominal pain
- Faintness, dizziness, or weakness
- Rapid breathing

How are ovarian cysts found?

Doctors most often find ovarian cysts during routine pelvic exams. The doctor may feel the swelling of a cyst on the ovary. Once a cyst is found, tests are done to help plan treatment. Tests include:

- **An ultrasound:** This test uses sound waves to create images of the body. With an ultrasound, the doctor can see the cyst.

- **A pregnancy test:** This test may be given to rule out pregnancy.

- **Hormone level tests:** Hormone levels may be checked to see if there are hormone-related problems.

- **A blood test:** This test is done to find out if the cyst may be cancerous. The test measures a substance in the blood called cancer-antigen 125 (CA-125). The amount of CA-125 is higher with ovarian cancer. But some ovarian cancers don't make enough CA-125 to be detected by the test. Some noncancerous diseases also raise CA-125 levels. Those diseases include uterine fibroids and endometriosis. Noncancerous causes of higher CA-125 are more common in women younger than 35. Ovarian cancer is very rare in this age group.

How are cysts treated?

Watchful waiting: If you have a cyst, you may be told to wait and have a second exam in one to three months. Your doctor will check to see if the cyst has changed in size. This is a common treatment option for women who fit these criteria:

- Are in their childbearing years, although it may be an option for postmenopausal women

- Have no symptoms
- Have a fluid-filled cyst

Surgery: Your doctor may want to remove the cyst if you are post-menopausal, or if the cyst follows these patterns:

- Doesn't go away after several menstrual cycles
- Gets larger
- Looks odd on the ultrasound
- Causes pain

The two main surgeries are as follows:

- **Laparoscopy:** Done if the cyst is small and looks benign (non-cancerous) on the ultrasound. While you are under general anesthesia, a very small cut is made above or below your navel. A small instrument that acts like a telescope is put into your abdomen. Then your doctor can remove the cyst.

- **Laparotomy:** Done if the cyst is large and may be cancerous. While you are under general anesthesia, larger incisions are made in the stomach to remove the cyst. The cyst is then tested for cancer. If it is cancerous, the doctor may need to take out the ovary and other tissues, like the uterus. If only one ovary is taken out, your body is still fertile and can still produce estrogen.

Birth control pills: If you keep forming functional cysts, your doctor may prescribe birth control pills to stop you from ovulating. If you don't ovulate, you are less likely to form new cysts. You can also use Depo-Provera. It is a hormone that is injected into muscle. It prevents ovulation for three months at a time.

Can ovarian cysts be prevented?

No, ovarian cysts cannot be prevented. The good news is that most cysts don't cause symptoms, are not cancerous, and go away on their own.

Talk to your doctor or nurse if you notice the following:

- Changes in your period
- Pain in the pelvic area
- Any of the major symptoms of cysts

When are women most likely to have ovarian cysts?

Most functional ovarian cysts occur during childbearing years. And most of those cysts are not cancerous. Women who are past menopause (ages 50–70) with ovarian cysts have a higher risk of ovarian cancer. At any age, if you think you have a cyst, see your doctor for a pelvic exam.

Section 20.2

Ovulation Pain (Mittelschmerz)

"Mittelschmerz," © 2013 A.D.A.M. Inc. Reprinted with permission.

Mittelschmerz is one-sided, lower abdominal pain that occurs in women at or around the time of an egg is released from the ovaries (ovulation).

Causes

About one in five women have mittelschmerz, or pain associated with ovulation. The pain may occur just before, during, or after ovulation.

There are several explanations for the cause of this pain. Just prior to ovulation, follicle growth may stretch the surface of the ovary, causing pain. At the time of ovulation, fluid or blood is released from the ruptured egg follicle and may cause irritation of the abdominal lining.

Symptoms

Mittelschmerz may be felt on one side one month, then switch to the opposite side the next month, or it may be felt on the same side for several months in succession.

Symptoms include lower-abdominal pain with these characteristics:

- One-sided
- Typically lasting minutes to a few hours, possibly as long as 24–48 hours
- Usually sharp, cramping, distinctive pain

- Severe (rare)

- May switch sides from month to month or from one episode to another

- Begins midway through the menstrual cycle

Exams and Tests

A pelvic examination shows no problems. Other tests (such as an abdominal ultrasound or transvaginal pelvic ultrasound) may be done to look for other causes of ovarian or pelvic pain, if the pain lasts a while.

Treatment

No treatment is usually necessary. Pain relievers (analgesics) may be needed in cases of prolonged or intense pain.

Outlook (Prognosis)

Mittelschmerz can be painful, but it is not harmful. It is not a sign of disease. In fact, women who feel this pain may be at an advantage when planning or trying to avoid pregnancy. Mittelschmerz pain is felt around the time of ovulation. A woman is most likely to become pregnant just before ovulation, on the day of ovulation, or immediately after ovulation.

Possible Complications

There are usually no complications.

When to Contact a Medical Professional

Call for an appointment with your health care provider if ovulation pain seems to change, lasts longer than usual, or occurs with vaginal bleeding.

Prevention

Birth control pills can be taken to prevent ovulation and help reduce ovulation-related pain.

Section 20.3

Polycystic Ovary Syndrome (PCOS)

Excerpted from "Polycystic Ovary Syndrome (PCOS) Fact Sheet,"
U.S. Department of Health and Human Services Office on Women's
Health (www.womenshealth.gov), March 17, 2010.

Editor's note—In January 2013, an independent panel convened
by the National Institutes of Health has concluded that the name of
a common hormone disorder in women, polycystic ovary syndrome
(PCOS), causes confusion and is a barrier to research progress and effective patient care. The current name focuses on a criterion—ovarian
cysts—that is neither necessary nor sufficient to diagnose the syndrome. In a report released January 23, 2013, the panel recommended
assigning a new name that more accurately reflects the disorder.

What is polycystic ovary syndrome (PCOS)?

Polycystic ovary syndrome (PCOS) is a health problem that can
affect a woman in these areas:

- Menstrual cycle
- Ability to have children
- Hormones
- Heart
- Blood vessels
- Appearance

With PCOS, women typically have the following:

- High levels of androgens, which are sometimes called male
  hormones, although females also make them
- Missed or irregular periods (monthly bleeding)
- Many small cysts (fluid-filled sacs) in their ovaries

218

How many women have PCOS?

Between 1 in 10 and 1 in 20 women of childbearing age has PCOS. As many as five million women in the United States may be affected. It can occur in girls as young as 11 years old.

What causes PCOS?

The cause of PCOS is unknown. But most experts think that several factors, including genetics, could play a role. Women with PCOS are more likely to have a mother or sister with PCOS.

A main underlying problem with PCOS is a hormonal imbalance. In women with PCOS, the ovaries make more androgens than normal. Androgens are male hormones that females also make. High levels of these hormones affect the development and release of eggs during ovulation.

Researchers also think insulin may be linked to PCOS. Insulin is a hormone that controls the change of sugar, starches, and other food into energy for the body to use or store. Many women with PCOS have too much insulin in their bodies because they have problems using it. Excess insulin appears to increase production of androgen. High androgen levels can lead to the following:

- Acne

- Excessive hair growth

- Weight gain

- Problems with ovulation

What are the symptoms of PCOS?

The symptoms of PCOS can vary from woman to woman. Some of the symptoms of PCOS include the following:

- Infertility (not able to get pregnant) because of not ovulating; in fact, PCOS is the most common cause of female infertility

- Infrequent, absent, and/or irregular menstrual periods

- Hirsutism—increased hair growth on the face, chest, stomach, back, thumbs, or toes

- Cysts on the ovaries

- Acne, oily skin, or dandruff

- Weight gain or obesity, usually with extra weight around the waist
- Male-pattern baldness or thinning hair
- Patches of skin on the neck, arms, breasts, or thighs that are thick and dark brown or black
- Skin tags—excess flaps of skin in the armpits or neck area
- Pelvic pain
- Anxiety or depression
- Sleep apnea, when breathing stops for short periods of time while asleep

Why do women with PCOS have trouble with their menstrual cycle and fertility?

The ovaries, where a woman's eggs are produced, have tiny fluid-filled sacs called follicles or cysts. As the egg grows, the follicle builds up fluid. When the egg matures, the follicle breaks open, the egg is released, and the egg travels through the fallopian tube to the uterus (womb) for fertilization. This is called ovulation.

In women with PCOS, the ovary doesn't make all of the hormones it needs for an egg to fully mature. The follicles may start to grow and build up fluid but ovulation does not occur. Instead, some follicles may remain as cysts. For these reasons, ovulation does not occur and the hormone progesterone is not made. Without progesterone, a woman's menstrual cycle is irregular or absent. Plus, the ovaries make male hormones, which also prevent ovulation.

Does PCOS change at menopause?

Yes and no. PCOS affects many systems in the body. So many symptoms may persist even though ovarian function and hormone levels change as a woman nears menopause. For instance, excessive hair growth continues, and male-pattern baldness or thinning hair gets worse after menopause. Also, the risks of complications (health problems) from PCOS, such as heart attack, stroke, and diabetes, increase as a woman gets older.

How do I know if I have PCOS?

There is no single test to diagnose PCOS. Your doctor will take the following steps to find out if you have PCOS or if something else is causing your symptoms.

Medical history: Your doctor will ask about your menstrual periods, weight changes, and other symptoms.

Physical exam: Your doctor will want to measure your blood pressure, body mass index (BMI), and waist size. He or she also will check the areas of increased hair growth. You should try to allow the natural hair to grow for a few days before the visit.

Pelvic exam: Your doctor might want to check to see if your ovaries are enlarged or swollen by the increased number of small cysts.

Blood tests: Your doctor may check the androgen hormone and glucose (sugar) levels in your blood.

Vaginal ultrasound (sonogram): Your doctor may perform a test that uses sound waves to take pictures of the pelvic area. It might be used to examine your ovaries for cysts and check the endometrium (lining of the womb). This lining may become thicker if your periods are not regular.

How is PCOS treated?

Because there is no cure for PCOS, it needs to be managed to prevent problems. Treatment goals are based on your symptoms, whether or not you want to become pregnant, and lowering your chances of getting heart disease and diabetes. Many women will need a combination of treatments to meet these goals. Some treatments for PCOS include these:

Lifestyle modification: Many women with PCOS are overweight or obese, which can cause health problems. You can help manage your PCOS by eating healthy and exercising to keep your weight at a healthy level. This helps to lower blood glucose (sugar) levels, improve the body's use of insulin, and normalize hormone levels in your body. Even a 10% loss in body weight can restore a normal period and make your cycle more regular.

Birth control pills: For women who don't want to get pregnant, birth control pills can control menstrual cycles, reduce male hormone levels, and help to clear acne.

Keep in mind that the menstrual cycle will become abnormal again if the pill is stopped. Women may also think about taking a pill that only has progesterone, like Provera, to control the menstrual cycle and reduce the risk of endometrial cancer. But progesterone alone does not help reduce acne and hair growth.

Diabetes medications: The medicine metformin (Glucophage) is used to treat type 2 diabetes. It has also been found to help with PCOS symptoms, though it isn't approved by the U.S Food and Drug Administration (FDA) for this use. Metformin affects the way insulin controls blood glucose (sugar) and lowers testosterone production. It slows the growth of abnormal hair and, after a few months of use, may help ovulation to return. Recent research has shown metformin to have other positive effects, such as decreased body mass and improved cholesterol levels.

Fertility medications: Lack of ovulation is usually the reason for fertility problems in women with PCOS. Several medications that stimulate ovulation can help women with PCOS become pregnant. Even so, other reasons for infertility in both the woman and man should be ruled out before fertility medications are used. Also, some fertility medications increase the risk for multiple births.

Another option is in vitro fertilization (IVF). IVF offers the best chance of becoming pregnant in any given cycle. It also gives doctors better control over the chance of multiple births. But IVF is very costly.

Surgery: "Ovarian drilling" is a surgery that may increase the chance of ovulation. It's sometimes used when a woman does not respond to fertility medicines. The doctor makes a very small cut above or below the navel (belly button) and inserts a small tool that acts like a telescope into the abdomen (stomach). This is called laparoscopy. The doctor then punctures the ovary with a small needle carrying an electric current to destroy a small portion of the ovary. This procedure carries a risk of developing scar tissue on the ovary. This surgery can lower male hormone levels and help with ovulation. But, these effects may only last a few months. This treatment doesn't help with loss of scalp hair or increased hair growth on other parts of the body.

Medicine for increased hair growth or extra male hormones: Medicines called anti-androgens may reduce hair growth and clear acne. Spironolactone (Aldactone), first used to treat high blood pressure, has been shown to reduce the impact of male hormones on hair growth in women. Finasteride (Propecia), a medicine taken by men for hair loss, has the same effect. Anti-androgens are often combined with birth control pills. These medications should not be taken if you are trying to become pregnant.

Before taking Aldactone, tell your doctor if you are pregnant or plan to become pregnant. Do not breastfeed while taking this medicine. Women who may become pregnant should not handle Propecia.

Other options include these:

- Vaniqa cream to reduce facial hair
- Laser hair removal or electrolysis to remove hair
- Hormonal treatment to keep new hair from growing

Other treatments: Some research has shown that bariatric (weight loss) surgery may be effective in resolving PCOS in morbidly obese women. Morbid obesity means having a BMI of more than 40, or a BMI of 35 to 40 with an obesity-related disease. The drug troglitazone was shown to help women with PCOS. But it was taken off the market because it caused liver problems. Similar drugs without the same side effect are being tested in small trials.

How does PCOS affect a woman while pregnant?

Women with PCOS appear to have higher rates of the following:

- Miscarriage
- Gestational diabetes
- Pregnancy-induced high blood pressure (preeclampsia)
- Premature delivery

Babies born to women with PCOS have a higher risk of spending time in a neonatal intensive care unit or of dying before, during, or shortly after birth. Most of the time, these problems occur in multiple-birth babies.

Researchers are studying whether the diabetes medicine metformin can prevent or reduce the chances of having problems while pregnant. Metformin also lowers male hormone levels and limits weight gain in women who are obese when they get pregnant.

Metformin is an FDA pregnancy category B drug. It does not appear to cause major birth defects or other problems in pregnant women. But there have only been a few studies of metformin use in pregnant women to confirm its safety. Also, metformin is passed through breast milk. Talk with your doctor about metformin use if you are pregnant, trying to become pregnant, or nursing.

Does PCOS put women at risk for other health problems?

Women with PCOS have greater chances of developing several serious health conditions, including life-threatening diseases. Recent studies discovered the following:

- More than 50% of women with PCOS will have diabetes or prediabetes (impaired glucose tolerance) before the age of 40.

- The risk of heart attack is four to seven times higher in women with PCOS than women of the same age without PCOS.

- Women with PCOS are at greater risk of having high blood pressure.

- Women with PCOS have high levels of LDL ("bad," low-density lipoprotein) cholesterol and low levels of HDL ("good," high-density lipoprotcin) cholesterol.

- Women with PCOS can develop sleep apnea. This is when breathing stops for short periods of time during sleep.

Women with PCOS may also develop anxiety and depression. It is important to talk to your doctor about treatment for these mental health conditions.

Women with PCOS are also at risk for endometrial cancer. Irregular menstrual periods and the lack of ovulation cause women to produce the hormone estrogen, but not the hormone progesterone. Progesterone causes the endometrium (lining of the womb) to shed each month as a menstrual period. Without progesterone, the endometrium becomes thick, which can cause heavy or irregular bleeding. Over time, this can lead to endometrial hyperplasia, when the lining grows too much, and cancer.

I have PCOS. What can I do to prevent complications?

If you have PCOS, get your symptoms under control at an earlier age to help reduce your chances of having complications like diabetes and heart disease. Talk to your doctor about treating all your symptoms, rather than focusing on just one aspect of your PCOS, such as problems getting pregnant. Also, talk to your doctor about getting tested for diabetes regularly.

How can I cope with the emotional effects of PCOS?

Having PCOS can be difficult. You may feel embarrassed by your appearance, worried about being able to get pregnant, or depressed.

Getting treatment for PCOS can help with these concerns and help boost your self-esteem. You may also want to look for support groups in your area or online to help you deal with the emotional effects of PCOS. You are not alone, and there are resources available for women with PCOS.

Chapter 21

Endometriosis

What is endometriosis?

Endometriosis is a common health problem in women. It gets its name from the word *endometrium*, the tissue that lines the uterus or womb. Endometriosis occurs when this tissue grows outside of the uterus on other organs or structures in the body.

Most often, endometriosis is found on the following:

- Ovaries
- Fallopian tubes
- Tissues that hold the uterus in place
- Outer surface of the uterus
- Lining of the pelvic cavity

Other sites for growths can include the vagina, cervix, vulva, bowel, bladder, or rectum. In rare cases, endometriosis has been found in other parts of the body, such as the lungs, brain, and skin.

What are the symptoms of endometriosis?

The most common symptom of endometriosis is pain in the lower abdomen or pelvis, or the lower back, mainly during menstrual periods.

Excerpted from "Endometriosis Fact Sheet," U.S. Department of Health and Human Services Office on Women's Health (www.womenshealth.gov), November 16, 2009.

The amount of pain a woman feels does not depend on how much endometriosis she has. Some women have no pain, even though their disease affects large areas. Other women with endometriosis have severe pain even though they have only a few small growths.

Symptoms of endometriosis can include the following:

• Very painful menstrual cramps; pain may get worse over time

• Chronic pain in the lower back and pelvis

• Pain during or after sex

• Intestinal pain

• Painful bowel movements or painful urination during menstrual periods

• Spotting or bleeding between menstrual periods

• Infertility or not being able to get pregnant

• Fatigue

• Diarrhea, constipation, bloating, or nausea, especially during menstrual periods

Recent research shows a link between other health problems in women with endometriosis and their families. Some of these include the following:

• Allergies, asthma, and chemical sensitivities

• Autoimmune diseases, in which the body's system that fights illness attacks itself instead

• Chronic fatigue syndrome (CFS) and fibromyalgia

• Being more likely to get infections and mononucleosis

• Mitral valve prolapse, a condition in which one of the heart's valves does not close as tightly as normal

• Frequent yeast infections

• Certain cancers, such as ovarian, breast, endocrine, kidney, thyroid, brain, and colon cancers, and melanoma and non-Hodgkin lymphoma

Why does endometriosis cause pain and health problems?

Growths of endometriosis are benign (not cancerous). But they still can cause many problems. Every month, hormones cause the lining of a woman's uterus to build up with tissue and blood vessels. If a woman does not get pregnant, the uterus sheds this tissue and blood. It comes out of the body through the vagina as her menstrual period.

Patches of endometriosis also respond to the hormones produced during the menstrual cycle. With the passage of time, the growths of endometriosis may expand by adding extra tissue and blood. The symptoms of endometriosis often get worse.

Tissue and blood that is shed into the body can cause inflammation, scar tissue, and pain. As endometrial tissue grows, it can cover or grow into the ovaries and block the fallopian tubes. Trapped blood in the ovaries can form cysts, or closed sacs. It also can cause inflammation and cause the body to form scar tissue and adhesions, tissue that sometimes binds organs together. This scar tissue may cause pelvic pain and make it hard for women to get pregnant. The growths can also cause problems in the intestines and bladder.

Who gets endometriosis?

More than five million women in the United States have endometriosis. It is one of the most common health problems for women. It can occur in any teen or woman who has menstrual periods, but it is most common in women in their thirties and forties.

The symptoms of endometriosis stop for a time during pregnancy. Symptoms also tend to decrease with menopause, when menstrual periods end for good. In some cases, women who take menopausal hormone therapy may still have symptoms of endometriosis.

What can raise my chances of getting endometriosis?

You might be more likely to get endometriosis if you have these criteria:

- Never had children
- Have menstrual periods that last more than seven days
- Have short menstrual cycles (27 days or less)
- Have a family member (mother, aunt, sister) with endometriosis
- Have a health problem that prevents normal passage of menstrual blood flow
- Have damaged cells in the pelvis from an infection

How can I reduce my chances of getting endometriosis?

There are no definite ways to lower your chances of getting endometriosis. Yet since the hormone estrogen is involved in thickening the lining of the uterus during the menstrual cycle, you can try to lower levels of estrogen in your body by doing the following:

- Exercising regularly
- Keeping a low amount of body fat
- Avoiding large amounts of alcohol and drinks with caffeine

Why is it important to find out if I have endometriosis?

The pain of endometriosis can interfere with your life. Studies show that women with endometriosis often skip school, work, and social events. This health problem can also get in the way of relationships with your partner, friends, children, and co-workers. Plus, endometriosis can make it hard for you to get pregnant.

Finding out that you have endometriosis is the first step in taking back your life. Many treatments can control the symptoms. Medicine can relieve your pain. When endometriosis causes fertility problems, surgery can boost your chances of getting pregnant.

How do I know that I have endometriosis?

If you have symptoms of this disease, talk with your doctor or your obstetrician/gynecologist. An ob/gyn has special training to diagnose and treat this condition. Sometimes endometriosis is mistaken for other health problems that cause pelvic pain and the exact cause might be hard to pinpoint.

The doctor will talk to you about your symptoms and health history. The doctor may also do these tests to check for clues of endometriosis:

Pelvic exam: Your doctor will perform a pelvic exam to feel for large cysts or scars behind your uterus. Smaller areas of endometriosis are hard to feel.

Ultrasound: Your doctor could perform an ultrasound, an imaging test to see if there are ovarian cysts from endometriosis. During a vaginal ultrasound, the doctor will insert a wand-shaped scanner into your vagina. During an ultrasound of your pelvis, a scanner is moved across your abdomen. Both tests use sound waves to make pictures of your reproductive organs. Magnetic resonance imaging (MRI) is another common imaging test that can produce a picture of the inside of your body.

Laparoscopy: The only way for your doctor to know for sure that you have endometriosis is to look inside your abdomen to see endometriosis tissue. He or she can do this through a minor surgery called laparoscopy. Sometimes doctors can diagnose endometriosis just by seeing the growths. Other times, they need to take a small sample of tissue and study it under a microscope.

If your doctor does not find signs of an ovarian cyst during an ultrasound, before doing a laparoscopy, your doctor may prescribe birth control pills to control your menstrual cycle. Sometimes this treatment helps lessen pelvic pain during your period. Some doctors may offer another treatment that blocks the menstrual cycle and lowers the amount of estrogen your body makes before doing a laparoscopy. This treatment is a medicine called a gonadotropin-releasing hormone (GnRH) agonist, which also may help pelvic pain. If your pain improves on this medicine, the doctor will likely think that you have endometriosis.

Laparoscopy is often recommended for diagnosis and treatment if the pelvic pain persists, even after taking birth control pills and pain medicine.

What causes endometriosis?

No one knows for sure what causes this disease, but experts have a number of theories:

- Since endometriosis runs in families, it may be carried in the genes, or some families have traits that make them more likely to get it.

- Endometrial tissue may move from the uterus to other body parts through the blood system or lymph system.

- If a woman has a faulty immune system it will fail to find and destroy endometrial tissue growing outside of the uterus. Recent research shows that immune system disorders and certain cancers are more common in women with endometriosis.

- The hormone estrogen appears to promote the growth of endometriosis. So, some research is looking at whether it is a disease of the endocrine system, the body's system of glands, hormones, and other secretions.

- Endometrial tissue has been found in abdominal scars and might have been moved there by mistake during a surgery.

- Small amounts of tissue from when a woman was an embryo might later become endometriosis.

- New research shows a link between dioxin exposure and getting endometriosis. Dioxin is a toxic chemical from the making of pesticides and the burning of wastes. More research is needed to find out whether man-made chemicals cause endometriosis.

- Endometrial tissue may back up into the abdomen through the fallopian tubes during a woman's monthly period. This transplanted tissue could grow outside of the uterus. However, most experts agree that this theory does not entirely explain why endometriosis develops.

How is endometriosis treated?

There is no cure for endometriosis, but there are many treatments for the pain and infertility that it causes. Talk with your doctor about what option is best for you. The treatment you choose will depend on your symptoms, age, and plans for getting pregnant.

Pain medication: For some women with mild symptoms, doctors may suggest taking over-the-counter medicines for pain. If these medicines don't help, doctors may prescribe stronger pain relievers.

Hormone treatment: When pain medicine is not enough, doctors often recommend hormone medicines to treat endometriosis. Only women who do not wish to become pregnant can use these drugs. Hormone treatment is best for women with small growths who do not have bad pain. Hormones come in many forms including pills, shots, and nasal sprays. Common hormones used for endometriosis include the following:

- **Birth control pills** decrease the amount of menstrual flow and prevent overgrowth of tissue that lines the uterus.

- **GnRH agonists and antagonists** greatly reduce the amount of estrogen in a woman's body, which stops the menstrual cycle. These drugs should not be used alone because they can cause side effects similar to those during menopause, such as hot flashes, bone loss, and vaginal dryness. Taking a low dose of progestin or estrogen along with these drugs can protect against these side effects.

- The hormone **progestin** can shrink spots of endometriosis by working against the effects of estrogen on the tissue.

- **Danazol** is a weak male hormone that lowers the levels of estrogen and progesterone in a woman's body. It is not often the first choice for treatment due to its side effects.

Surgery: Surgery is usually the best choice for women with severe endometriosis—many growths, a great deal of pain, or fertility problems. There are both minor and more complex surgeries that can help. Your doctor might suggest one of the following:

- **Laparoscopy** can be used to diagnose and treat endometriosis. During this surgery, doctors remove growths and scar tissue or burn them away. Women recover from laparoscopy much faster than from major abdominal surgery.

- **Laparotomy** or major abdominal surgery involves a much larger cut in the abdomen. This allows the doctor to reach and remove growths of endometriosis in the pelvis or abdomen.

- **Hysterectomy** is a surgery in which the doctor removes the uterus. Removing the ovaries as well can help ensure that endometriosis will not return. A woman cannot get pregnant after this surgery, so it should only be considered as a last resort.

How do I cope with a disease that has no cure?

It is important to get support to cope with endometriosis. Consider joining a support group to talk with other women who have endometriosis. It is also important to learn as much as you can about the disease. Talking with friends, family, and your doctor can help.

Chapter 22

Uterine Fibroids

What are fibroids?

Fibroids are muscular tumors that grow in the wall of the uterus (womb). Another medical term for fibroids is "leiomyoma" or just "myoma." Fibroids are almost always benign (not cancerous). Fibroids can grow as a single tumor, or there can be many in the uterus. They can be as small as an apple seed or as big as a grapefruit. In unusual cases they can become very large.

About 20% to 80% of women develop fibroids by the time they reach age 50. Fibroids are most common in women in their forties and early fifties. Not all women with fibroids have symptoms. Women who do have symptoms often find fibroids hard to live with. Some have pain and heavy menstrual bleeding. Fibroids also can put pressure on the bladder, causing frequent urination, or the rectum, causing rectal pressure. Should the fibroids get very large, they can cause the abdomen to enlarge, making a woman look pregnant.

Who gets fibroids?

There are factors that can increase a woman's risk of developing fibroids.

Excerpted from "Uterine Fibroids Fact Sheet," U.S. Department of Health and Human Services Office on Women's Health (www.womenshealth.gov), May 13, 2008.

- **Age:** Fibroids become more common as women age, especially during the thirties and forties through menopause. After menopause, fibroids usually shrink.

- **Family history:** Having a family member with fibroids increases your risk. If a woman's mother had fibroids, her risk of having them is about three times higher than average.

- **Ethnic origin:** African American women are more likely to develop fibroids than white women.

- **Obesity:** Women who are overweight are at higher risk for fibroids. For very heavy women, the risk is two to three times greater than average.

- **Eating habits:** Eating a lot of red meat (e.g., beef) and ham is linked with a higher risk of fibroids. Eating plenty of green vegetables seems to protect women from developing fibroids.

Where can fibroids grow?

Most fibroids grow in the wall of the uterus. Doctors put them into three groups based on where they grow:

- **Submucosal** fibroids grow into the uterine cavity.

- **Intramural** fibroids grow within the wall of the uterus.

- **Subserosal** fibroids grow on the outside of the uterus.

Some fibroids grow on stalks that grow out from the surface of the uterus or into the cavity of the uterus. They might look like mushrooms. These are called pedunculated fibroids.

What are the symptoms of fibroids?

Most fibroids do not cause any symptoms, but some women with fibroids can have the following:

- Heavy bleeding (which can be heavy enough to cause anemia) or painful periods

- Feeling of fullness in the pelvic area

- Enlargement of the lower abdomen

- Frequent urination

- Pain during sex

- Lower back pain

- Complications during pregnancy and labor, including a six-time greater risk of cesarean section

- Reproductive problems, such as infertility, which is very rare

What causes fibroids?

No one knows for sure what causes fibroids. Researchers think that more than one factor could play a role. These factors could be hormonal (affected by estrogen and progesterone levels) or genetic (runs in families).

We also don't know what causes fibroids to grow or shrink. We do know that they are under hormonal control. They grow rapidly during pregnancy, when hormone levels are high. They shrink when anti-hormone medication is used. They also stop growing or shrink once a woman reaches menopause.

Can fibroids turn into cancer?

Fibroids are almost always benign (not cancerous). Rarely (less than one in 1,000) a cancerous fibroid will occur. This is called leiomyosarcoma. Doctors think that these cancers do not arise from an already-existing fibroid. Having fibroids does not increase the risk of developing a cancerous fibroid. Having fibroids also does not increase a woman's chances of getting other forms of cancer in the uterus.

What if I become pregnant and have fibroids?

Women who have fibroids are more likely to have problems during pregnancy and delivery. This doesn't mean there will be problems. Most women with fibroids have normal pregnancies. The most common problems seen in women with fibroids are the following:

- **Cesarean section:** The risk of needing a c-section is six times greater for women with fibroids.

- **Baby is breech:** The baby is not positioned well for vaginal delivery.

- **Labor fails to progress**

- **Placental abruption:** The placenta breaks away from the wall of the uterus before delivery. When this happens, the fetus does not get enough oxygen.

- **Preterm delivery**

Talk to your obstetrician if you have fibroids and become pregnant. Most women who have fibroids and become pregnant do not need to see an ob/gyn who deals with high-risk pregnancies.

How do I know for sure that I have fibroids?

Your doctor may find that you have fibroids when you see her or him for a regular pelvic exam. The doctor can feel the fibroid with her or his fingers during an ordinary pelvic exam, as a (usually painless) lump or mass on the uterus. Often, a doctor will describe how small or how large the fibroids are by comparing their size to the size your uterus would be if you were pregnant. For example, you may be told that your fibroids have made your uterus the size it would be if you were 16 weeks pregnant. Or the fibroid might be compared to fruits, nuts, or a ball.

Your doctor can do imaging tests to confirm that you have fibroids. These are tests that create a "picture" of the inside of your body without surgery. These tests might include ultrasound, magnetic resonance imaging (MRI), X-rays, computed tomography (CT) scan, or a hysterosalpingogram (HSG) or sonohysterogram. An HSG involves injecting X-ray dye into the uterus and taking X-ray pictures. A sonohysterogram involves injecting water into the uterus and making ultrasound pictures.

You might also need surgery to know for sure if you have fibroids. There are two types of surgery to do this:

- **Laparoscopy:** The doctor inserts a long, thin scope into a tiny incision made in or near the navel. The scope has a bright light and a camera. This allows the doctor to view the uterus and other organs on a monitor during the procedure.

- **Hysteroscopy:** The doctor passes a long, thin scope with a light through the vagina and cervix into the uterus. No incision is needed.

What questions should I ask my doctor if I have fibroids?

- How many fibroids do I have?

- What size is my fibroid(s)?

- Where is my fibroid(s) located (outer surface, inner surface, or in the wall of the uterus)?

- Can I expect the fibroid(s) to grow larger?

- How rapidly have they grown (if they were known about already)?

- How will I know if the fibroid(s) is growing larger?

- What problems can the fibroid(s) cause?

- What tests or imaging studies are best for keeping track of the growth of my fibroids?

- What are my treatment options if my fibroid(s) becomes a problem?

- What are your views on treating fibroids with a hysterectomy versus other types of treatments?

How are fibroids treated?

Most women with fibroids do not have any symptoms. For women who do have symptoms, there are treatments that can help. Talk with your doctor about the best way to treat your fibroids. If you have fibroids but do not have any symptoms, you may not need treatment. Your doctor will check during your regular exams to see if they have grown.

Medications: If you have fibroids and have mild symptoms, your doctor may suggest taking medication. Over-the-counter drugs such as ibuprofen or acetaminophen can be used for mild pain. If you have heavy bleeding during your period, taking an iron supplement can keep you from getting anemia or correct it if you already are anemic.

Several drugs commonly used for birth control can be prescribed to help control symptoms of fibroids. Low-dose birth control pills do not make fibroids grow and can help control heavy bleeding. The same is true of progesterone-like injections (e.g., Depo-Provera). An IUD (intra-uterine device) called Mirena contains a small amount of progesterone-like medication, which can be used to control heavy bleeding as well as for birth control.

Other drugs used to treat fibroids are "gonadotropin-releasing hormone agonists" (GnRHa). These drugs, given by injection, nasal spray, or implanted, can temporarily shrink your fibroids. Sometimes they are used before surgery to make fibroids easier to remove. Side effects of GnRHas can include hot flashes, depression, not being able to sleep, decreased sex drive, and joint pain. Most women tolerate GnRHas quite well. Most women do not get a period when taking GnRHas. GnRHas can cause bone thinning, so their use is generally limited to six months or less. These drugs also are very expensive, and some insurance companies will cover only some or none of the cost.

Surgery: If you have fibroids with moderate or severe symptoms, surgery may be the best way to treat them.

- **Myomectomy** is surgery to remove fibroids without taking out the healthy tissue of the uterus. It is best for women who wish to have children after treatment for their fibroids or who wish to keep their uterus for other reasons. You can become pregnant after myomectomy. But if your fibroids were imbedded deeply in the uterus, you might need a cesarean section to deliver. It can be major surgery (involving cutting into the abdomen) or performed with laparoscopy or hysteroscopy.

- **Hysterectomy** is surgery to remove the uterus. This surgery is the only sure way to cure uterine fibroids. Fibroids are the most common reason that hysterectomy is performed. This surgery is used when a woman's fibroids are large, if she has heavy bleeding, is either near or past menopause, or does not want children. If the fibroids are large, a woman may need a hysterectomy that involves cutting into the abdomen to remove the uterus. If the fibroids are smaller, the doctor may be able to reach the uterus through the vagina, instead of making a cut in the abdomen. In some cases hysterectomy can be performed through the laparoscope. Removal of the ovaries and the cervix at the time of hysterectomy is usually optional. Although hysterectomy is usually quite safe, it does carry a significant risk of complications.

- **Endometrial ablation** is when the lining of the uterus is removed or destroyed to control very heavy bleeding. This can be done with laser, wire loops, boiling water, electric current, microwaves, freezing, and other methods. This procedure usually is considered minor surgery. Complications can occur, but are uncommon with most of the methods. About half of women who have this procedure have no more menstrual bleeding. About 3 in 10 women have much lighter bleeding. But a woman cannot have children after this surgery.

- **Myolysis** is when a needle is inserted into the fibroids, usually guided by laparoscopy, and electric current or freezing is used to destroy the fibroids.

- **Uterine fibroid embolization (UFE), or uterine artery embolization (UAE),** is when thin tube is threaded into the blood vessels that supply blood to the fibroid. Then, tiny plastic or gel particles are injected into the blood vessels. This blocks the blood

238

supply to the fibroid, causing it to shrink. UFE can be an out-patient or inpatient procedure. Complications, including early menopause, are uncommon but can occur. Studies suggest fibroids are not likely to grow back after UFE, but more long-term research is needed. Not all fibroids can be treated with UFE.

Are other treatments being developed for uterine fibroids?

Yes. Researchers are looking into other ways to treat uterine fibroids. The following methods are not yet standard treatments, so your doctor may not offer them or health insurance may not cover them.

- **MRI-guided ultrasound surgery** shrinks fibroids using a high-intensity ultrasound beam. The MRI scanner helps the doctor locate the fibroid, and the ultrasound sends out very hot sound waves to destroy the fibroid.

- Some health care providers use **lasers** to remove a fibroid or to cut off the blood supply to the fibroid, making it shrink.

- **Anti-hormonal drugs** being developed could provide symptom relief without bone-thinning side effects. These are promising treatments, but none are yet available or FDA approved.

Chapter 23

Disorders of the Cervix

Chapter Contents

Section 23.1

Cervical Dysplasia

© 2013 A.D.A.M. Inc. Reprinted with permission.

Cervical dysplasia refers is abnormal changes in the cells on the sur-face of the cervix that are seen underneath a microscope. The cervix is the lower part of the uterus (womb) that opens at the top of the vagina.

The changes are not cancer. However, they can lead to cancer of the cervix if not treated.

Causes

Cervical dysplasia is most often seen in women ages 25–35 but can develop at any age.

Most often, cervical dysplasia is caused by the human papilloma virus (HPV). HPV is a common virus that is spread through sexual contact. There are many different types of HPV. Some types lead to cervical dysplasia or cancer.

The following may increase your risk of cervical dysplasia:

- Having sex before age 18
- Having a baby before age 16
- Having multiple sexual partners
- Having other illnesses or using medications that suppress your immune system
- Smoking

Symptoms

There are usually no symptoms.

Exams and Tests

A pelvic examination is usually normal.

Cervical dysplasia that is seen on a Pap smear is called squamous intraepithelial lesion (SIL). These changes may be:

- low-grade (LSIL);
- high-grade (HSIL);
- possibly cancerous (malignant);
- atypical glandular cells (AGUS).

If a Pap smear shows abnormal cells or cervical dysplasia, you will need further testing:

- Follow-up Pap smears may be recommended if the condition is mild.
- Colposcopy-directed biopsy can confirm it.
- Cone biopsy or LEEP excision may be done after colposcopy.

Dysplasia that is seen on a biopsy of the cervix is called cervical intraepithelial neoplasia (CIN).

Some strains of human papillomavirus (HPV) are known to cause cervical cancer. An HPV DNA test can identify the high-risk types of HPV linked to such cancer. This may be done:

- as a screening test for women over age 30, or
- for women of any age who have a slightly abnormal Pap test result.

Treatment

Treatment depends on the degree of dysplasia. Mild dysplasia may go away without treatment.

You may only need careful observation by your doctor with repeat Pap smears every three to six months.

If the changes do not go away or get worse, treatment is necessary.

Treatment for moderate-to-severe dysplasia or mild dysplasia that does not go away may include:

- cryosurgery to freeze abnormal cells;
- laser therapy, which uses light to burn away abnormal tissue;
- LEEP (loop electrosurgical excision procedure), which uses electricity to remove abnormal tissue;
- surgery to remove the abnormal tissue (cone biopsy).

Rarely, a hysterectomy may be needed. If you have had dysplasia, you will need close follow-up, usually every three to six months or as recommended by your doctor.

Outlook (Prognosis)

Early diagnosis and prompt treatment will cure nearly all cases of cervical dysplasia. Sometimes, the condition returns.

Without treatment, severe cervical dysplasia may develop invasive cancer. It can take 10 or more years for cervical dysplasia to develop into cancer. The risk of cancer is lower for mild dysplasia.

When to Contact a Medical Professional

Call for an appointment with your health care provider if you are age 21 or older and have never had a pelvic examination and Pap smear.

Prevention

Ask your health care provider about the HPV vaccine. Girls who receive this vaccine before they become sexually active reduce their chance of getting cervical cancer by 70%.

You can reduce your risk of developing cervical dysplasia by taking the following steps:

- Do not smoke. Smoking increases your risk of developing more severe dysplasia and cancer.

- Get vaccinated for HPV between ages 9 and 26.

- Do not have sex until you are 18 or older.

- Practice safe sex, and use a condom.

- Practice monogamy, which means you only have one sexual partner at a time.

Section 23.2

Cervical Polyps

Cervical polyps are fingerlike growths on the lower part of the uterus that connects with the vagina (cervix).

Causes

The cause of cervical polyps is not completely understood. They may occur with:

- an abnormal response to increased levels of the female hormone, estrogen;
- chronic inflammation;
- clogged blood vessels in the cervix.

Cervical polyps are common, especially in women over age 20 who have had children. Polyps are rare in young women who have not started their period (menstruation).

Most women have only one polyp, but some women have two or three.

Symptoms

- Abnormally heavy periods (menorrhagia)
- Abnormal vaginal bleeding
  - After douching
  - After intercourse
  - After menopause
  - Between periods
- White or yellow mucus (leukorrhea)

Polyps may not cause symptoms.

Exams and Tests

During a pelvic examination, the health care provider will see smooth, red or purple, fingerlike growths on the cervix. A cervical biopsy will most often show cells that are consistent with a benign polyp. Rarely there may be abnormal, precancerous, or cancer cells in a polyp.

Treatment

The health care provider can remove polyps during a simple, outpatient procedure. Gentle twisting of a cervical polyp may remove it. Larger polyps may require removal with electrocautery.

Although most cervical polyps are not cancerous (benign), the removed tissue should be sent to a laboratory and checked further.

Outlook (Prognosis)

Typically, polyps are not cancerous (benign) and are easy to remove. Polyps do not usually grow back. Women who have polyps are at risk of growing more polyps.

Possible Complications

There may be bleeding and slight cramping for a few days after removal of a polyp. Some cervical cancers may first appear as a polyp. Certain uterine polyps may be associated with uterine cancer.

When to Contact a Medical Professional

Call for an appointment if you have:

- abnormal bleeding from the vagina, including bleeding after sex or between periods;

- abnormal discharge from the vagina;

- abnormally heavy periods.

Call your doctor or nurse to schedule regular gynecological exams. Ask how often you should receive a Pap smear.

Prevention

See your health care provider to treat infections as soon as possible.

Section 23.3

Cervicitis

© 2013 A.D.A.M. Inc. Reprinted with permission.

Cervicitis is swelling (inflammation) of the end of the uterus (cervix).

Causes

Cervicitis is most often caused by an infection, usually caught during sexual activity. Sexually transmitted infections (STIs) that can cause cervicitis include:

- chlamydia;

- gonorrhea;

- herpes virus (genital herpes);

- human papilloma virus (genital warts);

- trichomoniasis.

Cervicitis may sometimes be caused by:

- a device inserted into the pelvic area such as:

  - cervical cap;

  - device to support the uterus (pessary);

  - diaphragm;

- allergy to spermicides used for birth control;

- allergy to latex in condoms;

- exposure to a chemical.

Cervicitis is very common, affecting more than half of all women at some point during their adult life. Risks include:

- high-risk sexual behavior;

- history of STIs;

- many sexual partners;
- sex (intercourse) at an early age;
- sexual partners who have engaged in high-risk sexual behavior or have had an STI.

Bacteria (such as *Staphylococcus* and *Streptococcus*) and too much growth of normal bacteria in the vagina (bacterial vaginosis) can also cause cervicitis.

Symptoms

- Abnormal vaginal bleeding
  - After intercourse
  - After menopause
  - Between periods
- Unusual vaginal discharge
  - Does not go away
  - Gray, white, or yellow color
  - May have an odor
- Painful sexual intercourse
- Pain in the vagina
- Pressure or heaviness in the pelvis

Note: There may be no symptoms, so it is recommended that certain women be tested for chlamydia, even if they do not have symptoms.

Exams and Tests

A pelvic examination may show:
- discharge from the cervix;
- redness of the cervix;
- swelling (inflammation) of the walls of the vagina.

Tests:
- inspection of the discharge under a microscope (may show candidiasis, trichomoniasis, or bacterial vaginosis);

- Pap smear;

- tests for gonorrhea or chlamydia.

Rarely, colposcopy and biopsy of the cervix is necessary.

Treatment

Antibiotics are used to treat bacterial infections, such as chlamydia, gonorrhea, and others. Drugs called antivirals may be used to treat herpes infections.

Hormonal therapy (with estrogen or progesterone) may be used in women who have reached menopause (postmenopausal).

When these treatments have not worked or when cervicitis has been present for a long time, treatment may include:

- cryosurgery (freezing);

- electrocauterization;

- laser therapy.

Outlook (Prognosis)

Simple cervicitis usually heals with treatment if the cause is found and there is a treatment for that cause.

Cervicitis can last for months or years.

Possible Complications

Cervicitis may last for months to years. Cervicitis may lead to pain with intercourse (dyspareunia).

When to Contact a Medical Professional

Call your health care provider if you have symptoms of cervicitis.

Prevention

Here are some ways to reduce your risk of cervicitis:

- Avoid chemical irritants such as douches and deodorant tampons.

- Make sure that any foreign objects you insert into your vagina (such as tampons) are placed properly. Be sure to follow

instructions on how long to leave it inside, how often to change
it, or how often to clean it.

• Not having sexual intercourse (abstinence) is the only absolute
method of preventing sexually transmitted cervicitis. A monogamous sexual relationship with someone who is known to be free
of any STI can reduce the risk. Monogamous means you and
your partner do not have sex with any other people.

• You can greatly lower your risk of catching an STI by using a
condom every time you have sex. Condoms are available for both
men and women, but are most commonly worn by the man. A
condom must be used properly every time.

Chapter 24

Vaginal and Pelvic Infections

Chapter Contents

Section 24.1

Bacterial Vaginosis

"Bacterial Vaginosis," National Institute of Allergy and Infectious Diseases (www.niaid.nih.gov), August 1, 2008.

According to the Centers for Disease Control and Prevention (CDC), bacterial vaginosis (BV) is the most common cause of vaginitis symptoms among women of childbearing age. Health experts are not sure what role sexual activity plays in developing BV.

Cause

BV is a sign of a change in the growth of vaginal bacteria. The resulting chemical imbalance occurs when different types of bacteria outnumber the normal "good," or beneficial, ones. Instead of *Lactobacillus* (a type bacteria that normally lives in the vagina) being most common, increased numbers of bacteria such as *Gardnerella vaginalis*, *Bacteroides*, *Mobiluncus*, and *Mycoplasma hominis* inhabit the vaginas of women with BV.

Transmission

Although health experts are not sure what role sexual activity plays in developing BV, a change in sexual partners or having multiple sexual partners may increase a woman's chances of getting the infection. Using an IUD (intrauterine device) and douching also may increase her risk of getting BV.

Symptoms

The main symptom of BV is an abnormal, foul-smelling vaginal discharge. Some women describe it as a fish-like odor that is most noticeable after having sex.

Other symptoms may include the following:

- Thin vaginal discharge, usually white or gray in color

- Pain during urination

- Itching around the vagina

Some women who have signs of BV, such as increased levels of certain harmful bacteria, have no symptoms. A health care provider who sees these signs during a physical examination can confirm the diagnosis by doing lab tests of vaginal fluid.

Diagnosis and Treatment

A health care provider can examine a sample of vaginal fluid under a microscope, either stained or in special lighting, to look for bacteria associated with BV. Then, they can diagnose BV based on the following:

- Absence of lactobacilli bacteria

- Presence of numerous "clue cells" (cells from the vaginal lining that are coated with BV germs)

- Fishy odor

- Change from normal vaginal fluid

Health care providers use antibiotics such as metronidazole or clindamycin to treat women with BV. Generally, male sex partners will not be treated.

Complications

In most cases, BV causes no complications. There have been documented risks of BV, however, such as an association between BV and pelvic inflammatory disease (PID). PID is a serious disease in women that can cause infertility and tubal (ectopic) pregnancy.

BV also can cause other problems such as premature delivery and low-birth-weight babies. Therefore, some health experts recommend that all pregnant women who previously have delivered a premature baby be checked for BV, whether or not they have symptoms. A pregnant woman who has not delivered a premature baby should be treated if she has symptoms and laboratory evidence of BV.

BV also is associated with increased chances of getting one or more sexually transmitted diseases, including chlamydia, gonorrhea, or HIV infection.

Section 24.2

Pelvic Inflammatory Disease

Excerpted from "Pelvic Inflammatory Disease Fact Sheet,"
U.S. Department of Health and Human Services Office on Women's
Health (www.womenshealth.gov), May 18, 2010.

What is pelvic inflammatory disease (PID)?

Pelvic inflammatory disease is an infection of a woman's pelvic organs. The pelvic organs include the uterus (womb), fallopian tubes, ovaries, and cervix.

What causes PID?

A woman can get PID if bacteria (germs) move up from her vagina and infect her pelvic organs. Many different types of bacteria can cause PID. But most cases of PID are caused by bacteria that cause two common sexually transmitted infections (STIs)—gonorrhea and chlamydia. It can take from a few days to a few months for an infection to travel up from the vagina to the pelvic organs.

You can get PID without having an STI. Normal bacteria found in the vagina and on the cervix can sometimes cause PID. No one is sure why this happens.

How common is PID?

Each year in the United States, more than one million women have an episode of PID. More than 100,000 women become infertile each year because of PID. Also, many ectopic pregnancies that occur are due to problems from PID.

You're more likely to get PID if you fit these criteria:

- Have had an STI

- Are under 25 years of age and are having sex

- Have more than one sex partner

- Douche (douching can push bacteria into the pelvic organs and cause infection, as well as hide the signs of an infection)

- Have an IUD (you should get tested and treated for any infections before getting an IUD, which will lower your risk of getting PID)

How do I know if I have PID?

Many women don't know they have PID because they don't have any symptoms. For women who have them, symptoms can range from mild to severe. The most common symptom of PID is pain in your lower abdomen (stomach area). Other symptoms include the following:

- Fever (100.4° F or higher)
- Vaginal discharge that may smell foul
- Painful sex
- Painful urination
- Irregular periods (monthly bleeding)
- Pain in the upper right abdomen

PID can come on fast with extreme pain and fever, especially if it's caused by gonorrhea.

Are there any tests for PID?

If you think that you may have PID, see a doctor right away. If you have pain in your lower abdomen (stomach area), your doctor will perform a physical exam. This will include a pelvic (internal) exam. Your doctor will check for these symptoms:

- Abnormal discharge from your vagina or cervix
- Lumps called abscesses near your ovaries and tubes
- Tenderness or pain in your pelvic organs

Your doctor will also test you for STIs, including HIV and syphilis, urinary tract infection, and, if needed, pregnancy. If needed, your doctor may do other tests. These tests will help your doctor find out if you have PID, or if you have a different problem that looks like PID.

How is PID treated?

PID can be cured with antibiotics (drugs that kill bacteria). Most of the time, at least two antibiotics are used that work against a wide range of bacteria. Your doctor will work with you to find the best treatment for you. You must take all your medicine, even if your symptoms go away. This helps to make sure your infection is fully cured. You should see your doctor again two to three days after starting treatment to make sure the antibiotics are working.

Without treatment, PID can lead to severe problems like infertility, ectopic pregnancy, and chronic pelvic pain.

Any damage done to your pelvic organs before you start treatment likely cannot be undone. Still, don't put off getting treatment. If you do, you may not be able to have children. If you think you may have PID, see a doctor right away.

Your doctor may suggest going into the hospital to treat your PID if the following apply to you:

- Are very sick
- Are pregnant
- Don't respond to or cannot swallow pills (you will need intravenous—in the vein, or IV—antibiotics)
- Have an abscess (sore) in a tube or ovary

If you still have symptoms or if the abscess doesn't go away after treatment, you may need surgery. Problems caused by PID, such as constant pelvic pain and scarring, are often hard to treat. But sometimes they get better after surgery.

What if my partner is infected?

Even if your sex partner doesn't have any symptoms, she or he could still be infected with bacteria that can cause PID. Take steps to protect yourself from being infected again.

- Encourage your sex partner(s) to get treated, even if she or he doesn't have symptoms.
- Don't have sex with a partner who hasn't been treated.

My friend was told she can't get pregnant because she has PID. Is this true?

The more times you have PID, the more likely it is that you won't be able to get pregnant. When you have PID, bacteria infect the tubes or cause inflammation of the tubes. This turns normal tissue into scar tissue. Scar tissue can block your tubes and make it harder to get pregnant. Even having just a little scar tissue can keep you from getting pregnant without infertility treatment.

How can I keep myself from getting PID?

PID is most often caused by an STI that hasn't been treated. You can keep from getting PID by not getting an STI.

- The best way to prevent an STI is to not have sex of any kind.
- Have sex with one partner who doesn't have any STIs.
- Use condoms every time you have vaginal, anal, or oral sex. Read and follow the directions on the package. Condoms, when used the right way, can lower your chances of getting an STI.
- Don't douche. Douching removes some of the normal bacteria in the vagina that protect you from infection. This makes it easier for you to get an STI.
- If you're having sex, ask your doctor to test you for STIs. STIs are easier to treat if they are found early.
- Learn the common symptoms of STIs. If you think you might have an STI, see your doctor right away.

What should I do if I think I have an STI?

If you think you may have an STI, see a doctor right away. You may feel scared or shy about asking for information or help. Keep in mind, the sooner you seek treatment, the less likely the STI will cause you severe harm. And the sooner you tell your sex partner(s) that you have an STI, the less likely they are to infect you again or spread the disease to others.

To learn about STIs or get tested, contact your doctor, local health department, or an STI and family planning clinic. The American Social Health Association (ASHA) keeps lists of clinics and doctors who provide treatment for STIs. Call ASHA at 800-227-8922. You can get information from the phone line without leaving your name.

Section 24.3

Sexually Transmitted Diseases

Excerpted from "Sexually Transmitted Infections (STI) Fact Sheet," U.S. Department of Health and Human Services Office on Women's Health (www.womenshealth.gov), November 16, 2009.

What is a sexually transmitted infection?

An STI is an infection passed from person to person through intimate sexual contact. STIs are also called sexually transmitted diseases, or STDs.

How many people have STIs and who is infected?

In the United States about 19 million new infections are thought to occur each year. These infections affect men and women of all backgrounds and economic levels. But almost half of new infections are among young people ages 15 to 24. Women are also severely affected by STIs. They have more frequent and more serious health problems from STIs than men. African American women have especially high rates of infection.

How do you get an STI?

You can get an STI by having intimate sexual contact with someone who already has the infection. You can't tell if a person is infected because many STIs have no symptoms. But STIs can still be passed from person to person even if there are no symptoms. STIs are spread during vaginal, anal, or oral sex or during genital touching. So it's possible to get some STIs without having intercourse. Not all STIs are spread the same way.

Can STIs cause health problems?

Yes. Each STI causes different health problems. But overall, untreated STIs can cause cancer, pelvic inflammatory disease, infertility, pregnancy problems, widespread infection to other parts of the body, organ damage, and even death.

Having an STI also can put you at greater risk of getting HIV. For one, not stopping risky sexual behavior can lead to infection with other STIs, including HIV. Also, infection with some STIs makes it easier for you to get HIV if you are exposed.

What are the symptoms of STIs?

Many STIs have only mild or no symptoms at all. When symptoms do develop, they often are mistaken for something else, such as a urinary tract infection or yeast infection. This is why screening for STIs is so important. The STIs listed here are among the most common or harmful to women.

Bacterial vaginosis (BV): Most women have no symptoms. Women with symptoms may have the following:

- Vaginal itching

- Pain when urinating

- Discharge with a fishy odor

Chlamydia: Most women have no symptoms. Women with symptoms may have the following:

- Abnormal vaginal discharge

- Burning when urinating

- Bleeding between periods

Infections that are not treated, even if there are no symptoms, can lead to the following:

- Lower abdominal pain

- Low back pain

- Nausea

- Fever

- Pain during sex

Genital herpes: Some people may have no symptoms. During an "outbreak," the symptoms are clear:

- Small red bumps, blisters, or open sores where the virus entered the body, such as on the penis, vagina, or mouth

- Vaginal discharge
- Fever
- Headache
- Muscle aches
- Pain when urinating
- Itching, burning, or swollen glands in genital area
- Pain in legs, buttocks, or genital area

Symptoms may go away and then come back. Sores heal after two to four weeks.

Gonorrhea: Symptoms are often mild, but most women have no symptoms. If symptoms are present, they most often appear within 10 days of becoming infected. Symptoms are the following:

- Pain or burning when urinating
- Yellowish and sometimes bloody vaginal discharge
- Bleeding between periods
- Pain during sex
- Heavy bleeding during periods

Infection that occurs in the throat, eye, or anus also might have symptoms in these parts of the body.

Hepatitis B: Some women have no symptoms. Women with symptoms may have these:

- Low-grade fever
- Headache and muscle aches
- Tiredness
- Loss of appetite
- Upset stomach or vomiting
- Diarrhea
- Dark-colored urine and pale bowel movements
- Stomach pain
- Skin and whites of eyes turning yellow

HIV/AIDS: Some women may have no symptoms for 10 years or more. About half of people with HIV get flu-like symptoms about three to six weeks after becoming infected. Symptoms people can have for months or even years before the onset of AIDS include the following:

- Fevers and night sweats
- Feeling very tired
- Quick weight loss
- Headache
- Enlarged lymph nodes
- Diarrhea, vomiting, and upset stomach
- Mouth, genital, or anal sores
- Dry cough
- Rash or flaky skin
- Short-term memory loss

Women also might have these signs of HIV:

- Vaginal yeast infections and other vaginal infections, including STIs
- Pelvic inflammatory disease that does not get better with treatment
- Menstrual cycle changes

Human papillomavirus (HPV): Some women have no symptoms. Women with symptoms may have these:

- Visible warts in the genital area, including the thighs (warts can be raised or flat, alone or in groups, small or large, and sometimes they are cauliflower-shaped)
- Growths on the cervix and vagina that are often invisible

Pubic lice (sometimes called "crabs"): Symptoms include the following:

- Itching in the genital area
- Finding lice or lice eggs

Syphilis: Syphilis progresses in stages. Symptoms of the primary stage are the following:

- A single, painless sore appearing 10 to 90 days after infection. It can appear in the genital area, mouth, or other parts of the body. The sore goes away on its own.

- If the infection is not treated, it moves to the secondary stage. This stage starts three to six weeks after the sore appears. Symptoms of the secondary stage are the following:

  - Skin rash with rough, red or reddish-brown spots on the hands and feet that usually does not itch and clears on its own

  - Fever

  - Sore throat and swollen glands

  - Patchy hair loss

  - Headaches and muscle aches

  - Weight loss

  - Tiredness

- In the latent stage, symptoms go away but can come back. Without treatment, the infection may or may not move to the late stage. In the late stage, symptoms are related to damage to internal organs, such as the brain, nerves, eyes, heart, blood vessels, liver, bones, and joints. Some people may die.

Trichomoniasis (sometimes called "trich"): Many women do not have symptoms. Symptoms usually appear 5 to 28 days after exposure and can include the following:

- Yellow, green, or gray vaginal discharge (often foamy) with a strong odor

- Discomfort during sex and when urinating

- Itching or discomfort in the genital area

- Lower abdominal pain (rarely)

How do you get tested for STIs?

There is no one test for all STIs. Ask your doctor about getting tested for STIs. She or he can tell you what test(s) you might need and how it is done. Testing for STIs is also called STI screening. Testing (or screening) for STIs can involve the following:

- Pelvic and physical exam (your doctor can look for signs of infection, such as warts, rashes, discharge)

- Blood sample

- Urine sample

- Fluid or tissue sample (a swab is used to collect a sample that can be looked at under a microscope or sent to a lab for testing)

These methods are used for many kinds of tests. So if you have a pelvic exam and Pap test, for example, don't assume that you have been tested for STIs. Pap testing is mainly used to look for cell changes that could be cancer or precancer. Although a Pap test sample also can be used to perform tests for HPV, doing so isn't routine. And a Pap test does not test for other STIs. If you want to be tested for STIs, including HPV, you must ask.

You can get tested for STIs at your doctor's office or a clinic. But not all doctors offer the same tests. So it's important to discuss your sexual health history to find out what tests you need and where you can go to get tested.

Who needs to get tested for STIs?

If you are sexually active, talk to your doctor about STI screening. Which tests you might need and how often depend mainly on your sexual history and your partner's. Talking to your doctor about your sex life might seem too personal to share. But being open and honest is the only way your doctor can help take care of you. Also, don't assume you don't need to be tested for STIs if you have sex only with women. Talk to your doctor to find out what tests make sense for you.

How are STIs treated?

The treatment depends on the type of STI. For some STIs, treatment may involve taking medicine or getting a shot. For other STIs that can't be cured, like herpes, treatment can help to relieve the symptoms.

Only use medicines prescribed or suggested by your doctor. There are products sold over the internet that falsely claim to prevent or treat STIs. Some of these drugs claim to work better than the drugs your doctor will give you. But this is not true, and the safety of these products is not known.

What can I do to keep from getting an STI?

You can lower your risk of getting an STI with the following steps. The steps work best when used together. No single strategy can protect you from every single type of STI.

- **Don't have sex:** The surest way to keep from getting any STI is to practice abstinence. This means not having vaginal, oral, or anal sex. Keep in mind that some STIs, like genital herpes, can be spread without having intercourse.

- **Be faithful:** Having a sexual relationship with one partner who has been tested for STIs and is not infected is another way to lower your risk of getting infected. Be faithful to each other. This means you only have sex with each other and no one else.

- **Use condoms correctly and every time you have sex:** Use condoms for all types of sexual contact, even if intercourse does not take place. Use condoms from the very start to the very end of each sex act, and with every sex partner. A male latex condom offers the best protection. You can use a male polyurethane condom if you or your partner has a latex allergy. A dental dam might also offer some protection from some STIs.

- **Know that some methods of birth control, like birth control pills, shots, implants, or diaphragms, will not protect you from STIs:** If you use one of these methods, be sure to also use a condom correctly every time you have sex.

- **Talk with your sex partner(s) about STIs and using condoms before having sex:** It's up to you to set the ground rules and to make sure you are protected.

- **Don't assume you're at low risk for STIs if you have sex only with women:** Some common STIs are spread easily by skin-to-skin contact. Also, most women who have sex with women have had sex with men, too. So a woman can get an STI from a male partner and then pass it to a female partner.

- **Talk frankly with your doctor and your sex partner(s) about any STIs you or your partner has or has had:** Talk about symptoms, such as sores or discharge. Try not to be embarrassed. Your doctor is there to help you with any and all health problems. Also, being open with your doctor and partner will help you protect your health and the health of others.

- **Have a yearly pelvic exam:** Ask your doctor if you should be tested for STIs and how often you should be retested. Testing for many STIs is simple and often can be done during your checkup. The sooner an STI is found, the easier it is to treat.

- **Avoid using drugs or drinking too much alcohol:** These activities may lead to risky sexual behavior, such as not wearing a condom.

How do STIs affect pregnant women and their babies?

STIs can cause many of the same health problems in pregnant women as women who are not pregnant. But having an STI also can threaten the pregnancy and unborn baby's health. Having an STI during pregnancy can cause early labor, a woman's water to break early, and infection in the uterus after the birth.

Some STIs can be passed from a pregnant woman to the baby before and during the baby's birth. Some STIs, like syphilis, cross the placenta and infect the baby while it is in the uterus. Other STIs, like gonorrhea, chlamydia, hepatitis B, and genital herpes, can be passed from the mother to the baby during delivery as the baby passes through the birth canal. HIV can cross the placenta during pregnancy and infect the baby during the birth process.

The harmful effects to babies may include the following:

- Low birth weight
- Eye infection
- Pneumonia
- Infection in the baby's blood
- Brain damage
- Lack of coordination in body movements
- Blindness
- Deafness
- Acute hepatitis
- Meningitis
- Chronic liver disease
- Cirrhosis
- Stillbirth

Some of these problems can be prevented if the mother receives routine prenatal care, which includes screening tests for STIs starting early in pregnancy and repeated close to delivery, if needed. Other problems can be treated if the infection is found at birth.

In addition, some experts recommend that women who have had a premature delivery in the past be screened and treated for bacterial vaginosis at the first prenatal visit. Even if a woman has been tested for STIs in the past, she should be tested again when she becomes pregnant.

Chlamydia, gonorrhea, syphilis, trichomoniasis, and BV can be treated and cured with antibiotics during pregnancy. Viral STIs, such as genital herpes and HIV, have no cure. But antiviral medication may be appropriate for some pregnant woman with herpes to reduce symptoms. For women who have active genital herpes lesions at the onset of labor, a cesarean delivery (C-section) can lower the risk of passing the infection to the newborn. For women who are HIV positive, taking antiviral medicines during pregnancy can lower the risk of giving HIV to the newborn to less than 2%. C-section is also an option for some women with HIV. Women who test negative for hepatitis B may receive the hepatitis B vaccine during pregnancy.

Pregnant women also can take steps to lower their risk of getting an STI during pregnancy.

Do STIs affect breastfeeding?

If you have HIV, do not breastfeed. You can pass the virus to your baby.

Talk with your doctor, nurse, or a lactation consultant about the risk of passing the STI to your baby while breastfeeding. If you have chlamydia or gonorrhea, you can keep breastfeeding. If you have syphilis or herpes, you can keep breastfeeding as long as the sores are covered. Syphilis and herpes are spread through contact with sores and can be dangerous to your newborn. If you have sores on your nipple or areola, stop breastfeeding on that breast. Pump or hand express your milk from that breast until the sore clears. Pumping will help keep up your milk supply and prevent your breast from getting engorged or overly full. You can store your milk to give to your baby in a bottle for another feeding. But if parts of your breast pump that contact the milk also touch the sore(s) while pumping, you should throw the milk away.

If you are being treated for an STI, ask your doctor about the possible effects of the drug on your breastfeeding baby. Most treatments for STIs are safe to use while breastfeeding.

Section 24.4

Toxic Shock Syndrome

Toxic shock syndrome (TSS) is a serious but uncommon infection
caused by either *Staphylococcus aureus* bacteria or by *streptococcus*
bacteria.

Originally linked to the use of tampons, especially high-absorbency
ones and those that are not changed frequently, it's now also known
to be associated with the contraceptive sponge and diaphragm birth
control methods.

TSS also can arise from wounds secondary to minor trauma or
surgery incisions where bacteria have been able to enter the body and
cause the infection.

TSS also can affect anyone who has any type of staph infection,
including pneumonia, abscess, skin or wound infection, the blood infection septicemia, or the bone infection osteomyelitis.

Most often, streptococcal TSS appears after bacteria have invaded
areas of injured skin, such as cuts and scrapes, surgical wounds, and
even chickenpox blisters.

Symptoms of TSS can include sudden high fever, a faint feeling,
diarrhea, headache, a rash, and muscle aches. If you have these symptoms, call your doctor right away.

Symptoms

Toxic shock syndrome starts suddenly, often with high fever (temperature at least 102° F [38.8° C]), a rapid drop in blood pressure (with
lightheadedness or fainting), vomiting, diarrhea, headache, sore throat,
or muscle aches.

A sunburn-like rash may appear anywhere on the body, including
the palms of the hands and the soles of the feet. A person also might

have bloodshot eyes and an unusual redness under the eyelids or inside the mouth (and vagina in females). The area around an infected wound can become swollen, red, and tender, or may not even appear infected.

Other symptoms may include confusion or other mental changes, decreased urination, fatigue and weakness, and thirst.

If TSS is untreated, organs such as the liver and kidneys may begin to fail, and problems such as seizures, bleeding, and heart failure can develop.

Prevention

The bacteria that cause toxic shock syndrome can be carried on unwashed hands and prompt an infection anywhere on the body. So good hand washing is extremely important.

Women can reduce their risk of TSS by either avoiding tampons or alternating them with sanitary napkins. Women who use only tampons should choose ones with the lowest absorbency that will handle menstrual flow, and change the tampons frequently. On low-flow days, women should use pads instead of tampons.

Between menstrual periods, store tampons away from heat and moisture (where bacteria can grow)—for example, in a bedroom rather than in a bathroom closet.

Because _staphylococcus_ bacteria are often carried on hands, it's important for women to wash their hands thoroughly before and after inserting a tampon. If you have your menstrual period, be sure to take these precautions. Any female who has recovered from TSS should not use tampons.

Clean and bandage all skin wounds as quickly as possible. Call your doctor immediately whenever a wound becomes red, swollen, or tender, or if a fever begins.

Diagnosis and Treatment

TSS is a medical emergency. If you think you have TSS, call a doctor right away. Depending on the symptoms, a doctor may see you in the office or refer you to a hospital emergency department for immediate evaluation and testing.

If doctors suspect TSS, they will probably start intravenous (IV) fluids and antibiotics as soon as possible. They may take a sample from the suspected site of the infection, such as the skin, nose, or vagina, to check it for TSS. They may also take a blood sample.

Other blood tests can help monitor how various organs like the kidneys are working and check for other diseases that may be causing the symptoms.

Medical staff will remove tampons, contraceptive devices, or wound packing; clean any wounds; and, if there is a pocket of infection (an abscess), a doctor may need to drain pus from the infected area.

People with TSS typically need to stay in the hospital, often in the intensive care unit (ICU), for several days to closely monitor blood pressure, respiratory status, and to look for signs of other problems, such as organ damage.

TSS is a very rare illness. Although it can be fatal, if recognized and treated promptly it is usually curable.

When to Call the Doctor

Call your doctor immediately if you have any signs or symptoms of toxic shock syndrome. Once you realize that something is wrong, it's important to get medical attention right away. The sooner you get treatment, the better.

Section 24.5

Vaginal Yeast Infections

Excerpted from "Vaginal Yeast Infections Fact Sheet,"
U.S. Department of Health and Human Services Office on Women's
Health (www.womenshealth.gov), September 23, 2008.

What is a vaginal yeast infection?

A vaginal yeast infection is irritation of the vagina and the area around it called the vulva.

Yeast is a type of fungus. Yeast infections are caused by overgrowth of the fungus *Candida albicans*. Small amounts of yeast are always in the vagina. But when too much yeast grows, you can get an infection.

Yeast infections are very common. About 75% of women have one during their lives. And almost half of women have two or more vaginal yeast infections.

What are the signs of a vaginal yeast infection?

The most common symptom of a yeast infection is extreme itchiness in and around the vagina.

Other symptoms include the following:

- Burning, redness, and swelling of the vagina and the vulva
- Pain when passing urine
- Pain during sex
- Soreness
- A thick, white vaginal discharge that looks like cottage cheese and does not have a bad smell
- A rash on the vagina

You may only have a few of these symptoms. They may be mild or severe.

Should I call my doctor if I think I have a yeast infection?

Yes, you need to see your doctor to find out for sure if you have a yeast infection. The signs of a yeast infection are much like those of sexually transmitted infections like chlamydia and gonorrhea. So it's hard to be sure you have a yeast infection and not something more serious.

If you've had vaginal yeast infections before, talk to your doctor about using over-the-counter medicines.

How is a vaginal yeast infection diagnosed?

Your doctor will do a pelvic exam to look for swelling and discharge. Your doctor may also use a swab to take a fluid sample from your vagina. A quick look with a microscope or a lab test will show if yeast is causing the problem.

Why did I get a yeast infection?

Many things can raise your risk of a vaginal yeast infection, such as the following:

- Stress
- Lack of sleep
- Illness

- Poor eating habits, including eating extreme amounts of sugary foods

- Pregnancy

- Having your period

- Taking certain medicines, including birth control pills, antibiotics, and steroids

- Diseases such as poorly controlled diabetes and HIV/AIDS

- Hormonal changes during your periods

Can I get a yeast infection from having sex?

Yes, but it is rare. Most often, women don't get yeast infections from sex. The most common cause is a weak immune system.

How are yeast infections treated?

Yeast infections can be cured with antifungal medicines that come in these forms:

- Creams

- Tablets

- Ointments or suppositories that are inserted into the vagina

These products can be bought over the counter at the drug store or grocery store. Your doctor can also prescribe you a single dose of oral fluconazole. But do not use this drug if you are pregnant.

Infections that don't respond to these medicines are starting to be more common. Using antifungal medicines when you don't really have a yeast infection can raise your risk of getting a hard-to-treat infection in the future.

Is it safe to use over-the-counter medicines for yeast infections?

Yes, but always talk with your doctor before treating yourself for a vaginal yeast infection if any of these apply to you:

- Are pregnant

- Have never been diagnosed with a yeast infection

- Keep getting yeast infections

Studies show that two-thirds of women who buy these products don't really have a yeast infection. Using these medicines the wrong way may lead to a hard-to-treat infection. Plus, treating yourself for a yeast infection when you really have something else may worsen the problem. Certain STIs that go untreated can cause cancer, infertility, pregnancy problems, and other health problems.

If you decide to use these over-the-counter medicines, read and follow the directions carefully. Some creams and inserts may weaken condoms and diaphragms.

If I have a yeast infection, does my sexual partner need to be treated?

Yeast infections are not STIs, and health experts don't know for sure if they are transmitted sexually. About 12% to 15% of men get an itchy rash on the penis if they have unprotected sex with an infected woman. If this happens to your partner, he should see a doctor. Men who haven't been circumcised are at higher risk.

Lesbians may be at risk for spreading yeast infections to their partner(s). Research is still being done to know for sure. If your female partner has any symptoms, she should also be tested and treated.

How can I avoid getting another yeast infection?

To help prevent vaginal yeast infections, you can take the following precautions:

- Avoid douches.
- Avoid scented hygiene products like bubble bath, sprays, pads, and tampons.
- Change tampons and pads often during your period.
- Avoid tight underwear or clothes made of synthetic fibers.
- Wear cotton underwear and pantyhose with a cotton crotch.
- Change out of wet swimsuits and exercise clothes as soon as you can.
- Avoid hot tubs and very hot baths.

If you keep getting yeast infections, be sure and talk with your doctor. About 5% of women get four or more vaginal yeast infections in one year. This is called recurrent vulvovaginal candidiasis (RVVC). RVVC is more common in women with diabetes or weak immune systems. Doctors most often treat this problem with antifungal medicine for up to six months.

Chapter 25

Pelvic Floor Disorders

Chapter Contents

Section 25.1

Cystocele

"Cystocele (Fallen Bladder)," National Kidney and Urologic Diseases Information Clearinghouse, National Institute of Diabetes and Digestive and Kidney Diseases (www.kidney.niddk.nih.gov), June 29, 2012.

What is a cystocele?

A cystocele occurs when the wall between a woman's bladder and her vagina weakens and allows the bladder to droop into the vagina. This condition may cause discomfort and problems with emptying the bladder.

A bladder that has dropped from its normal position may cause two kinds of problems—unwanted urine leakage and incomplete emptying of the bladder. In some women, a fallen bladder stretches the opening into the urethra, causing urine leakage when the woman coughs, sneezes, laughs, or moves in any way that puts pressure on the bladder.

A cystocele is mild—grade 1—when the bladder droops only a short way into the vagina. With a more severe—grade 2—cystocele, the bladder sinks far enough to reach the opening of the vagina. The most advanced—grade 3—cystocele occurs when the bladder bulges out through the opening of the vagina.

What causes a cystocele?

A cystocele may result from muscle straining while giving birth. Other kinds of straining—such as heavy lifting or repeated straining during bowel movements—may also cause the bladder to fall. The hormone estrogen helps keep the muscles around the vagina strong. When women go through menopause—that is, when they stop having menstrual periods—their bodies stop making estrogen, so the muscles around the vagina and bladder may grow weak.

How is a cystocele diagnosed?

A doctor may be able to diagnose a grade 2 or grade 3 cystocele from a description of symptoms and from physical examination of the vagina because the fallen part of the bladder will be visible. A voiding cystourethrogram is a test that involves taking X-rays of the bladder during urination. This X-ray shows the shape of the bladder and lets the doctor see any problems that might block the normal flow of urine. Other tests may be needed to find or rule out problems in other parts of the urinary system.

How is a cystocele treated?

Treatment options range from no treatment for a mild cystocele to surgery for a serious cystocele. If a cystocele is not bothersome, the doctor may only recommend avoiding heavy lifting or straining that could cause the cystocele to worsen. If symptoms are moderately bothersome, the doctor may recommend a pessary—a device placed in the vagina to hold the bladder in place. Pessaries come in a variety of shapes and sizes to allow the doctor to find the most comfortable fit for the patient. Pessaries must be removed regularly to avoid infection or ulcers.

Large cystoceles may require surgery to move and keep the bladder in a more normal position. This operation may be performed by a gynecologist, a urologist, or a urogynecologist. The most common procedure for cystocele repair is for the surgeon to make an incision in the wall of the vagina and repair the area to tighten the layers of tissue that separate the organs, creating more support for the bladder. The patient may stay in the hospital for several days and take four to six weeks to recover fully.

Section 25.2

Rectocele

Reprinted with permission from the University of Michigan Bowel Control Program, http://www.med.umich.edu/bowelcontrol. © 2013 Regents of the University of Michigan. All rights reserved.

What is a rectocele?

A rectocele can be described as a bulge in the wall of the rectum into the vagina. The wall of the rectum becomes thin and weak. It may balloon out into the vagina when you have a bowel movement.

There are other structures that may also balloon into the vagina. The bladder bulging into the vagina is a cystocele. The small intestine pushing down on the vagina from above is an enterocele. The uterus bulging into the vagina is called uterine prolapse.

How does it occur?

The wall that lies between the rectum (front wall of the rectum) and the vagina (back wall of the vagina) is called the rectovaginal septum. The thinning of the rectovaginal septum and weakening of the pelvic support structures is the underlying cause of a rectocele.

The most common cause is childbirth and chronic constipation. The muscles and ligaments in the pelvis that hold up and support the female organs and vagina become stretched and weakened during straining. The more babies you have, the more the support tissues are stretched and weakened. Not everyone who has a baby will develop a rectocele. Some women have stronger supporting tissue in the pelvis and may not have as much of a problem as others.

Other conditions that can cause a rectocele include chronic constipation, a chronic cough, a lot of heavy lifting, and obesity. Older women may have this problem because the loss of female hormones causes the vaginal tissue to become weaker.

What are the symptoms?

There may not be any symptoms. If you do have symptoms, they may include:

- pelvic pressure in the rectal area;
- protrusion of the lower part of the vagina through the opening of the vagina;
- constipation and trapping of the stool, making it difficult to have a bowel movement (you may have to press on the lower part of your vagina to help push the stool out of your rectum; this is called splinting);
- a rapid urge to have a bowel movement after leaving the bathroom is caused by stool returning to the lower rectum that was trapped in the rectocele;
- incontinence especially after having a bowel movement.

How is it diagnosed?

Your health care provider will ask about your symptoms and perform a pelvic exam. Your provider will ask you to bear down, pushing like you are having a bowel movement so he or she can see how far the lower part of the vagina protrudes into the vagina and possibly outside of the vagina. Your provider will also ask you to contract the muscles of your pelvis (like you are stopping the stream in the middle of urinating) to determine the strength of your pelvic muscles. Your provider may also do a rectal exam. You may also be asked to have a defecography. A defecography is a special X-ray that looks at the pelvic organs while you are straining like you are trying to have a bowel movement.

How is it treated?

- If the rectocele is not causing any symptoms, it need not be treated (constipation should always be avoided; eating a diet rich in fiber and drinking six to eight glasses of decaffeinated fluid every day can assist in keeping bowel movements soft)

- Avoid prolonged straining (if the bowels will not completely empty after a bowel movement, get up and return later; a pessary— a ring that is inserted in the vagina—may be used to assist in supporting pelvic organs)

- Avoiding heavy lifting, and lifting correctly (with your legs, not with your waist or back)

- Treating a chronic cough or bronchitis

- Not smoking

- Avoiding too much weight gain

- Doing Kegel exercises, especially after you have a baby

- Splinting (this is inserting a tampon or two fingers inside the vagina and pushing back)

- Surgical repair may be indicated if the rectocele is severe; a rectocele repair may be performed through the anus, vagina, perineum (between the anus and vagina), the abdomen, or may be a combined repair

- Often a combination of nonsurgical and surgical treatments is needed to correct the problem

Section 25.3

Uterine Prolapse

Uterine prolapse is falling or sliding of the womb (uterus) from its normal position into the vaginal area.

Causes

Muscles, ligaments, and other structures hold the uterus in the pelvis. If these muscles and structures are weak, the uterus drops into the vaginal canal. This is called prolapse.

This condition is more common in women who have had one or more vaginal births.

Other things that can cause or lead to uterine prolapse include:

- normal aging;

- lack of estrogen after menopause;

- anything that puts pressure on the pelvic muscles, including chronic cough and obesity;

- pelvic tumor (rare).

Long-term constipation and the pushing associated with it can make this condition worse.

Symptoms

- Feeling like you are sitting on a small ball
- Difficult or painful sexual intercourse
- Frequent urination or a sudden urge to empty the bladder
- Low backache
- Uterus and cervix that stick out through the vaginal opening
- Repeated bladder infections
- Feeling of heaviness or pulling in the pelvis

- Vaginal bleeding
- Increased vaginal discharge

Many of the symptoms are worse when standing or sitting for long periods of time.

Exams and Tests

A pelvic examination is done while you are bearing down, as if you were trying to push out a baby. This shows your doctor how far your uterus has dropped.

- Uterine prolapse is mild when the cervix drops into the lower part of the vagina.
- Uterine prolapse is moderate when the cervix drops out of the vaginal opening.

The pelvic exam may also show that the bladder and front wall of the vagina (cystocele), or rectum and back wall of the vagina (rectocele), are entering the vagina. The urethra and bladder may also be lower in the pelvis than usual.

Treatment

Treatment is not necessary unless the symptoms bother you. Many women seek treatment by the time the uterus drops to the opening of the vagina.

Lifestyle changes: Weight loss is recommended in obese women with uterine prolapse. Heavy lifting or straining should be avoided, because they can worsen symptoms.

Coughing can also make symptoms worse. If you have a chronic cough, ask your doctor how to prevent or treat it. If you smoke, try to quit. Smoking can cause a chronic cough.

Vaginal pessary: Your doctor may recommend placing a rubber or plastic donut-shaped device, called a pessary, into the vagina. This device hold the uterus in place. It may be temporary or permanent. Vaginal pessaries are fitted for each individual woman. Some are similar to a diaphragm used for birth control.

Pessaries must be cleaned from time to time, sometimes by the doctor or nurse. Many women can be taught how to insert, clean, and remove the pessary herself.

Side effects of pessaries include:

- foul-smelling discharge from the vagina;

- irritation of the lining of the vagina;

- ulcers in the vagina;

- problems with normal sexual intercourse and penetration.

Surgery: Surgery should not be done until the prolapse symptoms are worse than the risks of having surgery. The specific type of surgery depends on:

- degree of prolapse;

- desire for future pregnancies;

- other medical conditions;

- the woman's desire to retain vaginal function;

- the woman's age and general health.

There are some surgical procedures that can be done without removing the uterus, such as a sacrospinous fixation. This procedure involves using nearby ligaments to support the uterus. Other procedures are available.

Often, a vaginal hysterectomy is used to correct uterine prolapse. Any sagging of the vaginal walls, urethra, bladder, or rectum can be surgically corrected at the same time.

Outlook (Prognosis)

Most women with mild uterine prolapse do not have bothersome symptoms and don't need treatment.

Vaginal pessaries can be effective for many women with uterine prolapse.

Surgery usually provides excellent results, however, some women may require treatment again in the future.

Possible Complications

Ulceration and infection of the cervix and vaginal walls may occur in severe cases of uterine prolapse.

Urinary tract infections and other urinary symptoms may occur because of a cystocele. Constipation and hemorrhoids may occur because of a rectocele.

When to Contact a Medical Professional

Call for an appointment with your health care provider if you have symptoms of uterine prolapse.

Prevention

Tightening the pelvic floor muscles using Kegel exercises helps to strengthen the muscles and reduces the risk of uterine prolapse.

Estrogen therapy, either vaginal or oral, in postmenopausal women may help maintain muscle tone in the vaginal area.

Weight loss and avoiding heavy lifting can decrease the risk for uterine prolapse.

Chapter 26

Vulval Disorders

Chapter Contents

Section 26.1

Vulvovaginitis

© 2013 A.D.A.M. Inc. Reprinted with permission.

Vulvovaginitis is inflammation or infection of the vulva and vagina.

Causes

Vulvovaginitis can affect women of all ages and is extremely common. It can be caused by bacteria, yeasts, viruses, and other parasites. Some sexually transmitted infections (STIs) can also cause vulvovaginitis, as can various chemicals found in bubble baths, soaps, and perfumes. Environmental factors such as poor hygiene and allergens may also cause this condition.

Candida albicans, which causes yeast infections, is one of the most common causes of vulvovaginitis in women of all ages. Antibiotic use can lead to yeast infections by killing the normal antifungal bacteria that live in the vagina. Yeast infections typically cause genital itching, a thick, white vaginal discharge, and other symptoms.

Another cause of vulvovaginitis is bacterial vaginosis, an overgrowth of certain types of bacteria in the vagina. Bacterial vaginosis may cause a thin, grey vaginal discharge and a fishy odor.

An STI called *Trichomonas* vaginitis infection is another common cause. This infection leads to genital itching, a vaginal odor, and a heavy vaginal discharge, which may be yellow-grey or green in color.

Bubble baths, soaps, vaginal contraceptives, feminine sprays, and perfumes can cause irritating itchy rashes in the genital area, while tight-fitting or nonabsorbent clothing sometimes cause heat rashes.

Irritated tissue is more susceptible to infection than normal tissue, and many infection-causing organisms thrive in environments that are warm, damp, and dark. Not only can these factors contribute to the cause of vulvovaginitis, they frequently prolong the recovery period.

A lack of estrogen in postmenopausal women can result in vaginal dryness and thinning of vaginal and vulvar skin, which may also lead to or worsen genital itching and burning.

Some skin conditions can cause itching and chronic irritation of the vulvar area. Foreign bodies, such as lost tampons, can also cause vulvar irritation and itching and strong-smelling discharge.

Nonspecific vulvovaginitis (where specific cause cannot be identified) can be seen in all age groups, but it occurs most commonly in young girls before puberty. Once puberty begins, the vagina becomes more acidic, which tends to help prevent infections.

Nonspecific vulvovaginitis can occur in girls with poor genital hygiene and is characterized by a foul-smelling, brownish-green discharge and irritation of the labia and vaginal opening. This condition is often associated with an overgrowth of a type of bacteria that is typically found in the stool. These bacteria are sometimes spread from the rectum to the vaginal area by wiping from back to front after using the bathroom.

Sexual abuse should be considered in girls with unusual infections and recurrent episodes of unexplained vulvovaginitis. *Neisseria gonorrhoeae*, the organism that causes gonorrhea, produces gonococcal vulvovaginitis in young girls who have sexual exposure. Gonorrhea-related vaginitis is considered a sexually transmitted illness. If lab tests confirm this diagnosis, young girls should be evaluated for sexual abuse.

Symptoms

- Irritation and itching of the genital area
- Inflammation (irritation, redness, and swelling) of the labia majora, labia minora, or perineal area
- Vaginal discharge
- Foul vaginal odor
- Discomfort or burning when urinating

Exams and Tests

If you have been diagnosed with a yeast infection in the past, you can try treatment with over-the-counter products. However, if your symptoms do not completely disappear in about a week, contact your health care provider. Many other infections have similar symptoms.

The health care provider will perform a pelvic examination. This may show red, tender areas on the vulva or vagina.

A wet prep (microscopic evaluation of vaginal discharge) is usually done to identify a vaginal infection or overgrowth of yeast or bacteria.

In some cases, a culture of the vaginal discharge may identify the organism causing the infection.

A biopsy of the irritated area on the vulva may be recommended if there are no signs of infection.

Treatment

Treatment depends on what is causing the infection. Treatment may include:

- antibiotics taken by mouth or applied to the skin;
- antifungal cream;
- antibacterial cream;
- cortisone cream;
- antihistamine, if the irritation is due to an allergic reaction;
- estrogen cream, if the irritation and inflammation is due to low levels of estrogen.

Proper cleansing is important and may help prevent irritation, particularly in those with infections caused by bacteria normally found in stool. Sitz baths may be recommended.

It is often helpful to allow more air to reach the genital area. Here are some tips:

- Wear cotton underwear (rather than nylon) or underwear that has a cotton lining in the crotch area. This increases air flow and decreases moisture.
- Do not wear pantyhose.
- Wear loose-fitting clothing.
- Remove underwear at bedtime.

Note: If a sexually transmitted infection is diagnosed, it is very important that any other sexual partners receive treatment, even if they do not have symptoms. If your sexual partner is infected but not treated, you risk becoming infected over and over again.

Outlook (Prognosis)

Proper treatment of an infection is usually very effective.

Possible Complications

- Discomfort that does not go away

- Skin infection (from scratching)

- Increased risk of getting HIV if you come into contact with the virus when you have a vaginal infection or irritation

When to Contact a Medical Professional

Call your health care provider if vulvovaginitis symptoms are present or if known vulvovaginitis does not respond to treatment.

Prevention

Use of a condom during sexual intercourse can prevent most sexually transmitted vaginal infections. Proper fitting and adequately absorbent clothing, combined with good hygiene of the genital area, also prevents many cases of noninfectious vulvovaginitis.

Children should be taught how to properly clean the genital area while bathing or showering. Proper wiping after using the toilet will also help (girls should always wipe from the front to the back to avoid introducing bacteria from the rectum to the vaginal area).

Hands should be washed thoroughly before and after using the bathroom.

Section 26.2

Vulvodynia

What is vulvodynia?

Vulvodynia is chronic pain or discomfort of the vulva, the area surrounding the vaginal opening. It is diagnosed when pain lasts for three months or longer without any evidence of other skin or gynecological disorders that might cause the pain. Up to 16% of women—roughly 13 million—will suffer with chronic vulvar pain at some point in their lives.

Do we know what causes it? Is it due to an infection?

We don't know what causes vulvodynia, although it is likely due to multiple factors. Some factors that may contribute are pelvic nerve damage, spasms or weakness of pelvic muscles, and genetic components such as susceptibility to inflammation. We do know that vulvodynia is not caused by active infection, the human papillomavirus (HPV), or other sexually transmitted diseases or cancer.

What are the symptoms of vulvodynia?

Women with vulvodynia often report having one or more of the following symptoms around the vulva:

- Burning
- Stinging
- Rawness
- Aching
- Throbbing
- Stabbing
- Soreness

Burning sensations are most common; however, the type and severity of symptoms are highly individual. More than half of women who suffer with chronic vulvar pain have other health problems, including interstitial cystitis, fibromyalgia, irritable bowel syndrome, chronic fatigue syndrome, and recurring yeast infections.

What triggers the pain?

Some women experience constant, generalized pain of the whole vulva area. Others have localized pain specific to one part of the vulva that may come and go. Vulvar pain may be triggered by sexual activity, tampon insertion or gynecological exams, or simply by wearing tight-fitting pants or sitting. Take note of what things make your pain better or worse and share this information with your health care professional, so he or she has a better sense of the location and intensity of your pain and how it impacts your overall and sexual health.

How is it diagnosed?

Vulvodynia is a "diagnosis of exclusion." That is, it is established after other potential causes of vulvar pain have been ruled out, including such things as yeast or bacterial infections. Most women see multiple health care providers before a correct diagnosis is made.

To diagnose vulvodynia, your doctor will first take a complete medical history, including the duration and intensity of the pain, sexual health, treatments already tried, and previous medical problems and pelvic/abdominal surgeries. A pelvic exam will follow. A cotton swab test that applies pressure to various parts of the vulva is often used, especially for women whose pain is provoked by pressure on the vulva. You will be asked to rate the extent of the pain at each site so your provider can map your pain.

It's important to talk openly with your health care professional about any difficulties you have exercising, using tampons, or having sexual intercourse, so he or she knows how the pain impacts your daily life.

What are the treatments for vulvodynia?

There is no cure for vulvodynia, but there are a variety of medications and nondrug therapies. Medications may include antidepressants, local anesthetics, and nerve blocks; treatments involve changes to your diet, counseling, and, in select cases, surgery. You might also want to ask about acupuncture, massage therapy, relaxation techniques, biofeedback, and cognitive behavioral therapy, which often are recommended as treatments for other conditions causing chronic pain. No single approach works for all women. It often takes time to find a treatment or combination of therapies that will adequately alleviate the pain.

What should I tell my partner?

Many women find it difficult, if not impossible, to engage in vaginal penetration due to the severity of what is sometimes described as "knife-like pain." Since this condition significantly affects your sexual relationship, it's important to educate your partner about this condition and how it affects you, both physically and psychologically. Be honest and open about how you feel, the steps you are taking to alleviate the pain, and ways your partner can support you. You may feel embarrassed to broach the subject, but it's important for your peace of mind and for your significant other to feel involved in the process. Counseling with a sexual therapist is often helpful for couples dealing with vulvodynia.

Chapter 27

Gynecological Procedures

Chapter Contents

Section 27.1

Common Gynecological Procedures

"Gynecology Surgery and Procedures 101" http://womenshealth.about.com/
od/surgeryforgyndiseases/a/gynprocedure101.htm. © 2013 Tracee Cornforth
(http://womenshealth.about.com/). Used with permission of About Inc., which
can be found online at www.about.com. All rights reserved.

Have you ever been to the gynecologist and been told you need a
procedure for further evaluation of a GYN problem? Millions of women
each year face the uncertainty of having a gynecological procedure or
surgery performed. Learn about these common GYN procedures and
surgeries before you need them and you'll be one step ahead when
your gynecologist says you need further evaluation of your problem.

1. **Colposcopy:** Colposcopy is a diagnostic tool used for further
    evaluation of abnormal Pap smears. This procedure provides a
    non-surgical way for your physician to visualize your cervix.

2. **Cryosurgery:** Cervical cryosurgery or cryotherapy is a gyneco-
    logical treatment that freezes a section of the cervix. Cryosur-
    gery destroys abnormal cervical cells that show changes that
    may lead to cancer. These changes are called precancerous
    cells. Your gynecologist may use the term *cervical dysplasia*
    to describe your condition.

3. **LEEP procedure:** The loop electrosurgical excision procedure
    (LEEP) is used when there is an indication of abnormal cells
    on the surface of the cervix.

4. **Hysteroscopy:** Hysteroscopy provides a way for your physician
    to look inside your uterus. A hysteroscope is a thin, telescope-like
    instrument that is inserted into the uterus through the vagina
    and cervix. This tool often helps a physician diagnose or treat a
    uterine problem.

5. **Pelvic laparoscopy:** Laparoscopy is usually performed under
    general anesthesia; however, it can be performed with other
    types of anesthesia that permit the patient to remain awake.

The typical pelvic laparoscopy involves a small (one-half- to three-quarter-inch) incision in the belly button or lower abdomen.

6. **D&C:** Often used to diagnose or treat abnormal uterine bleeding, the D&C is one of the most common GYN operative procedures. Dilation and curettage also provides important information about whether uterine cancer is present.

Section 27.2

Dilation and Curettage (D&C)

D and C is a procedure to scrape and collect the tissue (endometrium) from inside the uterus.

- Dilation ("D") is a widening of the cervix to allow instruments into the uterus.

- Curettage ("C") is the scraping of the walls of the uterus.

Description

D and C, also called uterine scraping, may be performed in the hospital or in a clinic while you are under general or local anesthesia.

The health care provider will insert an instrument called a speculum into the vagina. This holds open the vaginal canal. Numbing medicine may be applied to the opening to the uterus (cervix).

The cervical canal is widened, and a curette (a metal loop on the end of a long, thin handle) is passed through the opening into the uterus cavity. The health care provider gently scrapes the inner layer of tissue, called the endometrium. The tissue is collected for examination.

Why the Procedure Is Performed

This procedure may be done to:

- diagnose or rule out conditions such as uterine cancer;
- remove tissue after a miscarriage;
- treat heavy menstrual bleeding or irregular periods;
- perform a therapeutic or elective abortion.

Your health care provider may also recommend a D and C if you have:

- abnormal bleeding while on hormone replacement therapy;
- an embedded intrauterine device (IUD);
- bleeding after menopause;
- endometrial polyps;
- thickening of the uterus.

This list may not include all possible reasons for a D and C.

Risks

Risks related to D and C include:

- puncture of the uterus;
- scarring of the uterine lining (Asherman syndrome, may lead to infertility later);
- tear of the cervix.

Risks due to anesthesia include:

- reactions to medications,
- problems breathing.

Risks of any surgery include:

- bleeding,
- infection.

After the Procedure

A D and C has few risks. It can provide relief from bleeding and can help diagnose infection, cancer, and other diseases.

You may return to your normal activities as soon as you feel better, possibly even the same day.

You may have vaginal bleeding, pelvic cramps, and back pain for a few days after the procedure. You can usually manage pain well with medications. Avoid using tampons and having sexual intercourse for one to two weeks after the procedure.

Section 27.3

Hysterectomy

Excerpted from "Hysterectomy Fact Sheet," U.S. Department of Health and Human Services Office on Women's Health (www.womenshealth.gov), December 15, 2009.

What is a hysterectomy?

A hysterectomy is a surgery to remove a woman's uterus or womb. The uterus is where a baby grows when a woman is pregnant. The whole uterus or just part of it may be removed. After a hysterectomy, you no longer have menstrual periods and cannot become pregnant.

During the hysterectomy, your doctor also may remove your fallopian tubes and ovaries. The ovaries produce eggs and hormones. The fallopian tubes carry eggs from the ovaries to the uterus. The cervix is the lower end of the uterus that joins the vagina. These organs are located in a woman's lower abdomen.

If you have not yet reached menopause and you keep your ovaries during the hysterectomy, you may enter menopause at an earlier age than most women.

If your ovaries are removed during the hysterectomy, you will enter menopause if you have not already. You can talk with your doctor about ways to manage menopausal symptoms, such as hot flashes and vaginal dryness.

What are the types of hysterectomy?

- Partial, subtotal, or supracervical removes just the upper part of the uterus. The cervix is left in place.

- Total removes the whole uterus and the cervix.

- Radical removes the whole uterus, the tissue on both sides of the cervix, and the upper part of the vagina. This is done mostly when there is cancer present.

How is a hysterectomy performed?

There are different ways that your doctor can perform a hysterectomy. It will depend on your health history and the reason for your surgery.

- **Abdominal hysterectomy:** This is done through a five- to seven-inch incision, or cut, in the lower part of your belly. The cut may go either up and down, or across your belly, just above your pubic hair.

- **Vaginal hysterectomy:** This is done through a cut in the vagina. The doctor will take your uterus out through this incision and close it with stitches.

- **Laparoscopic hysterectomy:** A laparoscope is an instrument with a thin, lighted tube and small camera that allows your doctor to see your pelvic organs. Your doctor will make three to four small cuts in your belly and insert the laparoscope and other instruments. He or she will cut your uterus into smaller pieces and remove them through the incisions.

- **Laparoscopically assisted vaginal hysterectomy (LAVH):** Your doctor will remove your uterus through the vagina. The laparoscope is used to guide the procedure.

- **Robotic-assisted surgery:** Your doctor uses a special machine (robot) to do the surgery through small cuts in your belly, much like a laparoscopic hysterectomy. It is most often done when a patient has cancer or is very overweight and vaginal surgery is not safe.

Why do women have hysterectomies?

Hysterectomy may be needed if you have the following:

- **Cancer of the uterus, ovary, cervix, or endometrium:** Hysterectomy may be the best option if you have cancer in these organs. The endometrium is the tissue that lines the uterus. If you have precancerous changes of the cervix, you might be able to have a loop electrosurgical excision procedure (LEEP) to remove the cancerous cells. Other treatment options can include chemotherapy and radiation.

- **Fibroids:** Fibroids are noncancerous, muscular tumors that grow in the wall of the uterus. Many women with fibroids have only minor symptoms and do not need treatment. Fibroids also often shrink after menopause. In some women, fibroids can cause prolonged heavy bleeding or pain. Fibroids can be treated with medications. There are also procedures to remove the fibroids, such as uterine artery embolization, which blocks the blood supply to the tumors. Without blood, the fibroids shrink over time, which can reduce pain and heavy bleeding. Another procedure called myomectomy removes the tumors while leaving your uterus intact, but there is a risk that the tumors could come back. If medications or procedures to remove the fibroids have not helped, and a woman is either near or past menopause and does not want children, hysterectomy can cure problems from fibroids.

- **Endometriosis:** This health problem occurs when the tissue that lines the uterus grows outside the uterus on your ovaries, fallopian tubes, or other pelvic or abdominal organs. This can cause severe pain during menstrual periods, chronic pain in the lower back and pelvis, pain during or after sex, bleeding between periods, and other symptoms. You might need a hysterectomy when medications or less invasive surgery to remove the spots of endometriosis have not helped.

- **Prolapse of the uterus:** This is when the uterus slips from its usual place down into the vagina. This can lead to urinary and bowel problems and pelvic pressure. These problems might be helped for a time with an object called a vaginal pessary, which is inserted into the vagina to hold the womb in place.

- **Adenomyosis:** In this condition, the tissue that lines the uterus grows inside the walls of the uterus, which can cause severe pain. If other treatments have not helped, a hysterectomy is the only certain cure.

- **Chronic pelvic pain:** Surgery is a last resort for women who have chronic pelvic pain that clearly comes from the uterus. Many forms of pelvic pain are not cured by a hysterectomy, so it could be unnecessary and create new problems.

- **Abnormal vaginal bleeding:** Treatment depends on the cause. Changes in hormone levels, infection, cancer, or fibroids are some things that can cause abnormal bleeding. There are medications that can lighten heavy bleeding, correct irregular bleeding, and relieve pain. These include hormone medications, birth control pills, and nonsteroidal anti-inflammatory medications (NSAIDs). One procedure for abnormal bleeding is D&C, in which the lining and contents of the uterus are removed. Another procedure, endometrial ablation, also removes the lining of your uterus and can help stop heavy, prolonged bleeding. But it should not be used if you want to become pregnant or if you have gone through menopause.

Very rarely, hysterectomy is needed to control bleeding during a cesarean delivery following rare pregnancy complications. There are other methods doctors use to control bleeding in most of these cases, but hysterectomy is still needed for some women.

Keep in mind that there may be ways to treat your health problem without having this major surgery. Talk with your doctor about all of your treatment options.

How common are hysterectomies?

A hysterectomy is the second most common surgery among women in the United States. The most common surgery in women is childbirth by cesarean section delivery.

What should I do if I am told that I need a hysterectomy?

Ask about the possible risks of the surgery. Talk to your doctor about other treatment options, and ask about the risks of those treatments. Consider getting a second opinion from another doctor.

Keep in mind that every woman is different and every situation is different. A good treatment choice for one woman may not be good for another.

How long does it take to recover from a hysterectomy?

Recovering from a hysterectomy takes time. Most women stay in the hospital from one to two days for postsurgery care. Some women may stay longer, often when the hysterectomy is done because of cancer.

The time it takes for you to resume normal activities depends on the type of surgery. If you had abdominal surgery, recovery takes from four to six weeks. You will gradually be able to increase your activities.

If you had vaginal or laparoscopic surgery, recovery takes three to four weeks.

You should get plenty of rest and not lift heavy objects for a full six weeks after surgery. About six weeks after either surgery, you should be able to take tub baths and resume sexual intercourse. Research has found that women with a good sex life before hysterectomy can maintain it after the surgery.

What are the risks of having a hysterectomy?

Most women do not have health problems during or after the surgery, but some of the risks of a hysterectomy include the following:

- Injury to nearby organs, such as the bowel, urinary tract, bladder, rectum, or blood vessels
- Pain during sexual intercourse
- Early menopause, if the ovaries are removed
- Anesthesia problems, such as breathing or heart problems
- Allergic reactions to medicines
- Blood clots in the legs or lungs, which these can be fatal
- Infection
- Heavy bleeding

Do I still need to have Pap tests after a hysterectomy?

You will still need regular Pap tests to screen for cervical cancer if you had a partial hysterectomy and did not have your cervix removed, or if your hysterectomy was for cancer. Ask your doctor what is best for you and how often you should have Pap tests.

Even if you do not need Pap tests, all women who have had a hysterectomy should have regular pelvic exams and mammograms.

Part Four

Sexual and
Reproductive Concerns

Chapter 28

Understanding Your Sexuality

Sex and Sexuality

What do you know about sex? What do you know about sexuality? We hear about sex and sexuality almost every day, but much of what we hear is inaccurate and can be confusing. A basic understanding of sex and sexuality can help us sort out myth from fact and help us all enjoy our lives more.

We are all sexual. We are sexual from the day we are born until the day we die. Our sexuality affects who we are and how we express ourselves as sexual beings.

Our sexuality includes:

- our bodies, including our sexual and reproductive anatomy;

- our biological sex—male, female, or intersex;

- our gender—being a girl, boy, woman, man, or transgender;

- our gender identities—our comfort with and feelings about our gender;

- our sexual orientations—straight, lesbian, gay, bisexual;

- our sex drives;

- our sexual identity—the way we feel about our sex, gender, and sexual orientation.

The ways we experience and express our sexuality include:

- our body image—how we feel about our bodies;
- our desires, thoughts, fantasies, sexual pleasure, sexual preferences, and sexual dysfunction;
- our values, attitudes, beliefs, and ideals about life, love, and sexual relationships;
- our sexual behaviors—the ways we have sex including masturbation.

Our sexuality and the ways we experience and express it are influenced by:

- our biology;
- our emotional lives;
- our family lives;
- our culture and our status in our culture;
- our ethical, religious, and spiritual upbringing and experience.

Even though we spend our lifetimes as sexual beings, it's normal to have many questions about sex and sexuality. And this is good because the more we know about sex and sexuality, the better we are able to take charge of our sex lives and our sexual health.

Understanding Sexual Activity

- Sexual activity includes a wide range of behaviors.
- Some sexual activities are more common than others.
- Talking with a partner about sexual behaviors may seem difficult, but it can help increase closeness, trust, and pleasure.

Many of us find that sexual activity is an important way to connect with ourselves and other people. But even though sexual activity is very common and images of sex are all around us, people often have many questions about it. It is normal and common to have questions about sexual activity.

What is sexual activity?

Sexual activity is any voluntary sexual behavior we do. Some we do by ourselves, like masturbation. Other sexual activities we do with other people. Sexual activity is also called "sex play."

This chapter focuses on the kinds of sexual activity we do with other people.

What are some common sexual activities?

There are many common ways that people have sex. Here are just a few examples:

- Masturbation or mutual masturbation—people masturbating together

- Kissing—on the mouth, with the tongue, on body parts

- Massages—touching someone's body in an erotic way

- Touching a partner's nipples, breasts, or sex organs

- Sex talk—phone sex, cybersex, "talking dirty" during sex

- Rubbing bodies together—with or without clothing

- Watching or reading erotica

- Anal and vaginal intercourse

- Oral sex—stimulating a partner's sex organs with the mouth

- Using sex toys, alone or with a partner

What are some less common sexual activities?

Some sexual behaviors are less common. Here are some examples of less common sexual behaviors:

- SM (sadomasochism)—the use of domination and/or pain for sexual arousal

- BD (bondage and discipline)—sexual role play that includes elements of SM

- Paraphilia—one of a wide variety of uncommon sex practices that a person may find necessary for sexual arousal and orgasm

- Watersports—using urine or urination as a part of sex play

305

Why do people have sex?

One reason people have sex is to try to have children. But that is one of the least common reasons people say they're sexually active. There are many other reasons. Not all of them are good reasons. People choose to be sexually active to:

- express love, commitment, and caring;

- feel loved or cared for;

- experience physical pleasure;

- give someone else physical pleasure;

- fulfill curiosity;

- have fun;

- make up with their partners after a fight;

- relax;

- prove their masculinity or femininity;

- demonstrate power over a partner or allow a partner to demonstrate power;

- prove maturity;

- get even with another person.

Whatever the reason, having sex is sometimes a healthy choice, and sometimes it is not. People decide to have sex for different reasons. And we may have different reasons from day to day or at different times of our lives.

Our families and cultures shape our ideas of what is sexually acceptable. Negative messages we receive about certain reasons for having sex or for certain sexual activities can be very powerful. We may feel guilty or uncomfortable about the reasons we have sex. We may also feel that way about sex play that we enjoy or think we may enjoy. We may even fear discussing, learning about, or doing it.

Just because a sexual behavior isn't common or some people disapprove of it or the reasons people enjoy it, doesn't mean there is anything wrong with it. Many people enjoy less common kinds of sex play, but they are often less likely to discuss it with others. One way to think about uncommon sex play is this: if no one is hurt by the kind of sex someone might enjoy, then it is probably okay.

Am I ready for sex?

We all have sexual feelings. But we don't always engage in sexual activity when we have those feelings. When to have sex is a personal choice. Figuring out when you're ready for sex continues through life. People need to make decisions about sex in their teens, twenties, thirties, forties, fifties, and beyond—every time a sexual situation develops.

A good sex life is one that keeps in balance with everything you're about—your health, education and career goals, relationships with other people, and your feelings about yourself.

If you're considering having sex, ask yourself these questions:

- How clear can you be with your partner about what you do and don't want to happen?

- How will having sex will make you feel about yourself?

- How will sex affect you physically and emotionally?

- Are you considering having sex because you want to or because someone is pressuring you?

- Will sex change your relationship with your partner?

Sometimes it's helpful to talk these kinds of decisions through with someone you trust—a parent, a friend, a professional counselor, or someone else who cares about you and what will be good for you.

How do I talk with my partner about sex?

Talking about or showing our partners what feels good and what excites us can be an important part of a healthy and fulfilling sex life. Some people are able to share sexual desires and fantasies with a partner without embarrassment. For others, it is a bit more challenging.

But what turns you on might be very different from what turns on someone else. Discovering what feels good is part of what makes sex play fun and enjoyable. And our partners can only know what we like if we tell them or show them with our body language.

Taking a risk to suggest a new or different sexual activity may make us feel embarrassed, vulnerable, or silly. Whatever your feelings are, there are things you can do to help the conversation go more smoothly.

Here are some tips:

- Don't believe that your partner will think you are weird for suggesting a new sexual behavior. Often, these fears are worse than reality. You'll never know until you ask.

307

- Practice the conversation ahead of time. Predicting your partner's questions or concerns will help you feel more confident asking for what you want.

- Never pressure your partner into trying a sexual behavior that she or he is not comfortable with. It may take time to warm up to your ideas. Be patient!

- Always respect your partner's limits about what he or she wants to do and does not want to do.

- Ask your partner to share her or his desires. Maybe there is something your partner always wanted to try but hasn't had the courage to bring up.

- Don't think your partner is not attracted to you just because he or she says no to a behavior that you suggest. Remember, your partner is rejecting the behavior, not you.

It is common to be concerned about a partner's reaction when suggesting something new. But talking about what feels good and what is arousing can help sex partners have richer and more pleasurable sex lives. It also helps develop communication, trust, and openness in a relationship.

Sex and consent: It is important that partners are in agreement about shared sex play. Words, gestures, and actions are all ways people consent to sex. But it is important not to misunderstand your partner's intentions. If there is doubt or confusion about what you or your partner wants, stop and ask for clarity.

It is just as important for us to be able to stop sex play because we feel uncomfortable as it is for us to share our sexual desires by asking for what we want. Being able to talk about what you want is an important part of any healthy relationship.

Sex can also have legal consequences. Drugs or alcohol may impair a person's ability to agree to sex play. Do not have sex with someone who is too drunk or high to give consent. It is also illegal for adults to engage in sexual behaviors or sexually explicit discussions with minors. The age of consent varies from state to state. Making sure that someone is old enough and sober enough to agree to sex should be the first step before engaging in any sex play with another person.

How can I protect myself during sexual activity?

Infections can be passed during sex play from skin-to-skin contact or through the sharing of body fluids, especially:

- blood;

- semen;

- pre-cum;

- vaginal fluids.

Sexually active people can reduce their risk of infection during sex play by practicing safer sex.

Any sex play that allows semen to enter the vagina could lead to pregnancy. If you do not want to get pregnant or cause a pregnancy, be sure to use birth control.

Make sure to discuss safer sex with your partner before sex play starts. Also talk about birth control if pregnancy is possible. People are much more likely to take risks if they don't plan ahead.

Chapter 29

Female Sexual Dysfunction

Chapter Contents

Section 29.1

Sexual Dysfunction Basics in Women

So you're not in the mood. Or you're just not enjoying it anymore. Or sometimes, well, it hurts. And the thing is, these problems are bothering you or your partner or both of you. It's important to remember that sexual health issues—often referred to as sexual dysfunction by health care professionals—can affect women of all ages and at any stage of life.

Female Sexual Dysfunction Defined

Sexual dysfunction in women is not just one condition. Instead, sexual health experts have identified several types of female sexual dysfunction (FSD). These include:

- sexual desire disorders;
- sexual arousal disorders;
- orgasmic disorders;
- sexual pain disorders.

Just as there are different types of pneumonia, depression, and cancer, there also are different types of sexual disorders. Your diagnosis—and how you, your partner, and your health care professional approach treatment—depends on your symptoms.

The following list presents the different types of female sexual disorders and the definitions health care professionals use to diagnose them. Keep in mind that even if you think your sex life fits the description, if your condition doesn't bother you and you're just fine with your current sex life, then you do not have a disorder. Unless your sexual health issue causes distress, you don't necessarily need to "fix" it.

- **Hypoactive sexual desire disorder (HSDD):** The technical definition of HSDD is the persistent or recurrent lack (or absence) of sexual thoughts and desire for sexual activity. HSDD causes distress for the patient, may put a strain on relationships with partners, and is not due to the effects of a substance, including medications, or another medical condition. If you have HSDD, you simply aren't interested—or aren't as interested—in having sex as you once were. HSDD is undiagnosed for many women.

- **Subjective arousal disorder:** You don't feel sexually aroused or excited, and you don't get pleasure from sex, but you are still able to become lubricated.

- **Genital sexual arousal disorder:** You don't get physically aroused when your partner touches your genitals, but you can still become aroused from other sexual stimuli (for example, kissing, having your breasts stroked, touching your partner).

- **Combined genital and subjective arousal disorder:** As its name implies, this condition is a mix of both arousal disorders. Basically, nothing turns you on.

- **Persistent genital arousal disorder:** This is the opposite of the other three arousal disorders. You become physically aroused when nothing sexual is going on. Even having an orgasm doesn't make this feeling go away. The key here is that this constant arousal bothers you; you want it to go away.

- **Orgasmic disorder:** Put simply, despite being highly aroused and enjoying sex, you can't experience orgasm. This applies to women who have never experienced orgasm or to women who previously had orgasms but now no longer have them because of changes in their health, their medications, life circumstances, or relationships.

- **Dyspareunia:** This condition means pain with sex. Whether the pain occurs before, during, or after intercourse, if it interferes with your enjoyment of sex and your quality of life, it's a sexual disorder. Dyspareunia is more common than you might think. One study suggests that as many as 6 out of 10 women experience pain with intercourse.

- **Vaginismus:** This condition refers to a persistent or recurrent involuntary contraction of the muscles surrounding the vagina when penetration is attempted, making intercourse—or even inserting a tampon into your vagina—painful, if not impossible.

Questions to Ask Your Health Care Professional

1. I don't enjoy sex anymore, and I want to know why. Do you have experience diagnosing and treating sexual health problems?

2. Will you do a physical exam to help diagnose my sexual health issue? What types of tests will you perform?

3. Should my partner come to this or the next appointment with me?

4. Could a medication I am taking be causing my problem with sex?

5. Could a medication help make sex better?

6. How long will the medicine take to work?

7. Could counseling help?

8. Would physical therapy or other therapy help?

9. If I want to know more about my sexual health disorder, what resources and/or support groups would you recommend?

10. Will I need ongoing visits with you or another health care professional?

Getting the Diagnosis

If you have problems or concerns about sex and they are an issue for you—for whatever reason—it's time to see your health care professional. Only your health care professional can conduct the type of medical history and examination required to determine if you have a sexual disorder or if something else is going on. It is important that you are completely open and honest with your health care professional about your sexual history, including any sexual or physical abuse, sexually transmitted infections, problems with alcohol and/or drugs, and history of depression and/or anxiety.

Treating Sexual Dysfunction Disorders

There are numerous treatments for sexual disorders, including certain medications, surgical procedures, counseling, physical therapy, and lifestyle changes. You may need to see other health care professionals, such as a physical therapist or sex therapist. No matter what you and your health care professional decide, be patient. Most likely this health issue didn't occur overnight, and it may not improve overnight.

Section 29.2

Dyspareunia (Painful Intercourse)

Painful Sex

If you feel pain when you have sex, or even when you try to have sex, then you may have a condition called dyspareunia. You may be surprised to learn that many other women experience the same problem. In fact, at least 10% of women have experienced chronic pain in the genital area, and that number rises to 29% among postmenopausal women. Up to 60% of women who have dyspareunia say the pain is so bad they stopped having sex. Keep reading to learn the facts about painful sex, what causes it, and what your health care professional may be able to do to help you.

Causes of Painful Sex

Numerous conditions may cause painful sex. These include less lubrication related to declining estrogen levels just before and after menopause; tense pelvic floor muscles; vulvodynia, which is an oversensitivity of the nerves in the vulval area; endometriosis, in which the lining of the uterus grows outside the uterus; vaginismus, in which the vaginal muscles spasm, preventing anything from entering the vagina; and interstitial cystitis, or painful bladder syndrome, to name just a few conditions.

The most common cause of painful sex in premenopausal women is vulvodynia, defined as discomfort or burning pain in the vulvar area with no obvious cause. Vulvodynia can be generalized, in which you feel pain throughout the vulvar area for no apparent reason, or provoked, in which the pain occurs only when something touches the area.

Diagnosing Dyspareunia

Unfortunately, identifying the cause of your dyspareunia can be difficult. Many women see several doctors before they get a diagnosis and

315

some never get properly diagnosed. One online survey of 428 women with vulvar pain found that nearly half had visited four to nine health care providers about their pain, and more than half said their pain had not improved—or had gotten worse—since they began treatment. Another study found that only about half of women with chronic vulvar pain saw a health care provider at all, with a third of those women visiting five or more health care providers.

Dyspareunia and Relationships

As you might expect, if it hurts every time you try to have sex, the frequency with which you have sex will likely decline. That, in turn, may cause problems in your relationship. In one survey of 69 women with vulvar vestibulitis, a form of vulvodynia, 78% said their condition had changed their sexual life, particularly their interest in and satisfaction with sex. Most of the women said they were less able to sexually satisfy their partner and that their condition changed their relationship with their partners.

Questions to Ask Your Health Care Professional

1. What could be causing the pain I experience when I try to have sex?

2. Are there any lifestyle changes I can make?

3. Could an infection be causing the pain?

4. Why are you recommending this medication?

5. What are the potential side effects of this medication?

6. How long will the medicine take to work?

7. Is there anything I can do to maintain intimacy and a good relationship with my partner if I can't have sex?

8. When would surgery be an option?

9. Would physical therapy help?

10. Can you recommend a support group?

Dyspareunia and Mental Health

In that survey of 69 women mentioned earlier, 73% said they felt less sexually desirable, more than half said they felt less confident, and nearly half said they felt less feminine. The women were also highly frustrated, became depressed, had problems concentrating, and felt extremely stressed.

Treating Dyspareunia

Do bring your symptom to your health care provider's attention. When you visit your health care professional, expect a thorough physical examination to rule out a disease that might be causing your pain. Your health care professional may perform a comprehensive genital and pelvic examination. One test you may receive involves lightly touching the tip of a cotton swab to parts of your vulva to see if pain results. You will be asked to describe where it hurts, how much it hurts, and what the pain feels like.

Treatment for dyspareunia depends on your specific condition and your medical history. Your health care professional may prescribe low doses of an antidepressant or an anticonvulsant, both of which are used to treat nerve-related pain like that in vulvodynia. Other therapies may include topical anesthetics such as lidocaine and nerve blocks or trigger-point injections, in which the anesthetic is injected directly into the nerves or muscles. Additionally, some women may need surgery to remove painful areas at the entrance of the vagina. Hormone-containing vaginal cream may also be an option if your pain is related to menopausal vaginal dryness.

Because of pelvic muscle tightening or guarding that occurs in association with many cases of sexual pain, experts recommend you undergo physical therapy to address any muscle issues in your pelvic region. This may involve stretching and strengthening exercises as well as biofeedback to learn how to control the muscles in your pelvic area. You may also need psychotherapy to deal with issues related to your relationship and self-esteem.

When Sex Hurts

Between 25% and 45% of postmenopausal women find sex painful, a condition called dyspareunia.

While there are many causes, the most common reason for dyspareunia—painful sex—in women over 50 is vulvovaginal atrophy, a fancy name for a vulva and vagina that no longer have the beneficial effects from estrogen that they did prior to menopause.

As discussed earlier, lower estrogen levels significantly affect your vagina, impacting its ability to secrete lubricant, to expand and contract, and to grow new cells. Over time, blood flow diminishes, and the vagina and vulva can atrophy, or shrink as cells die off and aren't replaced.

The result? Soreness, burning after sex, pain during intercourse, and, sometimes, post-sex bleeding.

The good news is that vulvovaginal atrophy is very treatable. One of the best treatments doesn't involve medicine! Turns out that the more often you have sex, the less likely you are to develop atrophy or, at the very least, a serious case of it. That's because sex increases blood flow to the genitals, keeping them healthy.

Other treatments include:

Estrogen: As you might expect, if lack of estrogen is behind vulvovaginal atrophy, then giving back estrogen should help. Both systemic estrogens (oral pills and patches) and local estrogens (creams, rings, and tablets applied to the vulva and/or vagina) work. However, most major medical organizations recommend starting with the local approach first because it keeps the estrogen right where it's needed, limiting any effects on the rest of your body.

Studies on the estrogen ring, cream, and tablets find extremely high rates of improvement in dyspareunia, with up to 93% of women reporting significant improvement and between 57% and 75% saying that their sexual comfort was restored, depending on the approach used.

Side effects vary. Most estrogen products applied locally are associated with minimal side effects. However, each woman's response can differ. When using estrogen creams, pills, or rings, it is important to talk to your health care provider about any symptoms, such as: headache, stomach upset, bloating, nausea, weight changes, changes in sexual interest, breast tenderness, abdominal pain, back pain, respiratory infection, vaginal itching, or vaginal yeast infections. If you have had breast cancer or a family history of breast cancer, be sure to discuss your history with your health care professional, if you're considering using estrogen. Your health care professional likely has covered this topic with you already.

Non-medicated lubricants: If you'd rather not go the estrogen route, consider using some of the over-the-counter products designed to increase sexual comfort. Long-lasting vaginal moisturizers provide relief from vaginal dryness for up to four days.

Other Causes of Sexual Pain

Since many women over 50 do not experience vulvovaginal atrophy, women with sexual pain should be aware that there are other medical conditions that could be responsible for their symptoms. These include:

Vestibulodynia: Vestibulodynia is the most common cause of sexual pain in women under 50, but it can also affect older women. Women with this condition feel severe pain when any type of pressure or penetration is attempted at the entrance to the vagina (an area called the vestibule). It is treated with topical anesthetics, estrogen cream, antidepressants, antiepileptic drugs (often used for nerve-related pain), and physical therapy.

Vulvodynia: This condition involves stinging, burning, irritation, rawness, or pain on the vulva, the tissue that surrounds the vagina. The pain and irritation can occur even when nothing touches the area and is likely related to abnormal nerve firing. Vulvodynia is treated similarly to vestibulodynia.

Vaginismus or pelvic floor muscle dysfunction: In this condition, the vaginal and perineal muscles involuntarily spasm with attempted sexual activity. This can make vaginal entry very difficult or even impossible. Vaginismus can occur after a trauma (such as nonconsensual sex), or it can be related to underlying physical conditions, including musculoskeletal injuries or vestibulodynia. Vaginismus is often treated with dilator therapy (in which women are taught relaxation techniques while using progressive-sized dilators in their vagina) and physical therapy.

Urinary tract conditions, such as cystitis, or fungal infections can also cause pain upon intercourse, as can endometriosis, or a uterus that has "dropped" or prolapsed.

Time to Speak Up

Unfortunately, most women do not talk to their health care providers about sexual pain or problems, nor do their health care providers bring up the topic. In an international survey of 391 women by the Women's Sexual Health Foundation, fewer than 9% of women said their health care professionals had ever asked if they had sexual problems. Obviously, if you don't bring up the topic of sex with your health care professional, it won't get addressed. So speak up!

Section 29.3

Inhibited Sexual Desire

© 2013 A.D.A.M. Inc. Reprinted with permission.

Inhibited sexual desire (ISD) refers to a low level of sexual interest. A person with ISD will not start, or respond to their partner's desire for, sexual activity.

ISD can be primary (in which the person has never felt much sexual desire or interest), or secondary (in which the person used to feel sexual desire, but no longer does).

ISD can also relate to the partner (the person with ISD is interested in other people, but not his or her partner), or it can be general (the person with ISD isn't sexually interested in anyone). In the extreme form of sexual aversion, the person not only lacks sexual desire, but may find sex repulsive.

Sometimes, the sexual desire is not inhibited. The two partners have different sexual interest levels, even though both of their interest levels are within the normal range.

Someone can claim that his or her partner has ISD, when in fact they have overactive sexual desire and are very demanding sexually.

Causes

ISD is a very common sexual disorder. Often it occurs when one partner does not feel intimate or close to the other.

Communication problems, lack of affection, power struggles and conflicts, and not having enough time alone together are common factors. ISD also can occur in people who've had a very strict upbringing concerning sex, negative attitudes toward sex, or traumatic sexual experiences (such as rape, incest, or sexual abuse).

Illnesses and some medications can also contribute to ISD, especially when they cause fatigue, pain, or general feelings of malaise. A lack of certain hormones can sometimes be involved. Psychological conditions such as depression and excess stress can dampen sexual interest. Hormonal changes can also affect libido.

Commonly overlooked factors include insomnia or lack of sleep, which can lead to fatigue. ISD can also be associated with other sexual problems, and sometimes can be caused by them. For example, the woman who is unable to have an orgasm or has pain with intercourse, or the man who has erection problems (impotence) or retarded ejaculation, can lose interest in sex because they associate it with failure or it does not feel good.

People who were victims of childhood sexual abuse or rape, and those whose marriages lack emotional intimacy, are especially at risk for ISD.

Symptoms

The primary symptom is lack of sexual interest.

Exams and Tests

Most of the time, a medical exam and lab tests will not show a physical cause.

However, testosterone is the hormone that creates sexual desire in both men and women. Testosterone levels may be checked, especially in men who have ISD. Blood for such tests should be drawn before 10:00 a.m., when male hormone levels are at their highest.

Once physical causes have been ruled out, interviews with a sex therapy specialist may be helpful to reveal possible causes.

Treatment

Treatment must be targeted to the factors that may be lowering sexual interest. Often, there may be several such factors.

Some couples will need relationship or marital therapy before focusing on enhancing sexual activity. Some couples will need to be taught how to resolve conflicts and work through differences in nonsexual areas.

Communication training helps couples learn how to talk to one another, show empathy, resolve differences with sensitivity and respect for each other's feelings, learn how to express anger in a positive way, reserve time for activities together, and show affection, in order to encourage sexual desire.

Many couples will also need to focus on their sexual relationship. Through education and couple's assignments, they learn to increase the time they devote to sexual activity. Some couples will also need to focus on how they can sexually approach their partner in more interesting and desirable ways, and how to more gently and tactfully decline a sexual invitation.

Problems with sexual arousal or performance that affect sexual drive will need to be directly addressed. Some doctors recommend treating women with either cream or oral testosterone, often combined with estrogen, but there is no clear cut evidence yet. There are studies underway looking at the possible benefit of testosterone supplementation for women with decreased libido.

Outlook (Prognosis)

Disorders of sexual desire are often difficult to treat. They seem to be even more challenging to treat in men. For help, get a referral to someone who specializes in sex and marital therapy.

Possible Complications

When both partners have low sexual desire, sexual interest level will not be a problem in the relationship. Low sexual desire, however, may be a sign of the health of the relationship.

In other cases where there is an excellent and loving relationship, low sexual desire may cause a partner to feel hurt and rejected. This can lead to feelings of resentment and make the partners feel emotionally distant.

Sex is something that can either bring a relationship closer together, or slowly drive it apart. When one partner is much less interested in sex than the other partner, and this has become a source of conflict, they should get professional help before the relationship becomes further strained.

Prevention

One good way to prevent ISD is to set aside time for nonsexual intimacy. Couples who reserve time each week for talking and for a date alone without the kids will keep a closer relationship and are more likely to feel sexual interest.

Couples should also separate sex and affection, so that they won't be afraid that affection will always be seen as an invitation to have sex.

Reading books or taking courses in couple's communication, or reading books about massage, can also encourage feelings of closeness. For some people, reading novels or watching movies with romantic or sexual content also can encourage sexual desire.

Regularly setting aside "prime time," before exhaustion sets in, for both talking and sexual intimacy will improve closeness and sexual desire.

Section 29.4

Orgasmic Dysfunction

Orgasmic dysfunction is when a woman either can't reach orgasm or has difficulty reaching orgasm when she is sexually excited.

Causes, Incidence, and Risk Factors

The condition is called primary orgasmic dysfunction when a woman has never had an orgasm. This is the case in 10%–15% of women. It is called secondary orgasmic dysfunction when a woman has had at least one orgasm in the past, but is currently unable to have one. Surveys suggest that 33%–50% of women are dissatisfied with how often they reach orgasm.

Many factors can contribute to orgasmic dysfunction. They include:

- a history of sexual abuse or rape;

- boredom and monotony in sexual activity;

- certain prescription drugs, including fluoxetine (Prozac), paroxetine (Paxil), and sertraline (Zoloft);

- hormonal disorders, hormonal changes due to menopause, and chronic illnesses that affect general health and sexual interest;

- medical conditions that affect the nerve supply to the pelvis (such as multiple sclerosis, diabetic neuropathy, and spinal cord injury);

- negative attitudes toward sex (usually learned in childhood or adolescence);

- shyness or embarrassment about asking for whatever type of stimulation works best;

- strife or lack of emotional closeness within the relationship.

Prevention

A healthy attitude toward sex and education about sexual stimulation and response will minimize problems.

Couples who clearly communicate their sexual needs and desires, verbally or nonverbally, will experience orgasmic dysfunction less frequently.

It is also important to realize that sexual response is a complex coordination of the mind and the body, and both need to be functioning well for orgasms to happen.

Symptoms

The symptom of orgasmic dysfunction is being unable to reach orgasm, taking longer than you want to reach orgasm, or having only unsatisfying orgasms.

Signs and Tests

A complete medical history and physical examination needs to be done, but results are almost always normal. If the problem began after starting a medication, this should be discussed with the doctor who prescribed the drug. A qualified specialist in sex therapy may be helpful.

Treatment

Treatment can involve education, cognitive behavioral therapy, teaching orgasm by focusing on pleasurable stimulation, and directed masturbation.

Most women require clitoral stimulation to reach an orgasm. Incorporating this into sexual activity may be all that is necessary. If this doesn't solve the problem, then teaching the woman to masturbate may help her understand what she needs to become sexually excited.

A series of couple exercises to practice communication, more effective stimulation, and playfulness can help. If relationship difficulties play a role, treatment may include communication training and relationship enhancement work.

Medical problems, new medications, or untreated depression may need evaluation and treatment in order for orgasmic dysfunction to improve. The role of hormone supplementation in treating orgasmic dysfunction is controversial and the long-term risks remain unclear.

If other sexual dysfunctions (such as lack of interest and pain during intercourse) are happening at the same time, these need to be addressed as part of the treatment plan.

Expectations (Prognosis)

Women tend to have better results with treatment if their orgasmic dysfunction is due to another condition. Women with orgasmic dysfunction that is not due to another condition often do better when treatment involves learning sexual techniques or a method called desensitization, which gradually stops the response that causes lack of orgasms. Desensitization is helpful for women with significant sexual anxiety.

Improved orgasmic function is usually associated with being emotionally healthy and having a loving, affectionate relationship with a partner.

Complications

When sex is not enjoyable, it can become a chore rather than a mutually satisfying, intimate experience. When orgasmic dysfunction continues to happen, sexual desire usually declines, and eventually sex occurs less often. This can create resentment and conflict in the relationship.

Section 29.5

Vaginismus

© 2013 A.D.A.M. Inc. Reprinted with permission.

Vaginismus is an involuntary spasm of the muscles surrounding the vagina. The spasms close the vagina.

Causes

Vaginismus is a sexual problem. It has several possible causes, including:

- past sexual trauma or abuse;
- psychological factors;
- history of discomfort with sexual intercourse.

Sometimes no cause can be found.

Vaginismus is an uncommon condition. The exact number of women who have this problem is unknown.

Symptoms

The main symptoms are:

- difficult, painful, or impossible vaginal penetration during sex,
- vaginal pain during sexual intercourse or a pelvic exam.

Women with vaginismus often become anxious about sexual intercourse. However, this does not mean they cannot become sexually aroused. Many women with this condition can have orgasms when the clitoris is stimulated.

Exams and Tests

A pelvic exam can confirm the diagnosis of vaginismus. A medical history and complete physical exam are important to look for other causes of pain with sexual intercourse (dyspareunia).

Treatment

Treatment involves a combination of education, counseling, and exercises such as pelvic floor muscle contraction and relaxation (Kegel exercises).

Vaginal dilation exercises are recommended using plastic dilators. These should be done under the direction of a sex therapist or other health care provider. Therapy should involve the partner. It can gradually include more intimate contact, ultimately leading to intercourse.

Your health care provider should give you information about sexual anatomy, the sexual response cycle, and common myths about sex.

Outlook (Prognosis)

When women are treated by a specialist in sex therapy, success rates are generally very high.

Chapter 30

Birth Control

Chapter Contents

Section 30.1

Birth Control Methods and Effectiveness

Excerpted from "Birth Control Methods Fact Sheet," U.S. Department of Health and Human Services Office on Women's Health (www.womenshealth.gov), November 21, 2011.

All women and men can have control over when, and if, they become parents. Making choices about birth control, or contraception, isn't easy. To get started, learn about birth control methods. You can also talk with your doctor about the choices.

Before choosing a birth control method, think about the following:

- Your overall health

- How often you have sex

- The number of sex partners you have

- If you want to have children someday

- How well each method works to prevent pregnancy

- Possible side effects

- Your comfort level with using the method

Keep in mind, even the most effective birth control methods can fail. But your chances of getting pregnant are lowest if the method you choose always is used correctly and every time you have sex.

Methods of Birth Control

Continuous Abstinence

This means not having sex (vaginal, anal, or oral) at any time. It is the only sure way to prevent pregnancy and protect against sexually transmitted infections (STIs), including HIV.

Natural Family Planning/Rhythm Method

This method is when you do not have sex or use a barrier method on the days you are most fertile (most likely to become pregnant).

A woman who has a regular menstrual cycle has about nine or more days each month when she is able to get pregnant. These fertile days are about five days before and three days after ovulation, as well as the day of ovulation.

To have success with this method, you need to learn about your menstrual cycle. Then you can learn to predict which days you are fertile or "unsafe."

This method also involves checking your cervical mucus and recording your body temperature each day. Cervical mucus is the discharge from your vagina. You are most fertile when it is clear and slippery like raw egg whites. Use a basal thermometer to take your temperature and record it in a chart. Your temperature will rise 0.4 to 0.8° F on the first day of ovulation. You can talk with your doctor or a natural family planning instructor to learn how to record and understand this information.

Barrier Methods—Put up a Block, or Barrier, to Keep Sperm from Reaching the Egg

Contraceptive sponge: This barrier method is a soft, disk-shaped device with a loop for taking it out. It contains the spermicide non-oxynol-9, which kills sperm.

Before having sex, you wet the sponge and place it, loop side down, inside your vagina to cover the cervix. The sponge is effective for more than one act of intercourse for up to 24 hours. It needs to be left in for at least 6 hours after having sex to prevent pregnancy. It must then be taken out within 30 hours after it is inserted.

Diaphragm, cervical cap, and cervical shield: These barrier methods block the sperm from entering the cervix (the opening to your womb) and reaching the egg.

- The diaphragm is a shallow latex cup.

- The cervical cap is a thimble-shaped latex cup.

- The cervical shield is a silicone cup that has a one-way valve that creates suction and helps it fit against the cervix.

The diaphragm and cervical cap come in different sizes, and you need a doctor to "fit" you for one. The cervical shield comes in one size, and you will not need a fitting.

Before having sex, add spermicide (to block or kill sperm) to the device. Then place it inside your vagina to cover your cervix. You can buy spermicide gel or foam at a drug store.

All three of these barrier methods must be left in place for 6 to 8 hours after having sex to prevent pregnancy. The diaphragm should be taken out within 24 hours. The cap and shield should be taken out within 48 hours.

Female condom: This condom is worn by the woman inside her vagina. It keeps sperm from getting into her body. It is made of thin, flexible, man-made rubber and is packaged with a lubricant. It can be inserted up to eight hours before having sex. Use a new condom each time you have intercourse. And don't use it and a male condom at the same time.

Male condom: Male condoms are a thin sheath placed over an erect penis to keep sperm from entering a woman's body. Condoms can be made of latex, polyurethane, or "natural/lambskin." The natural kind do not protect against STIs. Condoms work best when used with a vaginal spermicide, which kills the sperm. And you need to use a new condom with each sex act.

Condoms can be the following:

- Lubricated, which can make sexual intercourse more comfortable

- Non-lubricated, which can also be used for oral sex; it is best to add lubrication to non-lubricated condoms if you use them for vaginal or anal sex

Keep condoms in a cool, dry place. If you keep them in a hot place (like a wallet or glove compartment), the latex breaks down. Then the condom can tear or break.

Hormonal Methods—Prevent Pregnancy by Interfering with Ovulation, Fertilization, and/or Implantation of the Fertilized Egg

Note: Women should wait three weeks after giving birth to begin using birth control that contains both estrogen and progestin. These methods increase the risk of dangerous blood clots that could form after giving birth. Women who delivered by cesarean section or have other risk factors for blood clots, such as obesity, history of blood clots, smoking, or preeclampsia, should wait six weeks.

Oral contraceptive—combined pill ("the pill"): The pill contains the hormones estrogen and progestin. It is taken daily to keep the ovaries from releasing an egg. The pill also causes changes in the lining of the uterus and the cervical mucus to keep the sperm from joining the egg.

Some women prefer the "extended cycle" pills. These have 12 weeks of pills that contain hormones (active) and 1 week of pills that don't contain hormones (inactive). While taking extended cycle pills, women only have their period three to four times a year.

Many types of oral contraceptives are available. Talk with your doctor about which is best for you.

Your doctor may advise you not to take the pill if the following are true of you:

- Are older than 35 and smoke

- Have a history of blood clots

- Have a history of breast, liver, or endometrial cancer

Antibiotics may reduce how well the pill works in some women. Talk to your doctor about a backup method of birth control if you need to take antibiotics.

The patch: Also called by its brand name, Ortho Evra, this skin patch is worn on the lower abdomen, buttocks, outer arm, or upper body. It releases the hormones progestin and estrogen into the bloodstream to stop the ovaries from releasing eggs in most women. It also thickens the cervical mucus, which keeps the sperm from joining with the egg. You put on a new patch once a week for three weeks. You don't use a patch the fourth week in order to have a period.

Shot/injection: The birth control shot often is called by its brand name Depo-Provera. With this method you get injections, or shots, of the hormone progestin in the buttocks or arm every three months. A new type is injected under the skin. The birth control shot stops the ovaries from releasing an egg in most women. It also causes changes in the cervix that keep the sperm from joining with the egg.

The shot should not be used more than two years in a row because it can cause a temporary loss of bone density. The loss increases the longer this method is used. The bone does start to grow after this method is stopped. But it may increase the risk of fracture and osteoporosis if used for a long time.

Vaginal ring: This is a thin, flexible ring that releases the hormones progestin and estrogen. It works by stopping the ovaries from releasing eggs. It also thickens the cervical mucus, which keeps the sperm from joining the egg.

It is commonly called NuvaRing, its brand name. You squeeze the ring between your thumb and index finger and insert it into your vagina. You wear the ring for three weeks, take it out for the week that you have your period, and then put in a new ring.

Implantable Devices—Devices That Are Inserted into the Body and Left in Place for a Few Years

Implantable rod: This is a matchstick-size, flexible rod that is put under the skin of the upper arm. It is often called by its brand name, Implanon. The rod releases a progestin, which causes changes in the lining of the uterus and the cervical mucus to keep the sperm from joining an egg. Less often, it stops the ovaries from releasing eggs. It is effective for up to three years.

Intrauterine devices, or IUDs: An IUD is a small device shaped like a *T* that goes in your uterus. There are two types:

- **Copper IUD:** The copper IUD goes by the brand name Para-Gard. It releases a small amount of copper into the uterus, which prevents the sperm from reaching and fertilizing the egg. If fertilization does occur, the IUD keeps the fertilized egg from implanting in the lining of the uterus. A doctor needs to put in your copper IUD. It can stay in your uterus for 5 to 10 years.

- **Hormonal IUD:** The hormonal IUD goes by the brand name Mirena. It is sometimes called an intrauterine system, or IUS. It releases progestin into the uterus, which keeps the ovaries from releasing an egg and causes the cervical mucus to thicken so sperm can't reach the egg. It also affects the ability of a fertilized egg to successfully implant in the uterus. A doctor needs to put in a hormonal IUD. It can stay in your uterus for up to five years.

Permanent Birth Control Methods—For People Who Are Sure They Never Want to Have a Child or Do Not Want More Children

Sterilization implant (Essure): Essure is the first nonsurgical method of sterilizing women. A thin tube is used to thread a tiny spring-like device through the vagina and uterus into each fallopian tube. The device works by causing scar tissue to form around the coil. This blocks the fallopian tubes and stops the egg and sperm from joining.

It can take about three months for the scar tissue to grow, so it's important to use another form of birth control during this time. Then you will have to return to your doctor for a test to see if scar tissue has fully blocked your tubes.

Surgical sterilization: For women, surgical sterilization closes the fallopian tubes by being cut, tied, or sealed. This stops the eggs from going down to the uterus where they can be fertilized. The surgery can be done a number of ways. Sometimes, a woman having cesarean birth has the procedure done at the same time, so as to avoid having additional surgery later.

For men, having a vasectomy keeps sperm from going to his penis, so his ejaculate never has any sperm in it. Sperm stays in the system after surgery for about three months. During that time, use a backup form of birth control to prevent pregnancy. A simple test can be done to check if all the sperm is gone; it is called a semen analysis.

Emergency Contraception—Used If a Woman's Primary Method of Birth Control Fails, Not as a Regular Method of Birth Control

Emergency contraception (Plan B One-Step or Next Choice, also called the "morning-after pill"): Emergency contraception keeps a woman from getting pregnant when she has had unprotected vaginal intercourse. "Unprotected" can mean that no method of birth control was used. It can also mean that a birth control method was used but it was used incorrectly or did not work (like a condom breaking). Or a woman may have forgotten to take her birth control pills. She also may have been abused or forced to have sex. These are just some of the reasons women may need emergency contraception.

Emergency contraception can be taken as a single-pill treatment or in two doses. A single-dose treatment works as well as two doses and does not have more side effects. It works by stopping the ovaries from releasing an egg or keeping the sperm from joining with the egg. For the best chances for it to work, take the pill as soon as possible after unprotected sex. It should be taken within 72 hours after having unprotected sex.

A single-pill dose or two-pill dose of emergency contraception is available over-the-counter (OTC) for women ages 17 and older.

Birth Control Effectiveness and Side Effects

All birth control methods work the best if used correctly and every time you have sex. Be sure you know the right way to use them. Sometimes doctors don't explain how to use a method because they assume you already know. Talk with your doctor if you have questions. They are used to talking about birth control, so don't feel embarrassed.

333

Some birth control methods can take time and practice to learn. For example, some people don't know you can put on a male condom "inside out." Also, not everyone knows you need to leave a little space at the tip of the condom for the sperm and fluid when a man ejaculates, or has an orgasm.

The following is a list of some birth control methods with their failure rates (the number of pregnancies expected per 100 women).

Sterilization surgery for women: Less than 1 pregnancy

Sterilization implant for women (Essure): Less than 1 pregnancy

Sterilization surgery for men: Less than 1 pregnancy

Implantable rod (Implanon): Less than 1 pregnancy (might not work as well for women who are overweight or obese)

Intrauterine device (ParaGard, Mirena): Less than 1 pregnancy

Shot/injection (Depo-Provera): Less than 1 pregnancy

Oral contraceptives (combination pill, or "the pill"): 5 pregnancies (being overweight may increase the chance of getting pregnant while using the pill)

Oral contraceptives (continuous/extended use, or "no-period pill"): 5 pregnancies (being overweight may increase the chance of getting pregnant while using the pill)

Oral contraceptives (progestin-only pill, or "mini-pill"): 5 pregnancies (being overweight may increase the chance of getting pregnant while using the pill)

Skin patch (Ortho Evra): 5 pregnancies (may not work as well in women weighing more than 198 pounds)

Vaginal ring (NuvaRing): 5 pregnancies

Male condom: 11–16 pregnancies

Diaphragm with spermicide: 15 pregnancies

Sponge with spermicide (Today Sponge): 16–32 pregnancies

Cervical cap with spermicide: 17–23 pregnancies

Female condom: 20 pregnancies

Natural family planning (rhythm method): 25 pregnancies

Spermicide alone: 30 pregnancies (it works best if used along with a barrier method, such as a condom)

Emergency contraception ("morning-after pill," Plan B One-Step, Next Choice): 1 pregnancy (it must be used within 72 hours of having unprotected sex); should not be used as regular birth control, only in emergencies

Methods of Acquiring Birth Control

Where you get birth control depends on what method you choose. You can buy these forms over the counter:

- Male condoms
- Female condoms
- Sponges
- Spermicides
- Emergency contraception pills (girls younger than 17 need a prescription)

You need a prescription for these forms:

- Oral contraceptives: the pill, the mini-pill
- Skin patch
- Vaginal ring
- Diaphragm (your doctor needs to fit one to your shape)
- Cervical cap
- Cervical shield
- Shot/injection (you get the shot at your doctor's office)
- IUD (inserted by a doctor)
- Implantable rod (inserted by a doctor)

You will need surgery or a medical procedure for the following:

- Sterilization, female and male

Foams or Gels to Prevent Pregnancy

You can buy spermicides over the counter. They work by killing sperm. They come in many forms. Spermicides are put in the vagina no more than one hour before having sex. If you use a film, suppository, or tablet, wait at least 15 minutes before having sex so the spermicide can dissolve. Do not douche or rinse out your vagina for at least six to eight hours after having sex. You will need to use more spermicide each time you have sex.

Spermicides work best if used along with a barrier method, such as a condom, diaphragm, or cervical cap. Some spermicides are made just for use with the diaphragm and cervical cap. Check the package to make sure you are buying what you need.

All spermicides contain sperm-killing chemicals. Some contain nonoxynol-9, which may raise your risk of HIV if you use it a lot. It irritates the tissue in the vagina and anus, so it can cause the HIV virus to enter the body more freely. Some women are sensitive to nonoxynol-9 and need to use spermicides without it. Medications for vaginal yeast infections may lower the effectiveness of spermicides. Also, spermicides do not protect against sexually transmitted infections.

Withdrawal as a Birth Control Method

Withdrawal as a birth control method is not very effective. Withdrawal is when a man takes his penis out of a woman's vagina (or "pulls out") before he ejaculates, or has an orgasm. This stops the sperm from going to the egg. "Pulling out" can be hard for a man to do. It takes a lot of self-control.

Even if you use withdrawal, sperm can be released before the man pulls out. When a man's penis first becomes erect, pre-ejaculate fluid may be on the tip of the penis. This fluid has sperm in it. So you could still get pregnant.

Withdrawal does not protect you from STIs or HIV.

Section 30.2

Emergency Contraception

Excerpted from "Emergency Contraception (Emergency Birth Control) Fact Sheet," U.S. Department of Health and Human Services Office on Women's Health (www.womenshealth.gov), November 21, 2011.

What is emergency contraception?

Emergency contraception, or emergency birth control, is used to help keep a woman from getting pregnant after she has had sex without using birth control or if the birth control method failed. If you are already pregnant, emergency contraception will not work.

Emergency contraception should not be used as regular birth control. Other birth control methods are much better at keeping women from becoming pregnant. Talk with your doctor to decide which one is right for you.

What are the types of emergency contraception and how do they work?

There are two types of emergency contraception.

Emergency contraceptive pills (ECPs): With ECPs, higher doses of the same hormones found in regular birth control pills stop pregnancy by keeping the egg from leaving the ovary or keeping the sperm from joining the egg. While it is possible that ECPs might work by keeping a fertilized egg from attaching to the uterus, the most up-to-date research suggests that ECPs do not work in this way. In the United States, there are two kinds of FDA-approved ECPs. One is called Plan B One-Step. The other is called Next Choice. However, when used in a certain way, some regular birth control pills also can be used as ECPs.

- **Plan B One-Step** is a progestin-only ECP. Plan B One-Step is like progestin-only birth control pills but contains higher levels of the hormone. Plan B One-Step is a one-pill emergency contraceptive available over the counter for people ages 17 and older. It must be taken within 72 hours of unprotected sex.

337

- **Next Choice** is also a progestin-only ECP. It is like progestin-only birth control pills but has higher levels of the hormone. Next Choice is two pills. The first pill should be taken as soon as possible within 72 hours of unprotected sex. The second pill should be taken 12 hours after the first pill. Next Choice is available over the counter for people ages 17 and older.

- **Higher dose of regular birth control pills** can sometimes be used as emergency contraception. The number of pills in a dose is different for each pill brand, and not all brands can be used for emergency contraception. For more information on birth control pills that can be used for emergency contraception, visit the Emergency Contraception website (not-2-late.com).

You should always take ECPs as soon as you can after having unprotected sex, but they can work up to five days later in some cases. However, if you use Plan B One-Step or Next Choice as emergency contraception, you should take your first pill within 72 hours of unprotected sex. Women who are breastfeeding or cannot take estrogen should use progestin-only ECPs (like Plan B One-Step). Some women feel sick and throw up after taking ECPs. If you throw up after taking ECPs, call your doctor or pharmacist.

Intrauterine device (IUD): The IUD is a small, T-shaped device placed into the uterus by a doctor within five days after having unprotected sex. The IUD works by keeping the sperm from joining the egg or keeping a fertilized egg from attaching to the uterus. Your doctor can remove the IUD after your next period. Or, it can be left in place for up to 10 years to use as your regular birth control method.

How well does emergency contraception work?

When used correctly, emergency contraceptive pills work very well at preventing pregnancy. Consider that about 8 in 100 women who have unprotected sex one time during the fertile part of their cycle will become pregnant. If these 100 women take progestin-only ECPs (like Plan B One-Step or Next Choice), about 1 will become pregnant. If 100 women take ECPs with estrogen and progestin, about 2 will become pregnant. The IUD works even better. Only 1 in 1,000 women who have an IUD put in after having unprotected sex will become pregnant.

The sooner you use emergency contraception after unprotected sex, the more likely it will prevent pregnancy. But you must use it correctly.

Does emergency contraception have side effects?

Some women feel sick and throw up after taking ECPs. Headache, dizziness, lower stomach cramps, irregular bleeding, breast tenderness, and fatigue also can occur. Progestin-only ECPs cause fewer side effects than combined pills that also contain estrogen. The over-the-counter drug Dramamine II can reduce the risk of feeling sick and throwing up. Take two of these pills 30 minutes before taking ECPs. If you throw up after taking ECPs, call your doctor or pharmacist.

IUD placement has risks of pelvic infection or harming the uterus. But these risks are quite rare. If the IUD is left in place to be used as birth control, it can cause side effects such as cramps and heavy bleeding during your period.

Will emergency contraception protect me from sexually transmitted infections (STIs)?

No. Emergency contraception can only lower the risk of becoming pregnant after having unprotected sex. Always use condoms to lower your risk of getting an STI.

How do I get emergency contraceptive pills?

You can get Plan B One-Step or Next Choice at drugstores and stores with a licensed pharmacist without a prescription for those 17 and older. Women and men must show proof of age to buy Plan B One-Step or Next Choice. If you are younger than 17 and need emergency contraception, you will need a prescription, so act quickly. Talk to your parents, your doctor, or visit a family planning clinic and ask for help. In some states (Alaska, California, Hawaii, Maine, Massachusetts, New Hampshire, New Mexico, Vermont, and Washington), some pharmacists can provide Plan B One-Step or Next Choice to women younger than 17 without a prescription. If you live in one of these states, call your pharmacy to see if this is an option for you.

Can I get emergency contraceptive pills before I need them?

Yes. Your doctor should bring up ECPs at your annual exam (when you have a Pap test). If your doctor does not talk about emergency contraception at your next exam, ask your doctor about it.

What do I need to do after I take emergency contraceptive pills?

After you have taken ECPs, your next period may come sooner or later than normal. Most women will get their period within seven days of the expected date. Your period also may be heavier, lighter, or more spotty than normal. If you do not get your period in three weeks or if you think you might be pregnant after taking ECPs, get a pregnancy test to find out for sure.

Use another birth control method if you have sex any time before your next period starts. Talk to your doctor about how to choose a birth control method that is right for you.

Are emergency contraceptive pills the same thing as the abortion pill?

No. Emergency contraception works before pregnancy begins. It will not work if a woman is already pregnant. Abortion takes place after a fertilized egg has attached to the uterus. The abortion pill (Mifeprex, also called RU-486) makes the uterus force out the egg, ending the pregnancy.

Chapter 31

Abortion

Chapter Contents

Section 31.1

Medical Abortion Procedures

Medical abortion procedures are available for terminating a pregnancy during the early weeks of the first trimester. For women seeking a medical abortion procedure, a sonogram is recommended to determine if the pregnancy is viable (uterine, non-ectopic pregnancy) and for accurate pregnancy dating.

Methotrexate and Misoprostol (MTX)

MTX is a medical abortion procedure used up to the first seven weeks (49 days) of pregnancy. This procedure is not as commonly used as in the past because of the availability of mifepristone.

- Methotrexate is given orally or by injection during the first office visit.

- Antibiotics are also given in order to prevent infection.

- Misoprostol tablets are given orally or inserted vaginally about three to seven days later. This can be done at home.

- This procedure will usually trigger contractions and expel the fetus. The process may take a few hours or as long as a few days.

- A physical exam is given a week later to ensure that the abortion procedure is complete and to check for complications.

- Methotrexate is primarily used in the treatment of cancer and rheumatoid arthritis because it attacks the most rapidly growing cells in the body. In the case of abortion, it causes the fetus and placenta to separate from the lining of the uterus. Using the drug for this purpose is not approved by the FDA [U.S. Food and Drug Administration].

The side effects and risks of methotrexate and misoprostol include the following:

- The procedure is unsuccessful approximately 5% of the time with the potential of requiring an additional surgical abortion procedure to complete the termination

- Cramping, nausea, diarrhea, heavy bleeding, fever

- Not advised for women who have anemia, bleeding disorders, liver or kidney disease, seizure disorder, acute inflammatory bowel disease, or use an intrauterine device (IUD)

Mifepristone (Mifeprex) and Misoprostol

Mifepristone (Mifeprex) and misoprostol is a medical abortion procedure used up to the first seven to nine weeks of pregnancy. It is also referred to as RU-486 or the abortion pill.

- A physical exam is first given in order to determine eligibility for this type of medical abortion procedure. You are not eligible if you have any of the following: ectopic pregnancy, ovarian mass, IUD, corticosteroid use, adrenal failure, anemia, bleeding disorders or use of blood thinners, asthma, liver or kidney problems, heart disease, or high blood pressure. You will be given antibiotics to prevent infection.

- Mifepristone is given orally during your first office visit. Mifepristone blocks progesterone from the uterine lining, causing the lining to break down, preventing the ability to continue a pregnancy.

- Misoprostol tablets are taken orally or inserted vaginally about 36 to 72 hours after taking the mifepristone. The tablets will cause contractions and expel the fetus. This process may take a few hours or as long as a few days.

- A physical exam is given two weeks later to ensure the abortion was complete and to check for complications.

The side effects and risks of Mifepristone and misoprostol include the following:

- The procedure is unsuccessful approximately 8%–10% of the time with the potential of requiring an additional surgical abortion procedure to complete the termination

- Cramping, nausea, vomiting diarrhea, heavy bleeding, infection

- Not advised for women who have anemia, bleeding disorders, liver or kidney disease, seizure disorder, acute inflammatory bowel disease, or use an intrauterine device (IUD)

Section 31.2

Surgical Abortion Procedures

"Surgical Abortion Procedures," © 2006 American Pregnancy Association (www.americanpregnancy.org). All rights reserved. Reprinted with permission. Reviewed by David A. Cooke, MD, FACP, February 2012.

The type of surgical abortion procedure used is based on the woman's stage of pregnancy. Before seeking a surgical abortion procedure, you should obtain a sonogram to determine if the pregnancy is viable (uterine, non-ectopic pregnancy) and for accurate pregnancy dating.

Aspiration

How is aspiration performed?

Aspiration is a surgical abortion procedure performed during the first 6 to 16 weeks gestation. It is also referred to as suction aspiration, suction curettage, or vacuum aspiration.

Your abortion provider will give you medication for pain and possibly sedation. You will lie on your back with your feet in stirrups and a speculum is inserted to open the vagina. A local anesthetic is administered to your cervix to numb it. Then a tenaculum (surgical instrument with long handles and a clamp at the end) is used to hold the cervix in place for the cervix to be dilated by absorbent rods that vary in size. The rods may also be put in a few days prior to the procedure. When the cervix is wide enough, a cannula, which is a long plastic tube connected to a suction device, is inserted into the uterus to suction out the fetus and placenta. The procedure usually lasts 10–15 minutes, but recovery can require staying at the clinic for a few hours. Your doctor will also give you antibiotics to help prevent infection.

What are the side effects and risks of suction aspiration?

Common side effects of the procedure include cramping, nausea, sweating, and feeling faint.

Less frequent side effects include possible heavy or prolong bleeding, blood clots, damage to the cervix, and perforation of the uterus. Infection due to retained products of conception or infection caused by an STD or bacteria being introduced to the uterus can cause fever, pain, abdominal tenderness, and possibly scar tissue.

Contact your health care provider immediately if your side effects persist or worsen.

Dilation and Evacuation (D & E)

How is dilation and evacuation performed?

Dilation and evacuation is a surgical abortion procedure performed after 16 weeks gestation. In most cases, 24 hours prior to the actual procedure, your abortion provider will insert laminaria or a synthetic dilator inside your cervix. When the procedure begins the next day, your abortion provider will use a tenaculum to keep the cervix and uterus in place and cone-shaped rods of increasing size are used to continue the dilation process. A numbing medication will be used on the cervix.

A shot may be given before the procedure begins to ensure fetal demise has occurred. Then a cannula (long tube) is inserted to begin removing tissue away from the lining. Then using a curette (surgical instrument shaped like a scoop or spoon), the lining is scraped to remove any residuals. If needed, forceps may be used to remove larger parts. The last step is usually a final suctioning to make sure the contents are completely removed.

The procedure normally takes between 15–30 minutes. The fetal remains are usually examined to ensure everything was removed and that the abortion was complete. An antibiotic will be given to help prevent infection.

What are the side effects and risks of dilation and evacuation?

Common side effects include nausea, bleeding, and cramping which may last for two weeks following the procedure. Although rare, the following are additional risks related to dilation and evacuation: damage to uterine lining or cervix, perforation of the uterus, infection, and blood clots.

Contact your health care provider immediately if your symptoms persist or worsen.

345

Dilation and Extraction

How is dilation and extraction performed?

The dilation and extraction procedure is used after 21 weeks gestation. The procedure is also known as D & X, intact D & X, intrauterine cranial decompression, and partial birth abortion. Two days before the procedure, laminaria is inserted vaginally to dilate the cervix. Your water should break on the third day and you should return to the clinic. The fetus is rotated and forceps are used to grasp and pull the legs, shoulders, and arms through the birth canal. A small incision is made at the base of the skull to allow a suction catheter inside. The catheter removes the cerebral material until the skull collapses. The fetus is then completely removed.

What are the side effects and risks related to dilation and extraction?

The side effects are the same as dilation and evacuation. However, there is an increased chance of emotional problems from the reality of more advanced fetal development.

Contact your health care provider immediately if your symptoms persist or worsen.

Chapter 32

Infertility and Infertility Treatment Options

What is infertility?

Infertility means not being able to get pregnant after one year of trying. Or six months, if a woman is 35 years of age or older. Women who can get pregnant but are unable to stay pregnant may also be infertile.

Pregnancy is the result of a process that has many steps. To get pregnant the following must occur:

- A woman's body must release an egg from one of her ovaries (ovulation).

- The egg must go through a fallopian tube toward the uterus (womb).

- A man's sperm must join with (fertilize) the egg along the way.

- The fertilized egg must attach to the inside of the uterus (implantation).

Infertility can happen if there are problems with any of these steps.

Is infertility a common problem?

Yes. About 10% of women (6.1 million) in the United States ages 15–44 years have difficulty getting pregnant or staying pregnant.

Excerpted from "Infertility FAQ's," Centers for Disease Control and Prevention (www.cdc.gov), April 19, 2012.

Is infertility just a woman's problem?

No, infertility is not always a woman's problem. Both women and men can have problems that cause infertility. About one-third of infertility cases are caused by women's problems. Another one-third of fertility problems are due to the man. The other cases are caused by a mixture of male and female problems or by unknown problems.

What causes infertility in men?

Infertility in men is most often caused by the following:

- A problem called varicocele happens when the veins on a man's testicle(s) are too large; this heats the testicles. The heat can affect the number or shape of the sperm.

- Other factors can cause a man to make too few sperm or none at all.

- Movement of the sperm can be a factor in infertility. This may be caused by the shape of the sperm. Sometimes injuries or other damage to the reproductive system block the sperm.

Sometimes a man is born with the problems that affect his sperm. Other times problems start later in life due to illness or injury. For example, cystic fibrosis often causes infertility in men.

What increases a man's risk of infertility?

A man's sperm can be changed by his overall health and lifestyle. Some things that may reduce the health or number of sperm include the following:

- Heavy alcohol use
- Drugs
- Smoking cigarettes
- Age
- Environmental toxins, including pesticides and lead
- Health problems such as mumps, serious conditions like kidney disease, or hormone problems
- Medicines
- Radiation treatment and chemotherapy for cancer

348

What causes infertility in women?

Most cases of female infertility are caused by problems with ovulation. Without ovulation, there are no eggs to be fertilized. Some signs that a woman is not ovulating normally include irregular or absent menstrual periods.

Ovulation problems are often caused by polycystic ovary syndrome (PCOS). PCOS is a hormone imbalance problem that can interfere with normal ovulation. PCOS is the most common cause of female infertility. Primary ovarian insufficiency (POI) is another cause of ovulation problems. POI occurs when a woman's ovaries stop working normally before she is 40. POI is not the same as early menopause.

Less common causes of fertility problems in women include the following:

- Blocked fallopian tubes due to pelvic inflammatory disease, endometriosis, or surgery for an ectopic pregnancy

- Physical problems with the uterus

- Uterine fibroids, which are non-cancerous clumps of tissue and muscle on the walls of the uterus

What things increase a woman's risk of infertility?

Many things can change a woman's ability to have a baby. These include the following:

- Age
- Smoking
- Excess alcohol use
- Stress
- Poor diet
- Athletic training
- Being overweight or underweight
- Sexually transmitted infections (STIs)
- Health problems that cause hormonal changes, such as polycystic ovary syndrome and primary ovarian insufficiency

How does age affect a woman's ability to have children?

Many women are waiting until their thirties and forties to have children. In fact, about 20% of women in the United States now have

349

their first child after age 35. So age is a growing cause of fertility problems. About one-third of couples in which the woman is older than 35 years have fertility problems.

Aging decreases a woman's chances of having a baby in the following ways:

- Her ovaries become less able to release eggs.
- She has a smaller number of eggs left.
- Her eggs are not as healthy.
- She is more likely to have health conditions that can cause fertility problems.
- She is more likely to have a miscarriage.

How long should women try to get pregnant before calling their doctors?

Most experts suggest at least one year. Women aged 35 years or older should see their doctors after six months of trying. A woman's chances of having a baby decrease rapidly every year after the age of 30.

Some health problems also increase the risk of infertility. So, women should talk to their doctors if they have the following:

- Irregular periods or no menstrual periods
- Very painful periods
- Endometriosis
- Pelvic inflammatory disease
- More than one miscarriage

It is a good idea for any woman to talk to a doctor before trying to get pregnant. Doctors can help you get your body ready for a healthy baby. They can also answer questions on fertility and give tips on conceiving.

How will doctors find out if a woman and her partner have fertility problems?

Doctors will do an infertility checkup. This involves a physical exam. The doctor will also ask for both partners' health and sexual histories. Sometimes this can find the problem. However, most of the time, the doctor will need to do more tests.

In men, doctors usually begin by testing the semen. They look at the number, shape, and movement of the sperm. Sometimes doctors also suggest testing the level of a man's hormones.

In women, the first step is to find out if she is ovulating each month. There are a few ways to do this. A woman can track her ovulation at home. Doctors can also check ovulation with blood tests. Or they can do an ultrasound of the ovaries. If ovulation is normal, there are other fertility tests available.

Some common tests of fertility in women include the following:

- **Hysterosalpingography:** This is an X-ray of the uterus and fallopian tubes. Doctors inject a special dye into the uterus through the vagina. Doctors can then watch to see if the dye moves freely through the uterus and fallopian tubes. This can help them find physical blocks that may be causing infertility. Blocks in the system can keep the egg from moving from the fallopian tube to the uterus. A block could also keep the sperm from reaching the egg.

- **Laparoscopy:** This is a minor surgery to see inside the abdomen. The doctor does this with a small tool with a light called a laparoscope. She or he makes a small cut in the lower abdomen and inserts the laparoscope. With the laparoscope, the doctor can check the ovaries, fallopian tubes, and uterus for disease and physical problems. Doctors can usually find scarring and endometriosis by laparoscopy.

Finding the cause of infertility can be a long and emotional process. It may take time to complete all the needed tests. So don't worry if the problem is not found right away.

How do doctors treat infertility?

Infertility can be treated with medicine, surgery, artificial insemination, or assisted reproductive technology. Many times these treatments are combined. In most cases infertility is treated with drugs or surgery. Doctors often treat infertility in men in the following ways:

- **Sexual problems:** Doctors can help men deal with impotence or premature ejaculation. Behavioral therapy and/or medicines can be used in these cases.

- **Too few sperm:** Sometimes surgery can correct the cause of the problem. In other cases, doctors surgically remove sperm directly from the male reproductive tract. Antibiotics can also be used to clear up infections affecting sperm count.

- **Sperm movement:** Sometimes semen has no sperm because of a block in the man's system. In some cases, surgery can correct the problem.

In women, some physical problems can also be corrected with surgery. A number of fertility medicines are used to treat women with ovulation problems. It is important to talk with your doctor about the pros and cons of these medicines. You should understand the possible dangers, benefits, and side effects.

What medicines are used to treat infertility in women?

Some common medicines used to treat infertility in women include the following:

- **Clomiphene citrate (Clomid):** This medicine causes ovulation by acting on the pituitary gland. It is often used in women who have PCOS or other problems with ovulation. This medicine is taken by mouth.

- **Human menopausal gonadotropin or hMG (Repronex, Pergonal):** This medicine is often used for women who don't ovulate due to problems with their pituitary gland—hMG acts directly on the ovaries to stimulate ovulation. It is an injected medicine.

- **Follicle-stimulating hormone or FSH (Gonal-F, Follistim):** FSH works much like hMG. It causes the ovaries to begin the process of ovulation. These medicines are usually injected.

- **Gonadotropin-releasing hormone (Gn-RH) analog:** These medicines are often used for women who don't ovulate regularly each month. Women who ovulate before the egg is ready can also use these medicines. Gn-RH analogs act on the pituitary gland to change when the body ovulates. These medicines are usually injected or given with a nasal spray.

- **Metformin (Glucophage):** Doctors use this medicine for women who have insulin resistance and/or PCOS. This drug helps lower the high levels of male hormones in women with these conditions. This helps the body to ovulate. Sometimes clomiphene citrate or FSH is combined with metformin. This medicine is usually taken by mouth.

- **Bromocriptine (Parlodel):** This medicine is used for women with ovulation problems due to high levels of prolactin. Prolactin is a hormone that causes milk production.

Many fertility drugs increase a woman's chance of having twins, triplets, or other multiples. Women who are pregnant with multiple fetuses have more problems during pregnancy. Multiple fetuses have a high risk of being born too early (prematurely). Premature babies are at a higher risk of health and developmental problems.

What is intrauterine insemination (IUI)?

Intrauterine insemination is an infertility treatment that is often called artificial insemination. In this procedure, the woman is injected with specially prepared sperm. Sometimes the woman is also treated with medicines that stimulate ovulation before IUI.

IUI is often used to treat the following:

• Mild male factor infertility

• Women who have problems with their cervical mucus

• Couples with unexplained infertility

What is assisted reproductive technology (ART)?

Assisted reproductive technology is a group of different methods used to help infertile couples. ART works by removing eggs from a woman's body. The eggs are then mixed with sperm to make embryos. The embryos are then put back in the woman's body. Success rates vary and depend on many factors.

The Centers for Disease Control and Prevention (CDC) collects success rates on ART for some fertility clinics. The average percentage of ART cycles that led to a live birth were the following in 2010:

• 42% in women younger than 35 years of age

• 32% in women aged 35–37 years

• 22% in women aged 38–40 years

• 12% in women aged 41–42 years

• 5% in women aged 43–44 years

ART can be expensive and time consuming. But it has allowed many couples to have children who otherwise would not have been conceived. The most common complication of ART is multiple fetuses. But this is a problem that can be prevented or minimized in several different ways.

What are the different types of ART?

Common methods of ART include the following:

- **In vitro fertilization (IVF)** means fertilization outside of the body. IVF is the most effective ART. It is often used when a woman's fallopian tubes are blocked or when a man produces too few sperm. Doctors treat the woman with a drug that causes the ovaries to produce multiple eggs. Once mature, the eggs are removed from the woman. They are put in a dish in the lab along with the man's sperm for fertilization. After three to five days, healthy embryos are implanted in the woman's uterus.

- **Zygote intrafallopian transfer (ZIFT) or tubal embryo transfer** is similar to IVF. Fertilization occurs in the laboratory. Then the very young embryo is transferred to the fallopian tube instead of the uterus.

- **Gamete intrafallopian transfer (GIFT)** involves transferring eggs and sperm into the woman's fallopian tube. So fertilization occurs in the woman's body. Few practices offer GIFT as an option.

- **Intracytoplasmic sperm injection (ICSI)** is often used for couples in which there are serious problems with the sperm. Sometimes it is also used for older couples or for those with failed IVF attempts. In ICSI, a single sperm is injected into a mature egg. Then the embryo is transferred to the uterus or fallopian tube.

ART procedures sometimes involve the use of donor eggs (eggs from another woman), donor sperm, or previously frozen embryos. Donor eggs are sometimes used for women who cannot produce eggs. Also, donor eggs or donor sperm is sometimes used when the woman or man has a genetic disease that can be passed on to the baby. An infertile woman or couple may also use donor embryos. These are embryos that were either created by couples in infertility treatment or were created from donor sperm and donor eggs. The donated embryo is transferred to the uterus. The child will not be genetically related to either parent.

Surrogacy: Women with no eggs or unhealthy eggs might also want to consider surrogacy. A surrogate is a woman who agrees to become pregnant using the man's sperm and her own egg. The child will be genetically related to the surrogate and the male partner. After birth, the surrogate will give up the baby for adoption by the parents.

Gestational carrier: Women with ovaries but no uterus may be able to use a gestational carrier. This may also be an option for women who shouldn't become pregnant because of a serious health problem. In this case, a woman uses her own egg. It is fertilized by the man's sperm and the embryo is placed inside the carrier's uterus. The carrier will not be related to the baby and gives him or her to the parents at birth.

Recent research by the Centers for Disease Control showed that ART babies are two to four times more likely to have certain kinds of birth defects. These may include heart and digestive system problems and cleft (divided into two pieces) lips or palate. Researchers don't know why this happens. The birth defects may not be due to the technology. Other factors, like the age of the parents, may be involved. More research is needed. The risk is relatively low, but parents should consider this when making the decision to use ART.

Chapter 33

Having a Healthy Pregnancy

Chapter Contents

Section 33.1

Preconception and Prenatal Care

Excerpted from "Prenatal Care Fact Sheet," U.S. Department
of Health and Human Services Office on Women's Health
(www.womenshealth.gov), March 6, 2009.

What is prenatal care?

Prenatal care is the health care you get while you are pregnant.
Take care of yourself and your baby by the following:

- Get **early** prenatal care. If you know you're pregnant, or think
  you might be, call your doctor to schedule a visit.

- Get **regular** prenatal care. Your doctor will schedule you for
  many checkups over the course of your pregnancy. Don't miss
  any—they are all important.

- Follow your doctor's advice.

Prenatal care can help keep you and your baby healthy. Babies of
mothers who do not get prenatal care are three times more likely to
have a low birth weight and five times more likely to die than those
born to mothers who do get care.

Doctors can spot health problems early when they see mothers regularly.
This allows doctors to treat them early. Early treatment can cure many
problems and prevent others. Doctors also can talk to pregnant women
about things they can do to give their unborn babies a healthy start to life.

I am thinking about getting pregnant. How can I take care of myself?

You should start taking care of yourself before you start trying to
get pregnant. This is called preconception health. It means knowing
how health conditions and risk factors could affect you or your unborn
baby if you become pregnant. For example, some foods, habits, and
medicines can harm your baby—even before he or she is conceived.
Some health problems also can affect pregnancy.

Talk to your doctor before pregnancy to learn what you can do to prepare your body. Women should prepare for pregnancy before becoming sexually active. Ideally, women should give themselves at least three months to prepare before getting pregnant.

The five most important things you can do before becoming pregnant are the following:

- Take 400 to 800 micrograms (400 to 800 mcg or 0.4 to 0.8 mg) of folic acid every day for at least three months before getting pregnant to lower your risk of some birth defects of the brain and spine. It's hard to get all the folic acid you need from foods alone. Taking a vitamin with folic acid is the best and easiest way to be sure you're getting enough.

- Stop smoking and drinking alcohol. Ask your doctor for help.

- If you have a medical condition, be sure it is under control. Some conditions include asthma, diabetes, depression, high blood pressure, obesity, thyroid disease, or epilepsy. Be sure your vaccinations are up to date.

- Talk to your doctor about any over-the-counter and prescription medicines you are using. These include dietary or herbal supplements. Some medicines are not safe during pregnancy. However, stopping medicines you need also can be harmful.

- Avoid contact with toxic substances or materials at work and at home that could be harmful. Stay away from chemicals and cat or rodent feces.

I'm pregnant. What should I do—or not do—to take care of myself and my unborn baby?

Follow these dos and don'ts to take care of yourself and the precious life growing inside you:

Health Care

- Get early and regular prenatal care. Your doctor will check to make sure you and the baby are healthy at each visit. If there are any problems, early action will help you and the baby.

- Take a multivitamin or prenatal vitamin with 400 to 800 micrograms of folic acid every day. Folic acid is most important in the early stages of pregnancy, but you should continue taking folic acid throughout pregnancy.

- Ask your doctor before stopping any medicines or starting any new medicines. Some medicines are not safe during pregnancy. Keep in mind that even over-the-counter medicines and herbal products may cause side effects or other problems. But not using medicines you need could also be harmful.

- Avoid X-rays. If you must have dental work or diagnostic tests, tell your dentist or doctor that you are pregnant so that extra care can be taken.

- Get a flu shot.

Food

- Eat a variety of healthy foods. Choose fruits, vegetables, whole grains, calcium-rich foods, and foods low in saturated fat. Also, make sure to drink plenty of fluids, especially water.

- Get all the nutrients you need each day, including iron. Getting enough iron prevents you from getting anemia, which is linked to preterm birth and low birth weight. Eating a variety of healthy foods will help you get the nutrients your baby needs. But ask your doctor if you need to take a daily prenatal vitamin or iron supplement to be sure you are getting enough.

- Protect yourself and your baby from food-borne illnesses, including toxoplasmosis and listeria. Wash fruits and vegetables before eating. Don't eat uncooked or undercooked meats or fish. Always handle, clean, cook, eat, and store foods properly.

- Don't eat fish with lots of mercury, including swordfish, king mackerel, shark, and tilefish.

Lifestyle

- Gain a healthy amount of weight. Your doctor can tell you how much weight gain you should aim for during pregnancy.

- Don't smoke, drink alcohol, or use drugs. These can cause long-term harm or death to your baby. Ask your doctor for help quitting.

- Unless your doctor tells you not to, try to get at least 2 hours and 30 minutes of moderate-intensity aerobic activity a week. It's best to spread out your workouts throughout the week. If you worked out regularly before pregnancy, you can keep up your activity level as long as your health doesn't change and you talk to your doctor about your activity level.

- Don't take very hot baths or use hot tubs or saunas.

- Get plenty of sleep and find ways to control stress.

- Get informed. Read books, watch videos, go to a childbirth class, and talk with moms you know.

- Ask your doctor about childbirth education classes for you and your partner to help you prepare for the birth of your baby.

Environmental

- Stay away from chemicals like insecticides, solvents (like some cleaners or paint thinners), lead, mercury, and paint (including paint fumes). Not all products have pregnancy warnings on their labels. If you're unsure if a product is safe, ask your doctor before using it.

- If you have a cat, ask your doctor about toxoplasmosis. This infection is caused by a parasite sometimes found in cat feces. If not treated, toxoplasmosis can cause birth defects. You can lower your risk of by avoiding cat litter and wearing gloves when gardening.

- Avoid contact with rodents, including pet rodents, and with their urine, droppings, or nesting material. Rodents can carry a virus that can be harmful or even deadly to your unborn baby.

- Take steps to avoid illness, such as washing hands frequently.

- Stay away from secondhand smoke.

How often should I see my doctor during pregnancy?

Your doctor will give you a schedule of all the doctor's visits you should have while pregnant. Most experts suggest you see your doctor at these times:

- About once each month for weeks 4 through 28

- Twice a month for weeks 28 through 36

- Weekly for weeks 36 to birth

If you are older than 35 or your pregnancy is high risk, you'll probably see your doctor more often.

What happens during prenatal visits?

During the first prenatal visit, you can expect your doctor to do the following:

- Ask about your health history including diseases, operations, or prior pregnancies

- Ask about your family's health history

- Do a complete physical exam, including a pelvic exam and Pap test

- Take your blood and urine for lab work

- Check your blood pressure, height, and weight

- Calculate your due date

- Answer your questions

At the first visit, you should ask questions and discuss any issues related to your pregnancy. Later prenatal visits will probably be shorter. Your doctor will check on your health and make sure the baby is growing as expected. Most prenatal visits will include these steps:

- Checking your blood pressure

- Measuring your weight gain

- Measuring your abdomen to check your baby's growth (once you begin to show)

- Checking the baby's heart rate

While you're pregnant, you also will have some routine tests. Some tests are suggested for all women. Other tests might be offered based on your age, health history, ethnic background, or the results of routine tests.

I am in my late thirties and I want to get pregnant. Should I do anything special?

As you age, you have an increasing chance of having a baby born with a birth defect. Yet most women in their late thirties and early forties have healthy babies. See your doctor regularly before you even start trying to get pregnant. She will be able to help you prepare your body for pregnancy. During your pregnancy, seeing your doctor regularly is very important. Because of your age, your doctor will probably suggest some extra tests to check on your baby's health.

More and more women are waiting until they are in their thirties and forties to have children. While many women of this age have no problems getting pregnant, fertility does decline with age. Women over

40 who don't get pregnant after six months of trying should see their doctors for a fertility evaluation.

Experts define infertility as the inability to become pregnant after trying for one year. If a woman keeps having miscarriages, it's also called infertility. If you think you or your partner may be infertile, talk to your doctor. Doctors are able to help many infertile couples go on to have healthy babies.

Where can I go to get free or reduced-cost prenatal care?

Women in every state can get help to pay for medical care during their pregnancies. This prenatal care can help you have a healthy baby. Programs give medical care, information, advice, and other services important for a healthy pregnancy.

To find out about the program in your state:

- Call 800-311-BABY (800-311-2229). This toll-free telephone number will connect you to the Health Department in your area code.

- For information in Spanish, call 800-504-7081.

- Contact your local Health Department.

Section 33.2

Pregnancy and Medicines

Excerpted from "Pregnancy and Medicines Fact Sheet,"
U.S. Department of Health and Human Services Office on Women's
Health (www.womenshealth.gov), April 14, 2010.

When deciding whether or not to use a medicine in pregnancy, you and your doctor need to talk about the medicine's benefits and risks.

There may be times during pregnancy when using medicine is a choice. Some of the medicine choices you and your doctor make while you are pregnant may differ from the choices you make when you are not pregnant. For example, if you get a cold, you may decide to "live with" your stuffy nose instead of using the "stuffy nose" medicine you use when you are not pregnant.

Other times, using medicine is not a choice—it is needed. Some women need to use medicines while they are pregnant. Sometimes, women need medicine for a few days or a couple of weeks to treat a problem like a bladder infection or strep throat. Other women need to use medicine every day to control long-term health problems like asthma, diabetes, depression, or seizures. Also, some women have a pregnancy problem that needs treatment with medicine.

Information on the Risks and Benefits of Medicine Use during Pregnancy

Doctors and nurses get information from medicine labels and packages, textbooks, and research journals. They also share knowledge with other doctors and nurses and talk to the people who make and sell medicines.

The U.S. Food and Drug Administration (FDA) is the part of our country's government that controls the medicines that can and can't be sold in the United States. Companies that make medicines usually have to show FDA doctors and scientists whether birth defects or other problems occur in baby animals when the medicine is given to pregnant animals. Most of the time, drugs are not studied in pregnant women.

The FDA works with the drug companies to make clear and complete medicine labels. But in most cases, there is not much information about how a medicine affects pregnant women and their growing babies.

To help doctors, the FDA created pregnancy letter categories to help explain what is known about using medicine during pregnancy. The letter category is listed in the label of a prescription medicine. The label states whether studies were done in pregnant women or pregnant animals and if so, what happened. Over-the-counter (OTC) medicines do not have a pregnancy letter category. Talk to your doctor and follow the instructions on the label before taking OTC medicines.

Prescription Medicines

The FDA chooses a medicine's letter category based on what is known about the medicine when used in pregnant women and animals.

Category A: In human studies, pregnant women used the medicine and their babies did not have any problems related to using the medicine. This includes folic acid and levothyroxine (thyroid hormone medicine).

Category B: In humans, there are no good studies. But in animal studies, pregnant animals received the medicine, and the babies did not show any problems related to the medicine, OR in animal studies, pregnant animals received the medicine, and some babies had problems, but in human studies, pregnant women used the medicine and their babies did not have any problems related to using the medicine. This includes the following:

- Some antibiotics like amoxicillin

- Zofran (ondansetron) for nausea

- Glucophage (metformin) for diabetes

- Some insulins used to treat diabetes such as regular and NPH insulin

Category C: In humans, there are no good studies. In animals, pregnant animals treated with the medicine had some babies with problems. However, sometimes the medicine may still help the human mothers and babies more than it might harm, OR no animal studies have been done, and there are no good studies in pregnant women.

- Diflucan (fluconazole) for yeast infections
- Ventolin (albuterol) for asthma
- Zoloft (sertraline) and Prozac (fluoxetine) for depression

Category D: Studies in humans and other reports show that when pregnant women use the medicine, some babies are born with problems related to the medicine. However, in some serious situations, the medicine may still help the mother and the baby more than it might harm.

- Paxil (paroxetine) for depression
- Lithium for bipolar disorder
- Dilantin (phenytoin) for epileptic seizures
- Some cancer chemotherapy

Category X: Studies or reports in humans or animals show that mothers using the medicine during pregnancy may have babies with problems related to the medicine. There are no situations where the medicine can help the mother or baby enough to make the risk of problems worth it. These medicines should never be used by pregnant women.

- Accutane (isotretinoin) for cystic acne
- Thalomid (thalidomide) for a type of skin disease

Medicine label information for prescription medicines is now changing, and the pregnancy part of the label will change over the next few years. As this prescription information is updated, it is added to an online information clearinghouse called DailyMed that gives up-to-date, free information to consumers and health care providers.

OTC Medicines

Things like caffeine, vitamins, and herbal remedies can affect the growing fetus. Talk with your doctor about cutting down on caffeine and ask which type of vitamin you should take. Never use an herbal product without talking to your doctor first.

All OTC medicines have a Drug Facts label. One section of the Drug Facts label is for pregnant women. With OTC medicines, the label usually tells a pregnant woman to speak with her doctor before using the medicine. Some OTC medicines are known to cause certain problems in pregnancy. The labels for these medicines give pregnant women facts about why and when they should not use the medicine.

Preconception

If you are not pregnant yet, you can help your chances for having a healthy baby by planning ahead. Schedule a pre-pregnancy checkup. At this visit, you can talk to your doctor about the medicines, vitamins, and herbs you use. It is very important that you keep treating your health problems while you are pregnant. Your doctor can tell you if you need to switch your medicine. Ask about vitamins for women who are trying to get pregnant. All women who can get pregnant should take a daily vitamin with folic acid (a B vitamin) to prevent birth defects of the brain and spinal cord.

Using Medicine during Pregnancy

Whether or not you should use medicine during pregnancy is a serious question to discuss with your doctor. Some health problems need treatment. Not using a medicine that you need could harm you and your baby. For example, a urinary tract infection (UTI) that is not treated may become a kidney infection. Kidney infections can cause preterm labor and low birth weight.

For women living with HIV, the Centers for Disease Control and Prevention (CDC) recommends using zidovudine (AZT) during pregnancy. Studies show that HIV -positive women who use AZT during pregnancy greatly lower the risk of passing HIV to their babies. If a diabetic woman does not use her medicine during pregnancy, she raises her risk for miscarriage, stillbirth, and some birth defects. If asthma and high blood pressure are not controlled during pregnancy, problems with the fetus may result.

Vitamins

Women who are pregnant should not take regular vitamins. They can contain doses that are too high. Ask about special vitamins for pregnant women that can help keep you and your baby healthy. These prenatal vitamins should contain at least 400–800 micrograms of folic acid. It is best to start taking these vitamins before you become pregnant or if you could become pregnant. Folic acid reduces the chance of a baby having a neural tube defect, like spina bifida, where the spine or brain does not form the right way. Iron can help prevent a low red blood cell count (anemia). It's important to take the vitamin dose prescribed by your doctor. Too many vitamins can harm your baby. For example, very high levels of vitamin A have been linked with severe birth defects.

Herbs, Minerals, or Amino Acids

No one is sure if these are safe for pregnant women, so it's best not to use them. Even some "natural" products may not be good for women who are pregnant or breastfeeding. Except for some vitamins, little is known about using dietary supplements while pregnant. Some herbal remedy labels claim that they will help with pregnancy. But most often there are no good studies to show if these claims are true or if the herb can cause harm to you or your baby. Talk with your doctor before using any herbal product or dietary supplement.

Pregnancy Exposure Registries

At this time, drugs are rarely tested for safety in pregnant women for fear of harming the unborn baby. Until this changes, pregnancy exposure registries help doctors and researchers learn how medicines affect pregnant mothers and their growing babies. A pregnancy exposure registry is a study that enrolls pregnant women who are using a certain medicine. The women sign up for the study while pregnant and are followed for a certain length of time after the baby is born. This type of study compares large groups of pregnant mothers and babies to look for medicine effects. A woman and her doctor can use registry results to make more informed choices about using medicine while pregnant.

If you are pregnant and are using a medicine or were using one when you got pregnant, check to see if there is a pregnancy exposure registry for that medicine. The Food and Drug Administration has a list of pregnancy exposure registries (at www.fda.gov/ScienceResearch/SpecialTopics/WomensHealthResearch/ucm134848.htm) that pregnant women can join.

Section 33.3

Nutrition and Fitness during Pregnancy

Excerpted from "Staying Healthy and Safe,"
U.S. Department of Health and Human Services Office on Women's
Health (www.womenshealth.gov), September 27, 2010.

Eating for Two

When pregnant, you need more protein, iron, calcium, and folic acid than you did before pregnancy. You also need more calories. But "eating for two" doesn't mean eating twice as much. Rather, it means that the foods you eat are the main source of nutrients for your baby. Sensible, balanced meals combined with regular physical fitness is still the best recipe for good health during your pregnancy.

Weight Gain

The amount of weight you should gain during pregnancy depends on your body mass index (BMI; see www.nhlbisupport.com/bmi/) before you became pregnant. The Institute of Medicine provides these guidelines:

- If you were at a normal weight before pregnancy, you should gain about 25 to 30 pounds.

- If you were underweight before pregnancy, you should gain between 28 and 40 pounds.

- If you were overweight before pregnancy, you should gain between 15 and 25 pounds.

- If you were obese before pregnancy, you should gain between 11 and 20 pounds.

Check with your doctor to find out how much weight gain during pregnancy is healthy for you. You should gain weight gradually during your pregnancy, with most of the weight gained in the last trimester. Generally, doctors suggest women gain weight at the following rate:

- Two to four pounds total during the first trimester
- Three to four pounds per month for the second and third trimesters

Where does the added weight go?
- Baby: 6 to 8 pounds
- Placenta: 1 1/2 pounds
- Amniotic fluid: 2 pounds
- Uterus growth: 2 pounds
- Breast growth: 2 pounds
- Your blood and body fluids: 8 pounds
- Your body's protein and fat: 7 pounds

Recent research shows that women who gain more than the recommended amount during pregnancy and who fail to lose this weight within six months after giving birth are at much higher risk of being obese nearly 10 years later. Findings from another large study suggest that gaining more weight than the recommended amount during pregnancy may raise your child's odds of being overweight in the future. If you find that you are gaining weight too quickly, try to cut back on foods with added sugars and solid fats. If you are not gaining enough weight, you can eat a little more from each food group.

Calorie Needs

Your calorie needs will depend on your weight gain goals. Most women need 300 calories a day more during at least the last six months of pregnancy than they do pre-pregnancy. Keep in mind that not all calories are equal. Your baby needs healthy foods that are packed with nutrients—not "empty calories" such as those found in soft drinks, candies, and desserts.

Although you want to be careful not to eat more than you need for a healthy pregnancy, make sure not to restrict your diet during pregnancy either. If you don't get the calories you need, your baby might not get the right amounts of protein, vitamins, and minerals. Low-calorie diets can break down a pregnant woman's stored fat. This can cause your body to make substances called ketones. Ketones can be found in the mother's blood and urine and are a sign of starvation. Constant production of ketones can result in a child with mental deficiencies.

Foods Good for Mom and Baby

A pregnant woman needs more of many important vitamins, minerals, and nutrients than she did before pregnancy. Making healthy food choices every day will help you give your baby what he or she needs to develop. The MyPlate for pregnant and breastfeeding women (at www.choosemyplate.gov/pregnancy-breastfeeding.html) can provide advice on what you need to eat. Use your personal MyPlate plan to guide your daily food choices.

Talk to your doctor if you have special diet needs for these reasons:

- **Diabetes:** Make sure you review your meal plan and insulin needs with your doctor. High blood glucose levels can be harmful to your baby.

- **Lactose intolerance:** Find out about low-lactose or reduced-lactose products and calcium supplements to ensure you are getting the calcium you need.

- **Vegetarian:** Ensure that you are getting enough protein, iron, vitamin B12, and vitamin D.

- **PKU:** Keep good control of phenylalanine levels in your diet.

Food Safety

Most foods are safe for pregnant women and their babies. But you will need to use caution or avoid eating certain foods. Follow these guidelines:

Clean, handle, cook, and chill food properly to prevent foodborne illness, including listeria and toxoplasmosis.

- Wash hands with soap after touching soil or raw meat.

- Keep raw meats, poultry, and seafood from touching other foods or surfaces.

- Cook meat completely.

- Wash produce before eating.

- Wash cooking utensils with hot, soapy water.

Do not eat the following:

- Refrigerated smoked seafood like whitefish, salmon, and mackerel

- Hot dogs or deli meats unless steaming hot

- Refrigerated meat spreads

- Unpasteurized milk or juices

- Store-made salads, such as chicken, egg, or tuna salad

- Unpasteurized soft cheeses, such as unpasteurized feta, Brie, queso blanco, queso fresco, and blue cheeses

- Shark, swordfish, king mackerel, or tilefish (also called golden or white snapper); these fish have high levels of mercury

- More than six ounces per week of white (albacore) tuna

- Herbs and plants used as medicines without your doctor's okay

- Raw sprouts of any kind

Fish Facts

Fish and shellfish can be an important part of a healthy diet. They are a great source of protein and heart-healthy omega-3 fatty acids. What's more, some researchers believe low fish intake may be linked to depression in women during and after pregnancy. Research also suggests that omega-3 fatty acids consumed by pregnant women may aid in babies' brain and eye development.

Women who are or may become pregnant and nursing mothers need 12 ounces of fish per week to reap the health benefits. Unfortunately, some pregnant and nursing women do not eat any fish because they worry about mercury in seafood. Mercury is a metal that at high levels can harm the brain of your unborn baby—even before it is conceived. Mercury mainly gets into our bodies by eating large, predatory fish. Yet many types of seafood have little or no mercury at all. So the risk of mercury exposure depends on the amount and type of seafood you eat.

Women who are nursing, pregnant, or who may become pregnant can safely eat a variety of cooked seafood but should steer clear of fish with high levels of mercury. Keep in mind that removing all fish from your diet will rob you of important omega-3 fatty acids. To reach 12 ounces while limiting exposure to mercury, follow these tips:

- Do not eat these fish that are high in mercury:
  - Swordfish
  - Tilefish
  - King mackerel
  - Shark

- Eat up to 6 ounces (about one serving) per week:

- Canned albacore or chunk white tuna (also sold as tuna steaks), which has more mercury than canned light tuna

- Eat up to 12 ounces (about two servings) per week of cooked* fish and shellfish with little or no mercury, such as the following:

  - Shrimp
  - Crab
  - Clams
  - Oysters
  - Scallops
  - Canned light tuna
  - Salmon
  - Pollock
  - Catfish
  - Cod
  - Tilapia

  *Don't eat uncooked fish or shellfish (such as clams, oysters, scallops), which includes refrigerated uncooked seafood labeled nova-style, lox, kippered, smoked, or jerky.

- Check before eating fish caught in local waters. State health departments have guidelines on fish from local waters. Or get local fish advisories at the U.S. Environmental Protection Agency (www.epa.gov). If you are unsure about the safety of a fish from local waters, only eat six ounces per week and don't eat any other fish that week.

- Eat a variety of cooked seafood rather than just a few types.

Foods supplemented with DHA/EPA (such as "omega-3 eggs") and prenatal vitamins supplemented with DHA are other sources of the type of omega-3 fatty acids found in seafood.

Vitamins and Minerals

In addition to making healthy food choices, ask your doctor about taking a prenatal vitamin and mineral supplement every day to be sure you are getting enough of the nutrients your baby needs. You also can check the label on the foods you buy to see how much of a certain nutrient the product contains. Women who are pregnant need more of these nutrients than women who are not pregnant:

- **Folic acid:** 400 to 800 micrograms (mcg; 0.4 to 0.8 mg) in the early stages of pregnancy, which is why all women who are capable of pregnancy should take a daily multivitamin that contains 400 to 800 mcg of folic acid (pregnant women should continue taking folic acid throughout pregnancy)

- **Iron:** 27 milligrams (mg)

- **Calcium:** 1,000 mg; 1,300 mg if 18 or younger

- **Vitamin A:** 770 mcg; 750 mcg if 18 or younger

- **Vitamin B12:** 2.6 mcg

Women who are pregnant also need to be sure to get enough vitamin D. The current recommendation for all adults younger than 71 (including pregnant and breastfeeding women) is 600 international units (IU) of vitamin D each day.

Keep in mind that taking too much of a supplement can be harmful. For example, very high levels of vitamin A can cause birth defects. For this reason, your daily prenatal vitamin should contain no more than 5,000 IU of vitamin A.

Don't Forget Fluids

All your body's systems need water. When you are pregnant, your body needs even more water to stay hydrated and support the life inside you. Water also helps prevent constipation, hemorrhoids, excessive swelling, and urinary tract or bladder infections. Not getting enough water can lead to premature or early labor.

Your body gets the water it needs through the fluids you drink and the foods you eat. How much fluid you need to drink each day depends on many factors, such as your activity level, the weather, and your size. Your body needs more fluids when it is hot and when you are physically active.

The Institute of Medicine recommends that pregnant women drink about 10 cups of fluids daily. Water, juices, coffee, tea, and soft drinks all count toward your fluid needs. But keep in mind that some beverages are high in sugar and "empty" calories. A good way to tell if your fluid intake is okay is if your urine is pale yellow or colorless and you rarely feel thirsty. Thirst is a sign that your body is on its way to dehydration. Don't wait until you feel thirsty to drink.

Alcohol: There is no known safe amount of alcohol a woman can drink while pregnant. When you are pregnant and you drink beer, wine, hard liquor, or other alcoholic beverages, alcohol gets into your blood. The alcohol in your blood gets into your baby's body through the umbilical cord. Alcohol can slow down the baby's growth, affect the baby's brain, and cause birth defects.

Caffeine: Moderate amounts of caffeine appear to be safe during pregnancy. Moderate means less than 200 mg of caffeine per day, which is the amount in about 12 ounces of coffee. Most caffeinated teas and soft drinks have much less caffeine. Some studies have shown a link between higher amounts of caffeine and miscarriage and preterm birth. But there is no solid proof that caffeine causes these problems. Ask your doctor whether drinking a limited amount of caffeine is okay for you.

Cravings

Many women have strong desires for specific foods during pregnancy. The desire for "pickles and ice cream" and other cravings might be caused by changes in nutritional needs during pregnancy. The fetus needs nourishment. And a woman's body absorbs and processes nutrients differently while pregnant. These changes help ensure normal development of the baby and fill the demands of breastfeeding once the baby is born.

Some women crave nonfood items such as clay, ice, laundry starch, or cornstarch. A desire to eat nonfood items is called pica. Eating nonfood items can be harmful. Talk to your doctor if you have these urges.

Keeping Fit

Fitness goes hand in hand with eating right to maintain your physical health and well-being during pregnancy. Pregnant or not, physical fitness helps keep the heart, bones, and mind healthy. Healthy pregnant women should get at least 2 hours and 30 minutes of moderate-intensity aerobic activity a week. It's best to spread your workouts throughout the week. If you regularly engage in vigorous-intensity aerobic activity or high amounts of activity, you can keep up your activity level as long as your health doesn't change and you talk to your doctor about your activity level throughout your pregnancy.

There are special benefits to physical activity during pregnancy:

- Exercise can ease and prevent aches and pains of pregnancy including constipation, varicose veins, backaches, and exhaustion.

- Active women seem to be better prepared for labor and delivery and recover more quickly.

- Exercise may lower the risk of preeclampsia and gestational diabetes during pregnancy.

- Fit women have an easier time getting back to a healthy weight after delivery.

- Regular exercise may improve sleep during pregnancy.

- Staying active can protect your emotional health. Pregnant women who exercise seem to have better self-esteem and a lower risk of depression and anxiety.

- Results from a recent, large study suggest that women who are physically active during pregnancy may lower their chances of preterm delivery.

Getting Started

For most healthy moms-to-be who do not have any pregnancy-related problems, exercise is a safe and valuable habit. Even so, talk to your doctor or midwife before exercising during pregnancy. If you have one of these conditions, your doctor will advise you not to exercise:

- Risk factors for preterm labor

- Vaginal bleeding

- Premature rupture of membranes (when your water breaks early, before labor)

Best Activity for Moms-to-Be

Low-impact activities at a moderate level of effort are comfortable and enjoyable for many pregnant women. Walking, swimming, dancing, cycling, and low-impact aerobics are some examples. These sports also are easy to take up, even if you are new to physical fitness.

Some higher intensity sports are safe for some pregnant women who were already doing them before becoming pregnant. If you jog, play racquet sports, or lift weights, you may continue with your doctor's okay.

Keep these points in mind when choosing a fitness plan:

- Avoid activities in which you can get hit in the abdomen like kickboxing, soccer, basketball, or ice hockey.

- Steer clear of activities in which you can fall like horseback riding, downhill skiing, and gymnastics.

- Do not scuba dive during pregnancy. Scuba diving can create gas bubbles in your baby's blood that can cause many health problems.

Tips for Safe and Healthy Physical Activity

Follow these tips for safe and healthy fitness:

- When you exercise, start slowly, progress gradually, and cool down slowly.

- You should be able to talk while exercising. If not, you may be overdoing it.

- Take frequent breaks.

- Don't exercise on your back after the first trimester. This can put too much pressure on an important vein and limit blood flow to the baby.

- Avoid jerky, bouncing, and high-impact movements. Connective tissues stretch much more easily during pregnancy.

- Be careful not to lose your balance. As your baby grows, your center of gravity shifts making you more prone to falls.

- Don't exercise at high altitudes (more than 6,000 feet). It can prevent your baby from getting enough oxygen.

- Make sure you drink lots of fluids before, during, and after exercising.

- Do not work out in extreme heat or humidity.

- If you feel uncomfortable, short of breath, or tired, take a break and take it easier when you exercise again.

Stop exercising and call your doctor as soon as possible if you have any of the following:

- Dizziness

- Headache

- Chest pain

- Calf pain or swelling

- Abdominal pain

- Blurred vision

- Fluid leaking from the vagina

- Vaginal bleeding

- Less fetal movement

- Contractions

Work Out Your Pelvic Floor (Kegel Exercises)

Your pelvic floor muscles support the rectum, vagina, and urethra in the pelvis. Toning these muscles with Kegel exercises will help you push during delivery and recover from birth. It also will help control bladder leakage and lower your chance of getting hemorrhoids.

Pelvic muscles are the same ones used to stop the flow of urine. You can be sure you are exercising the right muscles if when you squeeze them you stop urinating. Or you can put a finger into the vagina and squeeze. If you feel pressure around the finger, you've found the pelvic floor muscles. Try not to tighten your stomach, legs, or other muscles.

- Tighten the pelvic floor muscles for a count of three, then relax for a count of three.

- Repeat 10 to 15 times, three times a day.

- Start Kegel exercises lying down. This is the easiest position. When your muscles get stronger, you can do Kegel exercises sitting or standing as you like.

Chapter 34

The Birth of Your Baby

Chapter Contents

Section 34.1

Labor and Delivery Basics

Excerpted from "Labor and Birth," U.S. Department of Health and
Human Services Office on Women's Health (www.womenshealth.gov),
September 27, 2010.

Spot the Signs of Labor

As you approach your due date, you will be looking for any little
sign that labor is about to start. You might notice that your baby has
"dropped" or moved lower into your pelvis. This is called "lightening."
If you have a pelvic exam during your prenatal visit, your doctor might
report changes in your cervix that you cannot feel but that suggest your
body is getting ready. For some women, a flurry of energy and the im-
pulse to cook or clean, called "nesting," is a sign that labor is approaching.

Some signs suggest that labor will begin very soon. Call your doctor
or midwife if you have any of the following signs of labor. Call your
doctor even if it's weeks before your due date—you might be going into
preterm labor. Your doctor or midwife can decide if it's time to go to
the hospital or if you should be seen at the office first.

- You have contractions that become stronger at regular and
  increasingly shorter intervals.

- You have lower back pain and cramping that does not go away.

- Your water breaks (can be a large gush or a continuous trickle).

- You have a bloody (brownish or red-tinged) mucus discharge.
  This is probably the mucus plug that blocks the cervix. Losing
  your mucus plug usually means your cervix is dilating (opening
  up) and becoming thinner and softer (effacing). Labor could start
  right away or may still be days away.

Did my water break?

It's not always easy to know. If your water breaks, it could be a
gush or a slow trickle of amniotic fluid. Rupture of membranes is the
medical term for your water breaking. Let your doctor know the time

your water breaks and any color or odor. Also, call your doctor if you think your water broke but are not sure. An easy test can tell your doctor if the leaking fluid is urine (many pregnant women leak urine) or amniotic fluid. Often a woman will go into labor soon after her water breaks. When this doesn't happen, her doctor may want to induce (bring about) labor. This is because once your water breaks, your risk of getting an infection goes up as labor is delayed.

False Labor

Many women, especially first-time mothers-to-be, think they are in labor when they're not. This is called false labor. "Practice" contractions called Braxton Hicks contractions are common in the last weeks of pregnancy or earlier. The tightening of your uterus might startle you. Some might even be painful or take your breath away. It's no wonder that many women mistake Braxton Hicks contractions for the real thing. So don't feel embarrassed if you go to the hospital thinking you're in labor, only to be sent home.

So how can you tell if your contractions are true labor?

Time them. Use a watch or clock to keep track of the time one contraction starts to the time the next contraction starts, as well as how long each contraction lasts. With true labor, contractions become regular, stronger, and more frequent. Braxton Hicks contractions are not in a regular pattern, and they taper off and go away. Some women find that a change in activity, such as walking or lying down, makes Braxton Hicks contractions go away. This won't happen with true labor. Even with these guidelines, it can be hard to tell if labor is real. If you ever are unsure if contractions are true labor, call your doctor.

Stages of Labor

Labor occurs in three stages. When regular contractions begin, the baby moves down into the pelvis as the cervix both effaces (thins) and dilates (opens). How labor progresses and how long it lasts are different for every woman. But each stage features some milestones that are true for every woman.

First Stage

The first stage begins with the onset of labor and ends when the cervix is fully opened. It is the longest stage of labor, usually lasting about 12 to 19 hours. Many women spend the early part of this first stage at home. You might want to rest, watch TV, hang out with family, or even go for a walk. Most women can drink and eat during labor, which can provide needed energy later. Ask your doctor about eating during labor. While at home, time your contractions and keep your doctor up-to-date on your progress. Your doctor will tell you when to go to the hospital or birthing center.

At the hospital, your doctor will monitor the progress of your labor by periodically checking your cervix, as well as the baby's position and station (location in the birth canal). Most babies' heads enter the pelvis facing to one side and then rotate to face down. Sometimes, a baby will be facing up, toward the mother's abdomen. Intense back labor often goes along with this position. Your doctor might try to rotate the baby, or the baby might turn on its own.

As you near the end of the first stage of labor, contractions become longer, stronger, and closer together. Many of the positioning and relaxation tips you learned in childbirth class can help now. Try to find the most comfortable position during contractions and to let your muscles go limp between contractions.

Sometimes, medicines and other methods are used to help speed up labor that is progressing slowly. Many doctors will rupture the membranes. Although this practice is widely used, studies show that doing so during labor does not help shorten the length of labor.

Your doctor might want to use an electronic fetal monitor to see if blood supply to your baby is okay. For most women, this involves putting two straps around the mother's abdomen. One strap measures the strength and frequency of your contractions. The other strap records how the baby's heartbeat reacts to the contraction.

The most difficult phase of this first stage is the transition. Contractions are very powerful, with very little time to relax in between, as the cervix stretches the last few centimeters. The cervix is fully dilated when it reaches 10 centimeters.

Second Stage

The second stage involves pushing and delivery of your baby. It usually lasts 20 minutes to two hours. You will push hard during contractions and rest between contractions. A woman can give birth in many positions, such as squatting, sitting, kneeling, or lying back. You might find pushing to be easier or more comfortable one way, and you should be allowed to choose the birth position that feels best to you.

When the top of your baby's head fully appears (crowning), your doctor will tell you when to push and deliver your baby. Your doctor may make a small cut, called an episiotomy, to enlarge the vaginal opening. Most women in childbirth do not need episiotomy. Sometimes, forceps or suction is used to help guide the baby through the birth canal. This is called assisted vaginal delivery. After your baby is born, the umbilical cord is cut.

Third Stage

The third stage involves delivery of the placenta (afterbirth). It is the shortest stage, lasting 5 to 30 minutes. Contractions will begin 5 to 30 minutes after birth, signaling that it's time to deliver the placenta. You might have chills or shakiness. Labor is over once the placenta is delivered. Your doctor will repair the episiotomy and any tears you might have. Now you can rest and enjoy your newborn!

Managing Labor Pain

Virtually all women worry about how they will cope with the pain of labor and delivery. Childbirth is different for everyone. So no one can predict how you will feel.

Some women do fine with natural methods of pain relief alone. Many women blend natural methods with medications that relieve pain. Building a positive outlook on childbirth and managing fear may also help some women cope with the pain. It is important to realize that labor pain is not like pain due to illness or injury. Instead, it is caused by contractions of the uterus that are pushing your baby down and out of the birth canal. In other words, labor pain has a purpose.

Natural Methods of Pain Relief

Many natural methods help women to relax and make pain more manageable. Things women do to ease the pain include the following:

- Trying breathing and relaxation techniques

- Taking warm showers or baths

- Getting massages

- Using heat and cold, such as heat on lower back and cold wash-cloth on forehead

- Having the supportive care of a loved one, nurse, or doula

- Finding comfortable positions while in labor
- Using a labor ball
- Listening to music

Medical Methods of Pain Relief

While you're in labor, your doctor, midwife, or nurse should ask if you need pain relief. Nowadays women in labor have many pain relief options that work well and pose small risks when given by a trained and experienced doctor. Doctors also can use different methods for pain relief at different stages of labor. Still, not all options are available at every hospital and birthing center.

Keep in mind that rare but serious complications sometimes occur. Also, most medicines used to manage pain during labor pass freely into the placenta. Ask your doctor how pain relief methods might affect your baby or your ability to breastfeed after delivery.

Opioids: Also called narcotics, these medicines are given through a tube inserted in a vein or by injecting the medicine into a muscle. Opioids can make the pain bearable and don't affect your ability to push. After getting this kind of pain relief, you can still get an epidural or spinal block later.

- Opioids don't get rid of all the pain, and they are short-acting.
- They can make you feel sleepy and drowsy.
- They can cause nausea and vomiting.
- They can make you feel very itchy.
- Opioids cannot be given right before delivery because they may slow the baby's breathing and heart rate at birth.

Epidural and spinal blocks: An epidural involves placing a tube (catheter) into the lower back, into a small space below the spinal cord. Small doses of medicine can be given through the tube as needed throughout labor. With a spinal block, a small dose of medicine is given as a shot into the spinal fluid in the lower back. Spinal blocks usually are given only once during labor.

Epidural and spinal blocks allow most women to be awake and alert with very little pain during labor and childbirth. With epidural, pain relief starts 10 to 20 minutes after the medicine has been given. The degree of numbness you feel can be adjusted throughout your labor.

With spinal block, good pain relief starts right away, but it only lasts one to two hours.

- Although you can move, you might not be able to walk if the medicine used affects motor function.

- It can lower your blood pressure, which can slow your baby's heartbeat. Fluids given through IV are given to lower this risk.

- If the covering of the spinal cord is punctured, you can get a bad headache.

- You may experience backache for a few days after labor.

- Epidural can prolong the first and second stages of labor. If given late in labor or if too much medicine is used, it might be hard to push when the time comes. Studies show that epidural increases risk of assisted vaginal delivery.

Pudendal block: A doctor injects numbing medicine into the vagina and the nearby pudendal nerve. This nerve carries sensation to the lower part of your vagina and vulva.

This is only used late in labor, usually right before the baby's head comes out. With a pudendal block, you have some pain relief but remain awake, alert, and able to push the baby out.

- The baby is not affected by this medicine and it has very few disadvantages.

Inducing Labor

Sometimes, a doctor or midwife might need to induce (bring about) labor. The decision to induce labor often is made when a woman is past her due date but labor has not yet begun or when there is concern about the baby or mother's health. The doctor or midwife can use medicines and other methods to open a pregnant woman's cervix, stimulate contractions, and prepare for vaginal birth.

Elective labor induction has become more common in recent years. This is when labor is induced at term but for no medical reason. Some doctors may suggest elective induction due to a woman's discomfort, scheduling issues, or concern that waiting may lead to complications. But the benefits and harms of elective induction are not well understood. If your doctor suggests inducing labor, talk to your doctor about the possible harms and benefits for both mother and baby.

Cesarean Birth

Cesarean delivery, also called c-section, is surgery to deliver a baby. The baby is taken out through the mother's abdomen. Most cesarean births result in healthy babies and mothers. But c-section is major surgery and carries risks. Healing also takes longer than with vaginal birth.

Most healthy pregnant women with no risk factors for problems during labor or delivery have their babies vaginally. Still, the cesarean birth rate in the United States has risen greatly in recent decades. Today, nearly one in three women have babies by c-section in this country. The rate was one in five in 1995.

Public health experts think that many c-sections are unnecessary. So it is important for pregnant women to get the facts about c-sections before they deliver.

Your doctor might recommend a c-section if she or he thinks it is safer for you or your baby than vaginal birth. But most c-sections are done when unexpected problems happen during delivery.

Patient-Requested C-Section: Can a Woman Choose?

A growing number of women are asking their doctors for c-sections when there is no medical reason. But is it safe and ethical for doctors to allow women to choose c-section? The answer is unclear. Only more research on both types of deliveries will provide the answer.

Experts who believe c-sections should only be performed for medical reasons point to the risks. These include infection, dangerous bleeding, blood transfusions, and blood clots. Babies born by c-section have more breathing problems right after birth. Women who have c-sections stay at the hospital for longer than women who have vaginal births. Plus, recovery from this surgery takes longer and is often more painful than that after a vaginal birth. C-sections also increase the risk of problems in future pregnancies. Women who have had c-sections have a higher risk of uterine rupture. If the uterus ruptures, the life of the baby and mother is in danger.

Supporters of elective c-sections say that this surgery may protect a woman's pelvic organs, reduces the risk of bowel and bladder problems, and is as safe for the baby as vaginal delivery.

The C-Section Experience

Most c-sections are unplanned. So learning about c-sections is important for all women who are pregnant. Whether a c-section is planned or comes up during labor, it can be a positive birth experience for many women.

Before surgery: Cesarean delivery takes about 45 to 60 minutes. It takes place in an operating room. So if you were in a labor and delivery room, you will be moved to an operating room. A doctor will give you medicine through an epidural or spinal block, which will block the feeling of pain in part of your body but allow you to stay awake and alert. Medicine that makes you fall asleep and lose all awareness is usually only used in emergency situations. Your abdomen will be cleaned and prepped. You will have an IV for fluids and medicines. A nurse will insert a catheter to drain urine from your bladder. This is to protect the bladder from harm during surgery. Your heart rate, blood pressure, and breathing also will be monitored.

During surgery: The doctor will make two incisions. The first is about six inches long and goes through the skin, fat, and muscle. Most incisions are made side to side and low on the abdomen, called a bikini incision. Next, the doctor will make an incision to open the uterus. The opening is made just wide enough for the baby to fit through. One doctor will use a hand to support the baby while another doctor pushes the uterus to help push that baby out. Fluid will be suctioned out of your baby's mouth and nose. The doctor will hold up your baby for you to see. Once your baby is delivered, the umbilical cord is cut, and the placenta is removed. Then, the doctor cleans and stitches up the uterus and abdomen. The repair takes up most of the surgery time.

After surgery: You will be moved to a recovery room and monitored for a few hours. You might feel shaky, nauseated, and very sleepy. Later, you will be brought to a hospital room. When you and your baby are ready, you can hold, snuggle, and nurse your baby. C-section is major surgery, and recovery takes about six weeks (not counting the fatigue of new motherhood). In the weeks ahead, you will need to focus on healing, getting as much rest as possible, and bonding with your baby—nothing else. Be careful about taking on too much and accept help as needed.

Vaginal birth after c-section (VBAC): Some women who have delivered previous babies by c-section would like to have their next baby vaginally. This is called vaginal delivery after c-section, or VBAC. Today, VBAC is a reasonable and safe choice for most women with prior cesarean delivery, including some women who have had more than one cesarean delivery. Moreover, emerging evidence suggests that multiple c-sections can cause serious harm.

Choosing to try a VBAC is complex. If you are interested in a VBAC, talk to your doctor and read up on the subject. Only you and your doctor can decide what is best for you. VBACs and planned c-sections both have their benefits and risks. Learn the pros and cons and be aware of possible problems before you make your choice.

Section 34.2

Risks and Warning Signs of Premature Labor

"Premature Birth," Centers for Disease Control and Prevention
(www.cdc.gov), November 21, 2011.

More than a half million babies in the United States—that's one in every eight—are born premature each year. Premature birth is a birth that is at least three weeks before a baby's due date (less than 37 weeks—full term is 40 weeks).

Important growth and development occur throughout pregnancy—all the way through the final months and weeks. Although most babies born a few weeks early do well with no health consequences, some do have more health problems than full-term babies. For example, a baby born at 35 weeks is more likely to have jaundice, breathing problems, and longer hospital stays.

Most preterm deliveries happen spontaneously and without a known cause. Doctors sometimes decide to deliver a baby early because of concerns for the health of the mother or the baby. Medical intervention for an early delivery should only be considered when there is a medical reason to do so.

The more preterm a baby is born, the more severe his or her health problems are likely to be. Although babies born very preterm are a small percent of all births, preterm delivery is the most frequent cause of infant deaths. Some premature babies require special care and spend weeks or months hospitalized in a neonatal intensive care unit (NICU). Those who survive may face lifelong problems such as the following:

• Intellectual disabilities

388

- Cerebral palsy
- Breathing and respiratory problems
- Vision and hearing loss
- Feeding and digestive problems

Warning Signs of Preterm Labor

In most cases, preterm labor begins unexpectedly and with no known cause. The warning signs are the following:

- Contractions (abdomen tightens like a fist) every 10 minutes or more often
- Change in vaginal discharge (leaking fluid or bleeding from the vagina)
- Pelvic pressure—the feeling that the baby is pushing down
- Low, dull backache
- Cramps that feel like a menstrual period
- Abdominal cramps with or without diarrhea

Risk Factors

Even if a woman does everything "right" during pregnancy, she still can have a premature baby. There are some known risk factors for premature birth:

- Carrying more than one baby
- Having a previous preterm birth
- Black race
- Problems with the uterus or cervix
- Chronic health problems in the mother, such as high blood pressure, diabetes, and clotting disorders
- Certain infections during pregnancy
- Cigarette smoking, alcohol use, or illicit drug use during pregnancy

Preterm birth can happen to anyone, and most women who have a premature birth have no known risk factors. Birth is a complex and wonderful process. Fortunately, the outcome for most women is a full-term, healthy baby. More research still is needed to understand the risk factors for premature birth, such as how family history, genetics, infections, race and ethnicity, nutrition, and environment may interact to put some women at greater risk for a premature delivery.

Section 34.3

Maternal Health Benefits of Breastfeeding

Excerpted from "Your Guide to Breastfeeding," U.S. Department of Health and Human Services Office on Women's Health (www.womenshealth.gov), January 2011.

Mothers Benefit from Breastfeeding

Breastfeeding can make your life easier: Breastfeeding may take a little more effort than formula feeding at first. But it can make life easier once you and your baby settle into a good routine. When you breastfeed, there are no bottles and nipples to sterilize. You do not have to buy, measure, and mix formula. And there are no bottles to warm in the middle of the night.

Breastfeeding can save money: Formula and feeding supplies can cost well over $1,500 each year, depending on how much your baby eats. Breastfed babies are also sick less often, which can lower health care costs.

Breastfeeding can feel great: Physical contact is important to newborns. It can help them feel more secure, warm, and comforted. Mothers can benefit from this closeness, as well. Breastfeeding requires a mother to take some quiet relaxed time to bond. The skin-to-skin contact can boost the mother's oxytocin levels. Oxytocin is a hormone that helps milk flow and can calm the mother.

Breastfeeding can be good for the mother's health, too: Breastfeeding is linked to a lower risk of these health problems in women:

- Type 2 diabetes
- Breast cancer
- Ovarian cancer
- Postpartum depression

Experts are still looking at the effects of breastfeeding on osteoporosis and weight loss after birth. Many studies have reported greater weight loss for breastfeeding mothers than for those who don't. But more research is needed to understand if a strong link exists.

Nursing mothers miss less work: Breastfeeding mothers miss fewer days from work because their infants are sick less often.

Breastfeeding during an Emergency

When an emergency occurs, breastfeeding can save lives:

- Breastfeeding protects babies from the risks of a contaminated water supply.
- Breastfeeding can help protect against respiratory illnesses and diarrhea. These diseases can be fatal in populations displaced by disaster.
- Breast milk is the right temperature for babies and helps to prevent hypothermia when the body temperature drops too low.
- Breast milk is readily available without needing other supplies.

Breastfeeding Benefits Society

The nation benefits overall when mothers breastfeed. Recent research shows that if 90% of families breastfed exclusively for six months, nearly 1,000 deaths among infants could be prevented. The United States would also save $13 billion per year—medical care costs are lower for fully breastfed infants than for never-breastfed infants. Breastfed infants typically need fewer sick care visits, prescriptions, and hospitalizations.

Breastfeeding also contributes to a more productive workforce because mothers miss less work to care for sick infants. Employer medical costs are also lower.

Breastfeeding is also better for the environment. There is less trash and plastic waste compared to that produced by formula cans and bottle supplies.

Chapter 35

Recovering from Birth and Managing Postpartum Depression

Recovering from Birth

New mothers must take special care of their bodies after giving birth and while breastfeeding, too. Doing so will help you to regain your energy and strength. When you take care of yourself, you are able to best care for and enjoy your baby.

Getting Rest

The first few days at home after having your baby are a time for rest and recovery—physically and emotionally. You need to focus your energy on yourself and on getting to know your new baby. Even though you may be very excited and have requests for lots of visits from family and friends, try to limit visitors and get as much rest as possible. Don't expect to keep your house perfect. You may find that all you can do is eat, sleep, and care for your baby. And that is perfectly okay. Learn to pace yourself from the first day that you arrive back home. Try to lie down or nap while the baby naps. Don't try to do too much around the house. Allow others to help you and don't be afraid to ask for help with cleaning, laundry, meals, or with caring for the baby.

Excerpted from "Recovering from Birth," September 27, 2010, and "Depression during and after Pregnancy," March 6, 2009, U.S. Department of Health and Human Services Office on Women's Health (www.womenshealth.gov).

Physical Changes

After the birth of your baby, your doctor will talk with you about things you will experience as your body starts to recover.

- You will have vaginal discharge called lochia. It is the tissue and blood that lined your uterus during pregnancy. It is heavy and bright red at first, becoming lighter in flow and color until it goes aware after a few weeks.

- You might also have swelling in your legs and feet. You can reduce swelling by keeping your feet elevated when possible.

- You might feel constipated. Try to drink plenty of water and eat fresh fruits and vegetables.

- Menstrual-like cramping is common, especially if you are breastfeeding. Your breast milk will come in within three to six days after your delivery. Even if you are not breastfeeding, you can have milk leaking from your nipples, and your breasts might feel full, tender, or uncomfortable.

- Follow your doctor's instructions on how much activity, like climbing stairs or walking, you can do for the next few weeks.

Your doctor will check your recovery at your postpartum visit, about six weeks after birth. Ask about resuming normal activities, as well as eating and fitness plans to help you return to a healthy weight. Also ask your doctor about having sex and birth control. Your period could return in six to eight weeks, or sooner if you do not breastfeed. If you breastfeed, your period might not resume for many months. Still, using reliable birth control is the best way to prevent pregnancy until you want to have another baby.

Some women develop thyroid problems in the first year after giving birth. This is called postpartum thyroiditis. It often begins with overactive thyroid, which lasts two to four months. Most women then develop symptoms of an underactive thyroid, which can last up to a year. Thyroid problems are easy to overlook as many symptoms, such as fatigue, sleep problems, low energy, and changes in weight, are common after having a baby. Talk to your doctor if you have symptoms that do not go away. An underactive thyroid needs to be treated. In most cases, thyroid function returns to normal as the thyroid heals. But some women develop permanent underactive thyroid disease, called Hashimoto disease, and need lifelong treatment.

Regaining a Healthy Weight and Shape

The USDA's online, interactive tool at ChooseMyPlate.gov can help you choose foods based on your baby's nursing habits and your energy needs. You can learn how to do the following:

- Figure out how much you need to eat
- Choose healthy foods
- Get the vitamins and minerals you need

Both pregnancy and labor can affect a woman's body. After giving birth you will lose about 10 pounds right away and a little more as body fluid levels decrease. Don't expect or try to lose additional pregnancy weight right away. Gradual weight loss over several months is the safest way, especially if you are breastfeeding. Nursing mothers can safely lose a moderate amount of weight without affecting their milk supply or their babies' growth.

A healthy eating plan along with regular physical fitness might be all you need to return to a healthy weight. If you are not losing weight or losing weight too slowly, cut back on foods with added sugars and fats, like soft drinks, desserts, fried foods, fatty meats, and alcohol. Keep in mind, nursing mothers should avoid alcohol. By cutting back on "extras," you can focus on healthy, well-balanced food choices that will keep your energy level up and help you get the nutrients you and your baby need for good health. Make sure to talk to your doctor before you start any type of diet or exercise plan.

Feeling Blue

After childbirth you may feel sad, weepy, and overwhelmed for a few days. Many new mothers have the "baby blues" after giving birth. Changing hormones, anxiety about caring for the baby, and lack of sleep all affect your emotions.

Be patient with yourself. These feelings are normal and usually go away quickly. But if sadness lasts more than two weeks, go see your doctor. You might have a serious but treatable condition called postpartum depression. Postpartum depression can happen any time within the first year after birth.

Depression during and after Pregnancy

Depression is more than just feeling "blue" or "down in the dumps" for a few days. It's a serious illness that involves the brain. With depression, sad, anxious, or "empty" feelings don't go away and interfere with day-to-day life and routines. These feelings can be mild to severe. The good news is that most people with depression get better with treatment.

Depression is a common problem during and after pregnancy. About 13% of pregnant women and new mothers have depression.

How do I know if I have depression?

When you are pregnant or after you have a baby, you may be depressed and not know it. Some normal changes during and after pregnancy can cause symptoms similar to those of depression. But if you have any of the following symptoms of depression for more than two weeks, call your doctor:

- Feeling restless or moody
- Feeling sad, hopeless, and overwhelmed
- Crying a lot
- Having no energy or motivation
- Eating too little or too much
- Sleeping too little or too much
- Having trouble focusing or making decisions
- Having memory problems
- Feeling worthless and guilty
- Losing interest or pleasure in activities you used to enjoy
- Withdrawing from friends and family
- Having headaches, aches and pains, or stomach problems that don't go away

Your doctor can figure out if your symptoms are caused by depression or something else.

What causes depression? What about postpartum depression?

There is no single cause. Rather, depression likely results from a combination of factors:

- Depression is a mental illness that tends to run in families. Women with a family history of depression are more likely to have depression.

- Changes in brain chemistry or structure are believed to play a big role in depression.

- Stressful life events can trigger depression.

- Hormonal factors unique to women may contribute to depression in some women.

Depression after childbirth is called postpartum depression. Hormonal changes may trigger symptoms of postpartum depression. When you are pregnant, levels of the female hormones estrogen and progesterone increase greatly. In the first 24 hours after childbirth, hormone levels quickly return to normal. Researchers think the big change in hormone levels may lead to depression. This is much like the way smaller hormone changes can affect a woman's moods before she gets her period.

Levels of thyroid hormones may also drop after giving birth. The thyroid is a small gland in the neck that helps regulate how your body uses and stores energy from food. Low levels of thyroid hormones can cause symptoms of depression. A simple blood test can tell if this condition is causing your symptoms. If so, your doctor can prescribe thyroid medicine.

Other factors may play a role in postpartum depression. You may feel the following:

- Tired after delivery

- Tired from a lack of sleep or broken sleep

- Overwhelmed with a new baby

- Doubts about your ability to be a good mother

- Stress from changes in work and home routines

- An unrealistic need to be a perfect mom

- Loss of who you were before having the baby

- Less attractive

- A lack of free time

Are some women more at risk for depression during and after pregnancy?

Certain factors may increase your risk of depression during and after pregnancy:

- A personal history of depression or another mental illness
- A family history of depression or another mental illness
- A lack of support from family and friends
- Anxiety or negative feelings about the pregnancy
- Problems with a previous pregnancy or birth
- Marriage or money problems
- Stressful life events
- Young age
- Substance abuse

Women who are depressed during pregnancy have a greater risk of depression after giving birth.

What is the difference between "baby blues," postpartum depression, and postpartum psychosis?

Many women have the baby blues in the days after childbirth. The baby blues most often go away within a few days or a week. The symptoms are not severe and do not need treatment.

The symptoms of postpartum depression last longer and are more severe. Postpartum depression can begin anytime within the first year after childbirth. If you have postpartum depression, you may have any of the symptoms of depression listed in this chapter. Symptoms may also include the following:

- Thoughts of hurting the baby
- Thoughts of hurting yourself
- Not having any interest in the baby

Postpartum depression needs to be treated by a doctor.

Postpartum psychosis is rare. It occurs in about 1 to 4 out of every 1,000 births. It usually begins in the first two weeks after childbirth. Symptoms may include the following:

- Seeing things that aren't there
- Feeling confused
- Having rapid mood swings
- Trying to hurt yourself or your baby

What should I do if I have symptoms of depression during or after pregnancy?

Call your doctor in these situations:

- Your baby blues don't go away after two weeks.
- Symptoms of depression get more and more intense.
- Symptoms of depression begin any time after delivery, even many months later.
- It is hard for you to perform tasks at work or at home.
- You cannot care for yourself or your baby.
- You have thoughts of harming yourself or your baby.

Your doctor can ask you questions to test for depression. Your doctor can also refer you to a mental health professional who specializes in treating depression.

Some women don't tell anyone about their symptoms. They feel embarrassed, ashamed, or guilty about feeling depressed when they are supposed to be happy. They worry they will be viewed as unfit parents.

Any woman may become depressed during pregnancy or after having a baby. It doesn't mean you are a bad or "not together" mom. You and your baby don't have to suffer. There is help.

How is depression treated?

The two common types of treatment for depression are the following:

- **Talk therapy:** This involves talking to a therapist, psychologist, or social worker to learn to change how depression makes you think, feel, and act.
- **Medicine:** Your doctor can prescribe an antidepressant medicine. These medicines can help relieve symptoms of depression.

These treatment methods can be used alone or together. If you are depressed, your depression can affect your baby. Getting treatment is important for you and your baby. Talk with your doctor about the benefits and risks of taking medicine to treat depression when you are pregnant or breastfeeding.

Untreated depression can hurt you and your baby. Some women with depression have a hard time caring for themselves during pregnancy. Depression during pregnancy can raise certain risks:

- Problems during pregnancy or delivery

- Having a low-birth-weight baby

- Premature birth

Untreated postpartum depression can affect your ability to parent. As a result, you may feel guilty and lose confidence in yourself as a mother. These feelings can make your depression worse. Researchers believe postpartum depression in a mother can affect her baby. It can cause the baby to have the following:

- Delays in language development

- Problems with mother-child bonding

- Behavior problems

- Increased crying

It helps if your partner or another caregiver can help meet the baby's needs while you are depressed.

All children deserve the chance to have a healthy mom. And all moms deserve the chance to enjoy their life and their children. If you are feeling depressed during pregnancy or after having a baby, don't suffer alone. Please tell a loved one and call your doctor right away.

Chapter 36

Pregnancy Loss

Chapter Contents

Section 36.1

Ectopic Pregnancy

"Ectopic Pregnancy," January 2012, reprinted with permission from www.kidshealth.org. This information was provided by KidsHealth®, one of the largest resources online for medically reviewed health information written for parents, kids, and teens. For more articles like this, visit www.KidsHealth.org, or www.TeensHealth.org. Copyright © 1995–2012 The Nemours Foundation. All rights reserved.

Ectopic means "out of place." In a normal pregnancy, the fertilized egg implants and develops in the uterus. In most ectopic pregnancies, the egg settles in the fallopian tubes. This is why ectopic pregnancies are commonly called "tubal pregnancies." The egg can also implant in the ovary, abdomen, or the cervix, so you also might see these referred to as cervical or abdominal pregnancies.

None of these areas has as much space or nurturing tissue as a uterus for a pregnancy to develop. As the fetus grows, it will eventually burst the organ that contains it. This can cause severe bleeding and endanger the mother's life. A classical ectopic pregnancy does not develop into a live birth.

Signs and Symptoms

Ectopic pregnancy can be difficult to diagnose because symptoms often mirror those of a normal early pregnancy. These can include missed periods, breast tenderness, nausea, vomiting, fatigue, or frequent urination.

The first warning signs of an ectopic pregnancy are often pain or vaginal bleeding. There might be pain in the pelvis, abdomen, or even the shoulder or neck (if blood from a ruptured ectopic pregnancy builds up and irritates certain nerves). The pain can be mild or crampy early on, and can become sharp and stabbing. It may concentrate on one side of the pelvis.

Any of these additional symptoms can be seen with an ectopic pregnancy:

- Vaginal spotting
- Dizziness or fainting (caused by blood loss)
- Low blood pressure (also caused by blood loss)

• Lower back pain

What Causes an Ectopic Pregnancy?

An ectopic pregnancy results from a fertilized egg's inability to work its way quickly enough down the fallopian tube into the uterus. An infection or inflammation of the tube might have partially or entirely blocked it. Pelvic inflammatory disease (PID), which can be caused by gonorrhea or chlamydia, is a common cause of blockage of the fallopian tube.

Endometriosis (when cells from the lining of the uterus implant and grow elsewhere in the body) or scar tissue from previous abdominal or fallopian surgeries can also cause blockages. More rarely, birth defects or abnormal growths can alter the shape of the tube and disrupt the egg's progress.

Diagnosis

If you arrive in the emergency department complaining of abdominal pain, you'll likely be given a urine pregnancy test. Although these tests aren't sophisticated, they are fast—and speed can be crucial in treating ectopic pregnancy.

If you already know you're pregnant, or if the urine test comes back positive, you may have a quantitative hCG test. This blood test measures levels of the hormone human chorionic gonadotropin (hCG), which is produced by the placenta.

You may also have an ultrasound to look for a developing fetus in the uterus or elsewhere. Early in pregnancy, the ultrasound may be done using a wand-like device in your vagina. The doctor might give you a pelvic exam to locate the areas causing pain; to check for an enlarged, pregnant uterus; or to find any masses outside of the uterus.

Even with the best equipment, it's hard to see a pregnancy less than five weeks after the last menstrual period. If your doctor can't diagnose ectopic pregnancy but can't rule it out, he or she may ask you to return every few days for blood work and an ultrasound until it is clear whether or not there is an ectopic pregnancy.

Options for Treatment

Treatment of an ectopic pregnancy varies, depending on how medically stable the woman is and the size and location of the pregnancy.

An early ectopic pregnancy can sometimes be treated with an injection of methotrexate, which stops the growth of the embryo.

If the pregnancy is farther along, you'll likely need surgery to remove the abnormal pregnancy. In the past, this was a major operation, requiring a large incision across the pelvic area, and this can still be necessary in cases of emergency or extensive internal injury.

But sometimes ectopic tissue can be removed using laparoscopy, a less invasive surgical procedure. The surgeon makes small incisions in the lower abdomen and then inserts a tiny video camera and instruments through these incisions. The image from the camera is shown on a screen in the operating room, allowing the surgeon to see what's going on inside of your body without making large incisions. The ectopic tissue is then surgically removed and any damaged organs are repaired or removed.

Whatever your treatment, the doctor will want to see you regularly afterward to make sure your hCG levels return to zero. This may take several weeks. An elevated hCG could mean that some ectopic tissue was missed. This tissue may have to be removed using methotrexate or additional surgery.

What about Future Pregnancies?

Many women who have had an ectopic pregnancy will go on to have normal pregnancies in the future, but some will have difficulty becoming pregnant again. This difficulty is more common in women who also had fertility problems before the ectopic pregnancy. Your prognosis depends on your fertility before the ectopic pregnancy, as well as the extent of any damage incurred.

The likelihood of a repeat ectopic pregnancy increases with each subsequent ectopic pregnancy. Once you have had one ectopic pregnancy, you face an approximate 15% chance of having another.

Who's at Risk for an Ectopic Pregnancy?

While any woman can have an ectopic pregnancy, the risk is higher for women who are over 35 and those who have had:

- PID;
- a previous ectopic pregnancy;
- surgery on a fallopian tube;
- infertility problems or medication to stimulate ovulation.

Some birth control methods also can affect a woman's risk of ectopic pregnancy. Those who become pregnant while using an intrauterine device (IUD) might be more likely to have an ectopic pregnancy. Smoking and having multiple sexual partners also increase the risk of an ectopic pregnancy.

When to Call Your Doctor

If you believe you're at risk for an ectopic pregnancy, meet with your doctor to discuss your options before you become pregnant. You can help protect yourself against a future ectopic pregnancy by not smoking and by always using condoms when you're having sex but not trying to get pregnant. Condoms can protect against sexually transmitted infections (STDs) that can cause PID.

If you are pregnant and have any concerns about the pregnancy being ectopic, talk to your doctor—it's important to make sure it's detected early. You and your doctor might want to plan on checking your hormone levels or scheduling an early ultrasound to ensure that your pregnancy is developing normally.

Call your doctor immediately if you're pregnant and experiencing any pain, bleeding, or other symptoms of ectopic pregnancy. When it comes to detecting an ectopic pregnancy, the sooner it is found, the better.

Section 36.2

Miscarriage

Spontaneous abortion (SAB), or miscarriage, is the term used for a pregnancy that ends on its own, within the first 20 weeks of gestation. The medical name spontaneous abortion gives many women a negative feeling, so throughout this section we will refer to any type of spontaneous abortion or pregnancy loss under 20 weeks as miscarriage.

Miscarriage is the most common type of pregnancy loss, according to the American College of Obstetricians and Gynecologists (ACOG). Studies reveal that anywhere from 10%–25% of all clinically recognized pregnancies will end in miscarriage. Chemical pregnancies may account for 50%–75% of all miscarriages. This occurs when a pregnancy is lost shortly after implantation, resulting in bleeding that occurs around the time of her expected period. The woman may not realize that she conceived when she experiences a chemical pregnancy.

Most miscarriages occur during the first 13 weeks of pregnancy. Pregnancy can be such an exciting time, but with the great number of recognized miscarriages that occur, it is beneficial to be informed about miscarriage, in the unfortunate event that you find yourself or someone you know faced with one.

There can be many confusing terms and moments that accompany a miscarriage. There are different types of miscarriage, different treatments for each, and different statistics for what your chances are of having one. The following information gives a broad overview of miscarriage. This information is provided to help equip you with knowledge so that you might not feel so alone or lost if you face a possible miscarriage situation. As with most pregnancy complications, remember that the best person you can usually talk to and ask questions of is your health care provider.

Why Do Miscarriages Occur?

The reason for miscarriage is varied, and most often the cause cannot be identified. During the first trimester, the most common cause of miscarriage is chromosomal abnormality—meaning that something is not correct with the baby's chromosomes. Most chromosomal abnormalities are the cause of a damaged egg or sperm cell, or are due to a problem at the time that the zygote went through the division process. Other causes for miscarriage include (but are not limited to):

• hormonal problems, infections, or maternal health problems;

• lifestyle (i.e. smoking, drug use, malnutrition, excessive caffeine, and exposure to radiation or toxic substances);

• implantation of the egg into the uterine lining does not occur properly;

• maternal age;

• maternal trauma.

Factors that are not proven to cause miscarriage are sex, working outside the home (unless in a harmful environment), or moderate exercise.

What Are the Chances of Having a Miscarriage?

For women in their childbearing years, the chances of having a miscarriage can range from 10%–25%, and in most healthy women the average is about a 15%–20% chance.

• An increase in maternal age affects the chances of miscarriage.

• Women under the age of 35 years old have about a 15% chance of miscarriage.

• Women who are 35–45 years old have a 20%–35% chance of miscarriage.

• Women over the age of 45 can have up to a 50% chance of miscarriage.

• A woman who has had a previous miscarriage has a 25% chance of having another (only a slightly elevated risk than for someone who has not had a previous miscarriage).

What Are the Warning Signs of Miscarriage?

If you experience any or all of these symptoms, it is important to contact your health care provider or a medical facility to evaluate if you could be having a miscarriage:

- Mild to severe back pain (often worse than normal menstrual cramps)
- Weight loss
- White-pink mucus
- True contractions (very painful happening every 5–20 minutes)
- Brown or bright red bleeding with or without cramps (20%–30% of all pregnancies can experience some bleeding in early pregnancy, with about 50% of those resulting in normal pregnancies)
- Tissue with clot-like material passing from the vagina
- Sudden decrease in signs of pregnancy

The Different Types of Miscarriage

Miscarriage is often a process and not a single event. There are many different stages or types of miscarriage. There is also a lot of information to learn about healthy fetal development so that you might get a better idea of what is going on with your pregnancy. Understanding early fetal development and first trimester development can help you to know what things your health care provider is looking for when there is a possible miscarriage occurring.

Most of the time all types of miscarriage are just called miscarriage, but you may hear your health care provider refer to other terms or names of miscarriage such as:

Threatened miscarriage: Some degree of early pregnancy uterine bleeding accompanied by cramping or lower backache. The cervix remains closed. This bleeding is often the result of implantation.

Inevitable or incomplete miscarriage: Abdominal or back pain accompanied by bleeding with an open cervix. Miscarriage is inevitable when there is a dilation or effacement of the cervix and/or there is rupture of the membranes. Bleeding and cramps may persist if the miscarriage is not complete.

Complete miscarriage: A completed miscarriage is when the embryo or products of conception have emptied out of the uterus. Bleeding should subside quickly, as should any pain or cramping. A completed miscarriage can be confirmed by an ultrasound or by having a surgical curettage (D&C) performed.

Missed miscarriage: Women can experience a miscarriage without knowing it. A missed miscarriage is when embryonic death has occurred but there is not any expulsion of the embryo. It is not known why this occurs. Signs of this would be a loss of pregnancy symptoms and the absence of fetal heart tones found on an ultrasound.

Recurrent miscarriage (RM): Defined as three or more consecutive first-trimester miscarriages. This can affect 1% of couples trying to conceive.

Blighted ovum: Also called an anembryonic pregnancy. A fertilized egg implants into the uterine wall, but fetal development never begins. Often there is a gestational sac with or without a yolk sac, but there is an absence of fetal growth.

Ectopic pregnancy: A fertilized egg implants itself in places other than the uterus, most commonly the fallopian tube. Treatment is needed immediately to stop the development of the implanted egg. If not treated rapidly, this could end in serious maternal complications.

Molar pregnancy: The result of a genetic error during the fertilization process that leads to growth of abnormal tissue within the uterus. Molar pregnancies rarely involve a developing embryo, but often entail the most common symptoms of pregnancy including a missed period, positive pregnancy test, and severe nausea.

Treatment of Miscarriage

The main goal of treatment during or after a miscarriage is to prevent hemorrhaging and/or infection. The earlier you are in the pregnancy, the more likely that your body will expel all the fetal tissue by itself and will not require further medical procedures. If the body does not expel all the tissue, the most common procedure performed to stop bleeding and prevent infection is a dilation and curettage, known as a D&C. Drugs may be prescribed to help control bleeding after the D&C is performed. Bleeding should be monitored closely once you are at home; if you notice an increase in bleeding or the onset of chills or fever, it is best to call your physician immediately.

Prevention of Miscarriage

Since the cause of most miscarriages is due to chromosomal abnormalities, there is not much that can be done to prevent them. One vital step is to get as healthy as you can before conceiving to provide a healthy atmosphere for conception to occur.

- Exercise regularly

- Eat healthy

- Manage stress

- Keep weight within healthy limits

- Take folic acid daily

- Do not smoke

Once you find out that you are pregnant, again the goal is to be as healthy as possible, to provide a healthy environment for your baby to grow in:

- Keep your abdomen safe.

- Do not smoke or be around smoke.

- Do not drink alcohol.

- Check with your doctor before taking any over-the-counter medications.

- Limit or eliminate caffeine.

- Avoid environmental hazards such as radiation, infectious disease, and X-rays.

- Avoid contact sports or activities that have risk of injury.

Emotional Treatment

Unfortunately, miscarriage can affect anyone. Women are often left with unanswered questions regarding their physical recovery, their emotional recovery, and trying to conceive again. It is very important that women try to keep the lines of communication open with family, friends, and health care providers during this time.

Some helpful websites that address miscarriage and pregnancy loss include:

- www.angelfire.com

- www.mend.org

- www.aplacetoremember.com

Section 36.3

Stillbirth

Stillbirth: Trying to Understand

According the National Stillbirth Society, stillbirth is defined as the intrauterine death and subsequent delivery of a developing infant that occurs beyond 20 completed weeks of gestation.

Stillbirth occurs in about 1 in 160 pregnancies. The majority of stillbirths happen before labor, whereas a small percentage occurs during labor and delivery.

Why do stillbirths happen?

If you have had a stillbirth or are supporting someone through this difficult experience, you probably are in desperate need of knowing why this happened. An autopsy is normally the best way to diagnose a cause for stillbirth, but this is not always a standard procedure. Inquire about your hospitals procedures when handling stillborn babies and the cause of death. If normal procedure is not to have an autopsy, seek to find out how you can request one, if that's what you and your family desire.

The most common known causes of stillbirths include:

- **Placental problems:** Women with placental abruption, or a pregnancy-related form of high blood pressure called preeclampsia or pregnancy-induced hypertension, have twice the risk of abruption or stillbirth as unaffected women. Sometimes insufficient oxygen and nutrients can also contribute to a baby's death.

- **Birth defects:** Chromosomal disorders account for 15%–20% of all stillborn babies. Sometimes a baby has structural malformations that are not caused by chromosomal abnormalities, but can result from genetic, environmental, or unknown causes.

- **Growth restriction:** Babies who are small or not growing at an appropriate rate are at risk of death from asphyxia (lack of oxygen) both before and during birth, and from unknown causes.

- **Infections:** Bacterial infections between 24 and 27 weeks gestation can cause fetal deaths. These infections usually go unnoticed by the mother and may not be diagnosed until they cause serious complications.

- **Other infrequent causes of stillbirth include:** Umbilical cord accidents, trauma, maternal diabetes, high blood pressure, and postdate pregnancy (a pregnancy that lasts longer than 42 weeks)

Unfortunately, despite efforts to find out why, the cause cannot be determined in about one-third of stillbirths.

What are some factors that increase a mother's risk of stillbirth?

- Women 35 years old or older

- Malnutrition

- Inadequate prenatal care

- Smoking

- Alcohol and drug abuse

- African American ethnicity

How is a stillbirth diagnosis made?

Most women usually notice that their baby isn't very active and become worried about what this could mean. An ultrasound can confirm that the baby has died and in some cases determine the reason why.

Can stillbirth be prevented?

Improvements in medicine have decreased the number of stillbirths. Today women with high-risk pregnancies are carefully monitored through routine ultrasounds and/or fetal heart rate monitoring. If potential problems are identified, early delivery may be necessary. The following are steps you can take to help prevent stillbirth:

- A daily "kick count." Starting at 26–28 weeks of pregnancy, take time each day to record your baby's movements. If you familiarize yourself with what is normal for your baby, then you are more likely to notice when something does not feel right. If you notice a sudden decrease in movements, contact your health care provider. An ultrasound can normally confirm if there are any potential problems.

- Avoid drugs, alcohol, and smoking as these can increase your risk of stillbirth and other pregnancy complications.

- Contact your health care provider immediately if you have any vaginal bleeding in the second half of pregnancy.

- If you have had a previous stillbirth, future pregnancies should be monitored closely so that all necessary steps can be taken to prevent another loss.

Stillbirth: Surviving Emotionally

Stillbirth is one of the most devastating of losses, affecting over 25,000 families each year. Stillbirth touches families of all races, religion, and socioeconomic status. For many parents stillbirth is a loss that hits unexpectedly. In fact, up to half of all stillbirths occur in pregnancies that had seemed problem-free.

With any loss, grief can come in many different ways. The initial shock and numbness will eventually fade to other very intense emotions. The grieving process is different for everyone, with the one common thread being pain. Allowing yourself and others to experience this in individual ways can be vital to eventual healing.

What should I do if my baby has died?

As you are trying to cope with the heartbreaking news, you will also have to face an uncomfortable dilemma. If your baby has died before labor begins you will probably be given the choice of what type of birth you would prefer; this is not an easy decision to make. Giving birth naturally may give you a little more time to work through the shock and begin the grieving process. Generally, it is medically safe for the mother to continue carrying her baby until labor begins which is normally about two weeks after the baby has died. This lapse in time can have an effect on the baby's appearance at delivery and it is best to be prepared for this.

Some women prefer to be induced as soon as possible because it is emotionally difficult for some women to think of carrying their deceased baby in the womb. If labor has not started after two weeks, induction would become necessary to avoid dangerous blood clotting.

A cesarean is usually only recommended if complications arise during labor and delivery.

How will I recover physically after having a stillbirth?

After you give birth to a stillborn baby, your body needs time to heal as it would in any birthing situation. Your doctor will probably recommend taking it easy, to give your body time to heal. A few days after you get home from the hospital, your breasts may fill with milk. The milk will normally disperse within a few days but your breasts may feel sore and tender for awhile. This experience can be upsetting because it is a reminder of your loss. Try taking a warm bath to ease the discomfort. You may continue to bleed off and on for a few weeks. If you continue to bleed beyond three weeks, have a fever, or cramping, it is important to contact your health care provider.

Saying hello, goodbye, and making memories:

After the tests are completed, you will usually have the choice to spend time alone with your baby. You can find comfort in looking at, touching, and talking to your baby. Most parents find it helpful to make memories of this precious time that will last a lifetime. Here are a few ways you can make memories with your baby:

- You can give your baby a bath and dress them in a special outfit. Before leaving the hospital you can take a piece of this clothing to have as a keepsake.

- You can take pictures of your baby.

- The hospital staff can give you an imprint of handprints and/or footprints.

- You may want to take a lock of your baby's hair.

- It may seem odd at first but you can read a story or sing a lullaby to your baby.

- If you would like, the nurse can record your baby's measurements.

- You probably have also named your baby by now. Be sure to tell the hospital staff as soon as possible so all documents can have your baby's name listed.

- You can have your baby christened or blessed while in the hospital.

- A baptism certificate will also be given to you to keep.

You will be able to spend as much time as you need with your baby, but at some point you will need to say goodbye. This will probably be one of the most challenging things to do because it is so final. Allow yourself to cry; expressing emotion is natural in the grieving process. Having the keepsakes will remind you that a part of your baby will always be with you.

How do I tell people about our loss?

Telling family members and friends can be emotionally draining and overwhelming. You may want to have one family member be "in charge" of telling others about what has happened, about funeral arrangements, and ways they can help.

How can I help myself grieve?

The following are things you can do to help yourself get through this difficult time in your life.

- Talk to people about how you feel.
- Joining a support group may help you feel less isolated; it is good to know someone else understands what you are going through.
- Write about your feelings in a journal. You may want to write a letter to your baby.
- Make something for your baby such as an album, or plant a tree in the baby's memory, or anything that makes you feel that you have done something.

Healing will take time. Little by little the emptiness that you feel in your heart will lessen and you will learn to live your life again. You will have new dreams and hopes for the future and your outlook on life will change. This means you are beginning to accept your loss, not forget it.

What are my chances of having another stillbirth?

The chances of having another stillbirth are very small. In fact, most women will give birth to a healthy baby after experiencing a stillbirth.

When should we try again?

When to try again is something only you and your partner can decide. You will probably be physically ready before you are emotionally ready to start trying again. Future pregnancies will be tougher for you if you do not come to terms with your loss. Some professionals recommend you wait for at least a few months or up to a year before trying again as to give yourself time to grieve.

Part Five

Gynecological and High-Prevalence Cancers in Women

Chapter 37

Breast Cancer

A breast is made up of three main parts: glands, ducts, and connective tissue. The glands produce milk. The ducts are passages that carry milk to the nipple. The connective tissue (which consists of fibrous and fatty tissue) connects and holds everything together.

No breast is typical. What is normal for you may not be normal for another woman. Most women say their breasts feel lumpy or uneven. The way your breasts look and feel can be affected by getting your period, having children, losing or gaining weight, and taking certain medications. Breasts also tend to change as you age.

Lumps in the Breast

Many conditions can cause lumps in the breast, including cancer. But most breast lumps are caused by other medical conditions. The two most common causes of breast lumps are fibrocystic breast condition and cysts. Fibrocystic condition causes noncancerous changes in the breast that can make them lumpy, tender, and sore. Cysts are small fluid-filled sacs that can develop in the breast.

Common Kinds of Breast Cancer

There are different kinds of breast cancer. The kind of breast cancer depends on which cells in the breast turn into cancer. Breast cancer can begin in different parts of the breast, like the ducts or the lobes.

Excerpted from "Basic Information about Breast Cancer," Centers for Disease Control and Prevention (www.cdc.gov), September 17, 2012.

Common kinds of breast cancer are the following:

- **Ductal carcinoma:** The most common kind of breast cancer. It begins in the cells that line the milk ducts in the breast, also called the lining of the breast ducts.

    - **Ductal carcinoma in situ (DCIS):** The abnormal cancer cells are only in the lining of the milk ducts and have not spread to other tissues in the breast.

    - **Invasive ductal carcinoma:** The abnormal cancer cells break through the ducts and spread into other parts of the breast tissue. Invasive cancer cells can also spread to other parts of the body.

- **Lobular carcinoma:** In this kind of breast cancer, the cancer cells begin in the lobes, or lobules, of the breast. Lobules are the glands that make milk.

    - **Lobular carcinoma in situ (LCIS):** The cancer cells are found only in the breast lobules. Lobular carcinoma in situ, or LCIS, does not spread to other tissues.

    - **Invasive lobular carcinoma:** Cancer cells spread from the lobules to the breast tissues that are close by. These invasive cancer cells can also spread to other parts of the body.

Uncommon Kinds of Breast Cancer

There are several other less common kinds of breast cancer, such as Paget disease or inflammatory breast cancer. For more information, visit the National Cancer Institute's "Inflammatory Breast Cancer" (at www.cancer.gov/cancertopics/pdq/treatment/breast/Patient/page3) and "Paget Disease of the Nipple: Questions and Answers" (at www.cancer .gov/cancertopics/factsheet/sites-types/paget-breast).

Risk Factors

Research has found several risk factors that may increase your chances of getting breast cancer.

Reproductive risk factors are the following:

- Being younger when you first had your menstrual period

- Starting menopause at a later age

- Being older at the birth of your first child

- Never giving birth
- Not breastfeeding
- Long-term use of hormone-replacement therapy

Other risk factors are the following:

- Getting older
- Personal history of breast cancer or some non-cancerous breast diseases
- Family history of breast cancer (mother, sister, daughter)
- Treatment with radiation therapy to the breast/chest
- Being overweight (increases risk for breast cancer after menopause)
- Having changes in the breast cancer–related genes BRCA1 or BRCA2
- Drinking alcohol (more than one drink a day)
- Not getting regular exercise

Having a risk factor does not mean you will get the disease. Most women have some risk factors and most women do not get breast cancer. If you have breast cancer risk factors, talk with your doctor about ways you can lower your risk and about screening for breast cancer.

Prevention

You can help lower your risk of breast cancer in the following ways:

- Get screened for breast cancer regularly. By getting the necessary exams, you can increase your chances of finding out early on if you have breast cancer.
- Control your weight and exercise. Make healthy choices in the foods you eat and the kinds of drinks you have each day. Stay active. Learn more about keeping a healthy weight and ways to increase your physical activity.
- Know your family history of breast cancer. If you have a mother, sister, or daughter with breast cancer, ask your doctor what is your risk of getting breast cancer and how you can lower your risk.

- Find out the risks and benefits of hormone replacement therapy. Some women use hormone replacement therapy (HRT) to treat the symptoms of menopause. Ask your doctor about the risks and benefits of HRT and find out if hormone replacement therapy is right for you.

- Limit the amount of alcohol you drink.

Symptoms

Different people have different warning signs for breast cancer. Some people do not have any signs or symptoms at all. A person may find out they have breast cancer after a routine mammogram.

Some warning signs of breast cancer are as follows:

- New lump in the breast or underarm (armpit)

- Thickening or swelling of part of the breast

- Irritation or dimpling of breast skin

- Redness or flaky skin in the nipple area or the breast

- Pulling in of the nipple or pain in the nipple area

- Nipple discharge other than breast milk, including blood

- Any change in the size or the shape of the breast

- Pain in any area of the breast

Keep in mind that some of these warning signs can happen with other conditions that are not cancer. If you have any signs that worry you, be sure to see your doctor right away.

Screening

Kinds of Screening Tests

Breast cancer screening means checking a woman's breasts for cancer before there are signs or symptoms of the disease. Three main tests are used to screen the breasts for cancer. Talk to your doctor about which tests are right for you, and when you should have them.

- **Mammogram:** A mammogram is an X-ray of the breast. Mammograms are the best method to detect breast cancer early when it is easier to treat and before it is big enough to feel or cause symptoms. Having regular mammograms can lower the risk of dying from breast cancer. If you are age 50 to 74 years, be sure to have a screening mammogram every two years. If you are age 40–49 years, talk to your doctor about when and how often you should have a screening mammogram.

- **Clinical breast exam:** A clinical breast exam is an examination by a doctor or nurse, who uses his or her hands to feel for lumps or other changes.

- **Breast self-exam:** A breast self-exam is when you check your own breasts for lumps, changes in size or shape of the breast, or any other changes in the breasts or underarm (armpit).

Which tests to choose: Having a clinical breast exam or a breast self-exam have not been found to decrease risk of dying from breast cancer. Keep in mind that, at this time, the best way to find breast cancer is with a mammogram. If you choose to have clinical breast exams and to perform breast self-exams, be sure you also get regular mammograms.

Where Can I Go to Get Screened?

Most likely, you can get screened for breast cancer at a clinic, hospital, or doctor's office. If you want to be screened for breast cancer, call your doctor's office. They can help you schedule an appointment. Most health insurance companies pay for the cost of breast cancer screening tests.

The National Breast and Cervical Cancer Early Detection Program (NBCCEDP; at www.cdc.gov/cancer/nbccedp/) offers free or low-cost mammograms and education about breast cancer.

Diagnosis

Doctors often use additional tests to find or diagnose breast cancer.

- **Breast ultrasound:** A machine uses sound waves to make detailed pictures, called sonograms, of areas inside the breast.

- **Diagnostic mammogram:** If you have a problem in your breast, such as lumps, or if an area of the breast looks abnormal on a screening mammogram, doctors may have you get a diagnostic mammogram. This is a more detailed X-ray of the breast.

- **Magnetic resonance imaging (MRI):** A kind of body scan that uses a magnet linked to a computer. The MRI scan will make detailed pictures of areas inside the breast.

- **Biopsy:** This is a test that removes tissue or fluid from the breast to be looked at under a microscope and do more testing. There are different kinds of biopsies (for example, fine-needle aspiration, core biopsy, or open biopsy).

Staging

If breast cancer is diagnosed, tests are done to find out if cancer cells have spread within the breast or to other parts of the body. This process is called staging. Whether the cancer is only in the breast, is found in lymph nodes under your arm, or has spread outside the breast determines your stage of breast cancer. The type and stage of breast cancer tells doctors what kind of treatment will be needed.

Treatment

Breast cancer is treated in several ways. It depends on the kind of breast cancer and how far it has spread. Treatments include surgery, chemotherapy, hormonal therapy, biologic therapy, and radiation. People with breast cancer often get more than one kind of treatment.

- **Surgery:** Surgery is an operation where doctors cut out and remove cancer tissue.

- **Chemotherapy:** Chemotherapy uses special medicines or drugs to shrink or kill the cancer. The drugs can be pills you take or medicines given through an intravenous (IV) tube, or, sometimes, both.

- **Hormonal therapy:** Some cancers need certain hormones to grow. Hormonal treatment is used to block cancer cells from getting the hormones they need to grow.

- **Biological therapy:** This treatment works with your body's immune system to help it fight cancer or to control side effects from other cancer treatments. Side effects are how your body reacts to drugs or other treatments. Biological therapy is different from chemotherapy, which attacks cancer cells directly.

- **Radiation:** Radiation is the use of high-energy rays (similar to X-rays) to kill the cancer cells. The rays are aimed at the part of the body where the cancer is located.

It is common for doctors from different specialties to work together in treating breast cancer. Surgeons are doctors who perform operations.

Medical oncologists are doctors who treat cancers with medicines. Radiation oncologists are doctors who treat cancers with radiation.

For more information, visit the National Cancer Institute (NCI)– "Breast Cancer Treatment Option Overview" (at www.cancer.gov/cancertopics/pdq/treatment/breast/Patient/page5). This site can also help you find a doctor or treatment facility (www.cancer.gov/cancertopics/factsheet/Therapy/doctor-facility) that works in cancer care.

Complementary and Alternative Medicine

Complementary medicine is a group of medicines and practices that may be used in addition to the standard treatments for cancer. Alternative medicine means practices or medicines that are used instead of the usual, or standard, ways of treating cancer. Examples of complementary and alternative medicine are meditation, yoga, and dietary supplements like vitamins and herbs.

Complementary and alternative medicine does not treat breast cancer but may help lessen the side effects of the cancer treatments or of the cancer symptoms. It is important to note that many forms of complementary and alternative medicines have not been scientifically tested and may not be safe. Talk to your doctor before you start any kind of complementary or alternative medicine.

Which Treatment Is Right for Me?

Choosing which kind of treatment is right for you may be hard. If you have breast cancer, be sure to talk to your doctor about the treatment options available for your type and stage of cancer. Doctors can explain the risks and benefits of each treatment and their side effects.

Sometimes people get an opinion from more than one breast cancer doctor. This is called a "second opinion." Getting a second opinion may help you choose the treatment option that is right for you.

Chapter 38

Gynecological Cancers

Chapter Contents

Section 38.1

Cervical Cancer

Excerpted from "Cervical Cancer Fact Sheet," U.S. Department of Health and Human Services Office on Women's Health (www.womenshealth.gov), May 18, 2010.

What is cervical cancer?

Cancer is a disease that happens when body cells don't work right. The cells divide fast and grow out of control. These extra cells form a tumor. Cervical cancer is cancer in the cervix, the lower, narrow part of the uterus (womb). The uterus is the hollow, pear-shaped organ where a baby grows during a woman's pregnancy. The cervix forms a canal that opens into the vagina (birth canal), which leads to the outside of the body.

Most cases of cervical cancer are caused by the human papillomavirus (HPV). HPV is a virus that is passed from person to person through genital contact, most often during vaginal and anal sex. You are more likely to get HPV if you have multiple partners. However, any woman who has ever had genital contact with another person can get HPV. Most women infected with HPV will not get cervical cancer. But, you are more likely to develop cervical cancer if you smoke, have HIV or reduced immunity, or don't get regular Pap tests. Pap tests look for changes in the cervical cells that could become cancerous if not treated.

If the Pap test finds serious changes in the cells of the cervix, the doctor will suggest more powerful tests such as a colposcopy. This procedure uses a large microscope called a colposcope. This tool allows the doctor to look more closely at the cells of the vagina and cervix. This and other tests can help the doctor decide what areas should be tested for cancer.

Why should I be concerned about cervical cancer?

Cervical cancer is a disease that can be very serious. However, it is a disease that you can help prevent. Cervical cancer happens when normal cells in the cervix change into cancer cells. This normally takes several years to happen, but it can also happen in a very short period of time.

How can I help prevent cervical cancer?

Two kinds of vaccines (Cervarix and Gardasil) can protect girls and young women against the types of HPV that cause most cervical cancers. Cervarix and Gardasil are licensed, safe, and effective for females ages 9 through 26 years. The Centers for Disease Control and Prevention (CDC) recommended that all girls who are 11 or 12 years old get three doses (shots) of either brand of HPV vaccine to protect against cervical cancer and precancer. (Gardasil also protects against most genital warts.) Girls and young women ages 13 through 26 should get all three doses of an HPV vaccine if they have not received all doses yet. It is very important to get all three doses.

Gardasil is also licensed, safe, and effective for males ages 9 through 26 years. Boys and young men may choose to get this vaccine to prevent genital warts.

People who have already had sexual contact before getting all three doses of an HPV vaccine might still benefit, but only if they were not infected with the HPV types included in the vaccine they received. The best way to be sure that a person gets the most benefit from HPV vaccination is to complete all three doses before sexual activity begins. Ask your doctor which brand of the vaccine is best for you.

The vaccine does not replace the need to wear condoms to lower your risk of getting other types of HPV and other sexually transmitted infections. Women who have had the HPV vaccine still need to have regular Pap tests. By getting regular Pap tests and pelvic exams, your doctor can find and treat any changing cells before they turn into cancer. Practicing safer sex is also very important. Here are additional things you can do to help protect yourself against HPV and cervical cancer.

- Don't have sex. The best way to prevent any STI is to not have vaginal, oral, or anal sex.

- Be faithful. Having sex with just one partner can also lower your risk. That means that you only have sex with each other and no one else.

- Use condoms. HPV can occur in both female and male genital areas that are not covered by condoms. However, research has shown that condom use is linked to lower cervical cancer rates. Protect yourself with a condom every time you have vaginal, anal, or oral sex.

How often should I get a Pap test?

Follow these guidelines:

- Have a Pap test every two years starting at age 21. Women 30 and older who have had three normal Pap tests in a row can now have one every three years.

- If you are older than 65, you may be able to stop having Pap tests. Discuss your needs with your doctor.

- If you had your cervix taken out as part of a hysterectomy, you may not need further Pap tests if the surgery was not due to cancer. Talk to your doctor.

- Talk with your doctor or nurse about when to begin testing, how often you should be tested, and when you can stop.

Section 38.2

Ovarian Cancer

Excerpted from "Basic Information about Ovarian Cancer," Centers for Disease Control and Prevention (www.cdc.gov), June 28, 2012.

When cancer starts in the ovaries, it is called ovarian cancer. Women have two ovaries that are located in the pelvis, one on each side of the uterus. The ovaries make female hormones and produce eggs. Ovarian cancer causes more deaths than any other cancer of the female reproductive system. But when ovarian cancer is found in its early stages, treatment is most effective.

Ovarian Cancer Risk Factors

There is no way to know for sure if you will get ovarian cancer. Most women get it without being at high risk. However, several factors may increase a woman's risk for ovarian cancer:

- Being middle-aged or older

- Having close family members (such as your mother, sister, aunt, or grandmother) on either your mother's or your father's side, who have had ovarian cancer

- Having a genetic mutation (abnormality) called BRCA1 or BRCA2
- Having had breast, uterine, or colorectal (colon) cancer
- Having an Eastern European (Ashkenazi) Jewish background
- Having never given birth or having had trouble getting pregnant
- Having endometriosis (a condition where tissue from the lining of the uterus grows elsewhere in the body)

In addition, some studies suggest that women who take estrogen by itself (without progesterone) for 10 or more years may have an increased risk of ovarian cancer.

If one or more of these factors is true for you, it does not mean you will get ovarian cancer. But you should speak with your doctor about your risk.

Ovarian Cancer Prevention

There is no known way to prevent ovarian cancer. But these things may lower your chance of getting ovarian cancer:

- Having used birth control pills for more than five years
- Having had a tubal ligation (getting your tubes tied), both ovaries removed, or a hysterectomy (an operation in which the uterus, and sometimes the cervix, is removed)
- Having given birth

Symptoms of Ovarian Cancer

Ovarian cancer may cause one or more of these signs and symptoms:

- Vaginal bleeding or discharge from your vagina that is not normal for you
- Pain in the pelvic or abdominal area (the area below your stomach and between your hip bones)
- Back pain
- Bloating, which is when the area below your stomach swells or feels full
- Feeling full quickly while eating
- A change in your bathroom habits, such as having to pass urine very badly or very often, constipation, or diarrhea

431

Pay attention to your body, and know what is normal for you. If you have vaginal bleeding that is not normal for you, see a doctor right away. Also see a doctor if you have any of the other signs for two weeks or longer and they are not normal for you. These symptoms may be caused by something other than cancer, but the only way to know is to see a doctor. The earlier ovarian cancer is found and treated, the more likely treatment will be effective.

Ovarian Cancer Screening

Screening is when a test is used to look for a disease before there are any symptoms. Cancer screening tests are effective when they can detect disease early. Detecting disease early can lead to more effective treatment. Diagnostic tests are used when a person has symptoms. The purpose of diagnostic tests is to find out, or diagnose, what is causing the symptoms. Diagnostic tests also may be used to check a person who is considered at high risk for cancer.

There is no simple and reliable way to screen for ovarian cancer in women who do not have any signs or symptoms. The Pap test does not check for ovarian cancer. The only cancer the Pap test screens for is cervical cancer. Since there is no simple and reliable way to screen for any gynecologic cancers except for cervical cancer, it is especially important to recognize warning signs and learn what you can do to reduce your risk.

Here is what you can do:

• Pay attention to your body, and know what is normal for you.

• If you notice any changes in your body that are not normal for you and could be a sign of ovarian cancer, talk to your doctor about them and ask about possible causes, such as ovarian cancer.

Ask your doctor if you should have a test, such as a rectovaginal pelvic exam, a transvaginal ultrasound, or a CA-125 blood test if the following apply to you:

• You have any unexplained signs or symptoms of ovarian cancer (these tests sometimes help find or rule out ovarian cancer)

• You have had breast, uterine, or colorectal cancer; or a close relative has had ovarian cancer

Ovarian Cancer Treatment

If your doctor says that you have ovarian cancer, ask to be referred to a gynecologic oncologist—a doctor who has been trained to treat cancers of a woman's reproductive system. This doctor will work with you to create a treatment plan.

Types of Treatment

There are several ways to treat ovarian cancer. The treatment depends on the type of ovarian cancer and how far it has spread. Treatments include surgery, chemotherapy, and/or radiation.

- **Surgery:** Doctors remove cancer tissue in an operation.

- **Chemotherapy:** Chemotherapy involves the use of drugs to stop or slow the growth of cancer cells. Chemotherapy may cause side effects, but these often get better or go away when chemotherapy is over. Chemotherapy drugs may be given in several forms, including pills or through an IV (intravenous) injection.

- **Radiation:** Radiation uses high-energy rays (similar to X-rays) to try to kill the cancer cells and stop them from spreading. The rays are aimed at the part of the body where the cancer is.

Different treatments may be provided by different doctors on your medical team.

Section 38.3

Uterine Cancer

Excerpted from "Basic Information about Uterine Cancer," Centers for
Disease Control and Prevention (www.cdc.gov), August 28, 2012.

When cancer starts in the uterus, it is called uterine cancer. The
uterus is the pear-shaped organ in a woman's pelvis (the area below
your stomach and in between your hip bones). The uterus, also called
the womb, is where the baby grows when a woman is pregnant. All
women are at risk for uterine cancer, but the risk increases with age.

Uterine Cancer Risk Factors

There is no way to know for sure if you will get uterine cancer. Some
women get it without being at high risk. However, several factors may
increase the chance that you will get uterine cancer, including if the
following are true of you:

- Are older than 50

- Are obese (have an abnormally high, unhealthy amount of body fat)

- Take estrogen by itself (without progesterone) for hormone
  replacement during menopause

- Have had trouble getting pregnant, or have had fewer than five
  periods in a year before starting menopause

- Take tamoxifen, a drug used to treat certain types of breast cancer

- Have close family members who have had uterine, colon, or ovarian cancer

If one or more of these things is true for you, it does not mean you
will get uterine cancer. But you should speak with your doctor to see
if he or she recommends more frequent exams.

Uterine Cancer Prevention

There is no known way to prevent uterine cancer. But these things
may reduce your chance of getting uterine cancer:

- Using birth control pills
- Maintaining a healthy weight and being physically active
- Taking progesterone, if you are taking estrogen

Ask your doctor about how often you should be checked for uterine cancer, especially if you think that you have factors that increase your chance of getting it.

Symptoms of Uterine Cancer

Uterine cancer may cause vaginal discharge or bleeding that is not normal for you. Bleeding may be abnormal because of how heavy it is or when it happens, such as after you have gone through menopause, between periods, or any other bleeding that is longer or heavier than is normal for you. Uterine cancer may also cause other symptoms, such as pain or pressure in your pelvis.

If you have bleeding that is not normal for you, especially if you have already gone through menopause, see a doctor right away. Also see a doctor if you have any other signs or symptoms for two weeks or longer.

Uterine Cancer Screening

Screening is when a test is used to look for a disease before there are any symptoms. Diagnostic tests are used when a person has symptoms. The purpose of diagnostic tests is to find out, or diagnose, what is causing the symptoms. Diagnostic tests also may be used to check a person who is considered at high risk for cancer.

There are no simple and reliable ways to test for uterine cancer in women who do not have any signs or symptoms. The Pap test does not screen for uterine cancer. The only cancer the Pap test screens for is cervical cancer. It is especially important to recognize warning signs and learn what you can do to reduce your risk.

If you have symptoms or believe you may be at high risk for uterine cancer, your doctor may perform an endometrial biopsy or a transvaginal ultrasound. These tests can be used to help diagnose or rule out uterine cancer. Your doctor may do this test in his or her office or may refer you to another doctor. The doctor might perform more tests if the endometrial biopsy does not provide enough information, or if symptoms continue.

Uterine Cancer Treatment

If your doctor says that you have uterine cancer, ask to be referred to a gynecologic oncologist—a doctor who has been trained to treat cancers like this. This doctor will work with you to create a treatment plan.

Types of Treatment

There are several ways to treat uterine cancer. The type of treatment a woman receives depends on the type of uterine cancer and how far it has spread. Treatments include surgery, chemotherapy, and/or radiation.

- **Surgery:** Doctors remove cancer tissue in an operation.

- **Radiation:** Radiation uses high-energy rays (similar to X-rays) to try to kill the cancer cells and stop them from spreading. The rays are aimed at the part of the body where the cancer is.

- **Hormone therapy:** Hormone therapy removes hormones or blocks their action and stops cancer cells from growing. Hormones are substances made by glands in the body and circulated in the bloodstream.

- **Chemotherapy:** Chemotherapy involves the use of drugs to stop or slow the growth of cancer cells. Chemotherapy may cause side effects, but these often get better or go away when chemotherapy is over. Chemotherapy drugs may be given in several forms, including pills or through an IV (intravenous) injection.

Different treatments may be provided by different doctors on your medical team.

Section 38.4

Vaginal and Vulvar Cancers

Excerpted from "Basic Information about Vaginal and
Vulvar Cancers," Centers for Disease Control and Prevention
(www.cdc.gov), June 28, 2012.

When cancer starts in the vagina, it is called vaginal cancer. The
vagina, also called the birth canal, is the hollow, tube-like channel
between the bottom of the uterus and the outside of the body.

When cancer forms in the vulva, it is vulvar cancer. The vulva is
the outer part of the female genital organs. It has two folds of skin,
called the labia. Vulvar cancer most often occurs on the inner edges
of the labia.

Vaginal and Vulvar Cancers Risk Factors

There is no way to know for sure if you will get vaginal or vulvar
cancer. Some women get these cancers without being at high risk.
However, several factors may increase the chance that you will get
vaginal or vulvar cancer, including if the following are true of you:

- Have HPV

- Have had cervical precancer or cervical cancer

- Have a condition that weakens your immune system (such as
  HIV), making it hard for your body to fight off health problems

- Smoke

- Have chronic vulvar itching or burning

If one or more of these things is true for you, it does not mean you
will get vaginal or vulvar cancer. But you should speak with your doctor to see if he or she recommends more frequent exams.

Vaginal and Vulvar Cancers Prevention

The human papillomavirus (HPV) is a common virus with more
than 100 different kinds or types. More than 30 of the types can be

passed from one person to another during sex. Almost all cervical cancers and some vaginal and vulvar cancers are caused by HPV.

There is a vaccine that protects against the types of HPV that most often cause cervical, vaginal, and vulvar cancers. It is given in a series of three shots. The vaccine is recommended for 11- and 12-year-old girls. It is also recommended for girls and women aged 13 through 26 who did not get any or all of the shots when they were younger. (Note: The vaccine can be given to girls beginning at age 9.)

Symptoms of Vaginal and Vulvar Cancers

Early on, most vaginal cancers do not cause signs and symptoms. But if there are symptoms, they may include the following:

• Vaginal discharge or bleeding that is not normal for you (the bleeding may be abnormal because of how heavy it is, or when it happens, such as bleeding after you have gone through menopause; bleeding between periods; or any other bleeding that is longer or heavier than is normal for you)

• A change in bathroom habits, such as having blood in the stool or urine; going to the bathroom more often than usual; or feeling constipated

• Pain in your pelvis, the area below your stomach and in between your hip bones, especially when you pass urine or have sex

Many women who have vulvar cancer have the following signs and symptoms:

• Itching, burning, or bleeding on the vulva that does not go away

• Changes in the color of the skin of the vulva, so that it looks redder or whiter than is normal for you

• Skin changes in the vulva, including what looks like a rash or warts

• Sores, lumps, or ulcers on the vulva that do not go away

• Pain in your pelvis, especially when you urinate or have sex

It is important for you to pay attention to your body and know what is normal for you. If you have vaginal bleeding that is not normal for you, see a doctor right away. Also see a doctor if you have any of the other symptoms for two weeks or longer and they are not normal for you. Symptoms may be caused by something other than cancer, but the only way to know is to see your doctor.

Vaginal and Vulvar Cancers Screening

Screening is when a test is used to look for a disease before there are any symptoms. Cancer screening tests are effective when they can detect disease early. Detecting disease early can lead to more effective treatment. Diagnostic tests are used when a person has symptoms. The purpose of diagnostic tests is to find out, or diagnose, what is causing the symptoms. Diagnostic tests also may be used to check a person who is considered at high risk for cancer.

There is no simple and reliable way to test for vaginal or vulvar cancers in women who do not have any signs or symptoms. The Pap test does not screen for vaginal or vulvar cancers. It is especially important to recognize warning signs, and learn what you can do to reduce your risk.

Here are steps you can take:

- Pay attention to your body, and know what is normal for you.

- If you notice any changes in your body that are not normal for you and could be a sign of either vaginal or vulvar cancer, talk to your doctor about them and ask about possible causes.

- Visit your doctor regularly for a checkup. During your checkup, your doctor may perform a pelvic examination to look for signs of vaginal and vulvar cancer.

When vaginal and vulvar cancers are found early, treatment is most effective.

If your doctor says that you have vaginal or vulvar cancer, ask to be referred to a gynecologic oncologist—a doctor who has been trained to treat cancers like these. This doctor will work with you to create a treatment plan.

Chapter 39

Colon and Rectal Cancers

What is colorectal cancer?

Cancer is a group of diseases in which there is abnormal and uncontrolled growth of cells in the body. If left untreated, malignant (or cancerous) cells can spread to other parts of the body.

"Colorectal" refers to the colon and rectum, which together make up the large intestine. Colorectal cancer can begin anywhere in the large intestine. The majority of colorectal cancers begin as polyps—abnormal growths—inside the colon or rectum that may become cancers over a long period of time.

How does colorectal cancer affect the U.S. population?

Of cancers that affect both men and women, colorectal cancer is the second leading cancer killer in the United States. In 2008, 142,950 adults were diagnosed with colorectal cancer, and 52,857 adults died of the disease.

What causes colorectal cancer, and who is at risk of developing it?

The exact cause of most colorectal cancers is not yet known. About 75% of colorectal cancers occur in people with no known risk factors.

"Frequently Asked Questions about Colorectal Cancer," Centers for Disease Control and Prevention (www.cdc.gov), March 5, 2012.

Some conditions that may increase a person's risk of developing colorectal cancer include having the following:

- A personal or family history of colorectal polyps or colorectal cancer

- Inflammatory bowel disease (ulcerative colitis or Crohn disease)

- A genetic syndrome such as familial adenomatous polyposis (FAP) or hereditary non-polyposis colorectal cancer (Lynch syndrome)—just 5% of colorectal cancers are linked to these genetic syndromes

What are the symptoms of colorectal cancer?

Colorectal polyps and colorectal cancer don't always cause symptoms, especially at first. Someone could have polyps or colorectal cancer and not know it. That is why getting screened regularly for colorectal cancer is so important.

If there are symptoms, they may include the following:

- Blood in or on your stool (bowel movement)

- Stomach pain, aches, or cramps that don't go away

- Losing weight and you don't know why

If you have any of these symptoms, talk to your doctor. These symptoms may be caused by something other than cancer. However, the only way to know what is causing them is to see your doctor.

Is there anything I can do to reduce my risk for colorectal cancer?

There is strong scientific evidence that having regular screening tests for colorectal cancer beginning at age 50 reduces deaths from colorectal cancer. Screening tests can find precancerous polyps (abnormal growths) in the colon and rectum, and polyps can be removed before they turn into cancer.

Studies have also shown that increased physical activity and maintaining a healthy weight can decrease the risk for colorectal cancer. Evidence is less clear about other ways to prevent colorectal cancer.

Research is underway to determine whether dietary changes may decrease the risk for colorectal cancer. Currently, there is no consensus on the role of diet in preventing colorectal cancer, but medical experts recommend a diet low in animal fats and high in fruits, vegetables, and whole grain products to reduce the risk of other chronic diseases, such as coronary artery disease and diabetes. This diet also may reduce the risk of colorectal cancer. In addition, researchers are examining the role of certain medications and supplements, including aspirin, calcium, vitamin D, and selenium, in preventing colorectal cancer.

Overall, the most effective way to reduce your risk of colorectal cancer is by having regular colorectal cancer screening tests beginning at age 50.

What is cancer screening?

Screening is when a test is used to look for a disease before there are any symptoms. Cancer screening tests, including those for colorectal cancer, are effective when they can detect disease early. Detecting disease early can lead to more effective treatment. (Diagnostic tests are used when a person has symptoms and are intended to find out what is causing the symptoms.)

Why should I get screened for colorectal cancer?

Screening for colorectal cancer saves lives. Screening tests can find polyps, so they can be removed before they turn into cancer. Screening tests also can find colorectal cancer early, when treatment works best and the chance for a full recovery is very high. Having regular screening tests beginning at age 50 could save your life.

What are the screening tests for colorectal cancer?

Several screening tests can be used to find polyps or colorectal cancer. Each can be used alone. Sometimes they are used in combination with each other. The U.S. Preventive Services Task Force recommends colorectal cancer screening for men and women aged 50–75 using high-sensitivity fecal occult blood testing (FOBT), sigmoidoscopy, or colonoscopy. Talk to your doctor about which test or tests are right for you. The decision to be screened after age 75 should be made on an individual basis. If you are older than 75, ask your doctor if you should be screened.

- **High-sensitivity FOBT (stool test):** There are two types of FOBT. One uses the chemical guaiac to detect blood. The other, a fecal immunochemical test (FIT), uses antibodies to detect blood in the stool. You receive a test kit from your health care provider.

At home, you use a stick or brush to obtain a small amount of stool. You return the test kit to the doctor or a lab, where the stool samples are checked for anything unusual. This test should be repeated once a year.

- **Flexible sigmoidoscopy:** For this test, the health care provider puts a short, thin, flexible, lighted tube into your rectum. The doctor checks for polyps or cancer inside the rectum and lower third of the colon. This test should occur every five years.

- **Colonoscopy:** This is similar to flexible sigmoidoscopy, except the doctor uses a longer, thin, flexible, lighted tube to check for polyps or cancer inside the rectum and the entire colon. During the test, the doctor can find and remove most polyps and some cancers. Colonoscopy also is used as a follow-up test if anything unusual is found during one of the other screening tests. A colonoscopy should be performed every 10 years.

What about other colorectal cancer screening tests?

Although these tests are not recommended by the U.S. Preventive Services Task Force, they are used in some settings, and other groups may recommend them. Many insurance plans don't cover these tests, and if anything unusual is found during the test, you likely will need a follow-up colonoscopy.

- **Double-contrast barium enema:** You receive an enema with a liquid called barium, followed by an air enema. The barium and air create an outline around your colon, allowing the doctor to see the outline of your colon on an X-ray.

- **Virtual colonoscopy:** Uses X-rays and computers to produce images of the entire colon which are displayed on a computer screen.

- **Stool DNA test:** You collect an entire bowel movement and send it to a lab to be checked for cancer cells.

How do I know which screening test is right for me?

Scientific data do not currently suggest that there is a single "best test" for any one person. Each test has advantages and disadvantages. Patients and their doctors are encouraged to discuss the benefits and potential risks associated with each screening option as they decide which test to use and how often to be tested.

Is colorectal cancer screening covered by insurance?

Most insurance plans help pay for colorectal cancer screening tests for people aged 50 or older. Many plans also help pay for screening tests for people younger than 50 who are at increased risk for colorectal cancer. Check with your health insurance provider to determine your colorectal cancer screening benefits.

What are the Medicare Preventive Service benefits for colorectal cancer screening?

People with Medicare who are aged 50 or older are eligible for colorectal cancer screening. There is no minimum age for colonoscopy. For information about Medicare's coverage related to colorectal cancer screening, call the Centers for Medicare and Medicaid Services at 800-MEDICARE (800-633-4227) (TTY users should call 877-486-2048) or visit the Medicare website (www.medicare.gov).

Chapter 40

Lung Cancer

Lung cancer is the leading cause of cancer death and the second most diagnosed cancer in both men and women in the United States. In 2008, 14% of all cancer diagnoses and 28% of all cancer deaths were due to lung cancer. After increasing for decades, lung cancer incidence and mortality among men and women are decreasing, paralleling decreases in cigarette smoking.

Lung cancer begins in the lungs and may spread to lymph nodes or other organs in the body, such as the brain. Cancer from other organs may spread to the lungs. When cancer cells spread from one organ to another, they are called metastases.

Lung cancers usually are grouped into two main types called small cell and non-small cell. These types of lung cancer grow differently and are treated differently. Non-small cell lung cancer is more common than small cell lung cancer.

Cigarette smoking is the number one cause of lung cancer. Lung cancer also can be caused by using other types of tobacco (such as pipes or cigars), breathing secondhand smoke, being exposed to substances such as asbestos or radon at home or work, and having a family history of lung cancer.

Excerpted from "Basic Information about Lung Cancer," Centers for Disease Control and Prevention (www.cdc.gov), 2011–2012.

Risk Factors

Research has found several risk factors for lung cancer. A risk factor is anything (for example, a behavior or a characteristic) that increases the chance of getting a disease. Different risk factors change risk by different amounts.

Examples of risk factors for lung cancer include the following:

- Smoking tobacco and being around others' smoke

- Exposures at home or work (such as radon gas or asbestos)

- Personal history (such as having radiation therapy or a family history of lung cancer)

We know a lot about risk factors, but they don't tell us everything. Some people who get cancer don't seem to have any known risk factors. Other people have one or more risk factors and do not get cancer. If a person has several risk factors and develops lung cancer, we don't know how much each risk factor contributed to the cancer.

Smoking and Secondhand Smoke

Cigarette smoking is the number one risk factor for lung cancer. In the United States, cigarette smoking causes about 90% of lung cancers. Tobacco smoke is a toxic mix of more than 7,000 chemicals. Many are poisons. At least 70 are known to cause cancer in people or animals. People who smoke are 15 to 30 times more likely to get lung cancer or die from lung cancer than people who do not smoke. Even smoking a few cigarettes a day or smoking occasionally increases the risk of lung cancer. The more years a person smokes and the more cigarettes smoked each day, the more risk goes up.

People who quit smoking have a lower risk of lung cancer than if they had continued to smoke, but their risk is higher than the risk for people who never smoked. Quitting smoking at any age can lower the risk of lung cancer. For help quitting, visit Quit Smoking (at www.cdc.gov/tobacco/quit_smoking) or call 800-QUIT-NOW (800-784-8669); TTY 800-332-8615.

Smoking can cause cancer almost anywhere in the body. Smoking causes cancer of the mouth, nose, throat, voice box (larynx), esophagus, bladder, kidney, pancreas, cervix, stomach, blood, and bone marrow (acute myeloid leukemia).

Using other tobacco products such as cigars or pipes also increases the risk for lung cancer.

Smoke from other people's cigarettes, pipes, or cigars (second-hand smoke) also causes lung cancer. When a person breathes in secondhand smoke, it is like he or she is smoking. Two out of five adults who don't smoke and half of children in the United States are exposed to secondhand smoke. Every year in the United States, about 3,000 people who never smoked die from lung cancer due to secondhand smoke.

Exposures at Home and Work That May Cause Lung Cancer

Several exposures in the home or workplace may cause lung cancer:

- Radon is a naturally occurring gas that comes from rocks and dirt and can get trapped in houses and buildings. It cannot be seen, tasted, or smelled. According to the U.S. Environmental Protection Agency (EPA), radon causes about 20,000 cases of lung cancer each year, making it the second-leading cause of lung cancer. Nearly one out of every 15 homes in the United States is estimated to have high radon levels. The EPA recommends testing homes for radon and using proven methods to reduce high radon levels. For more information, read "A Citizen's Guide to Radon" (at www.epa.gov/radon/pubs/citguide.html).

- Examples of substances found at some workplaces that increase risk include asbestos, arsenic, diesel exhaust, and some forms of silica and chromium. For many of these substances, the risk of getting lung cancer is even higher for those who also smoke.

Family History

Risk of lung cancer may be higher if a person's parents, siblings, or children have had lung cancer. This increased risk could come from one or more things. They may share behaviors, like smoking. They may live in the same place where there are carcinogens such as radon. They may have inherited increased risk in their genes.

Radiation Therapy to the Chest

Cancer survivors who had radiation therapy to the chest are at higher risk of lung cancer. Patients at highest risk include those treated for Hodgkin disease and women with breast cancer treated with radiation after a mastectomy (but not a lumpectomy).

Diet

Scientists are studying many different foods and dietary supplements to see whether they increase the risk of getting lung cancer. There is much we still need to know. We do know that smokers who take beta-carotene supplements have increased risk of lung cancer. Also, arsenic in drinking water (primarily from private wells) can increase the risk of lung cancer.

Prevention

There may be several ways to reduce your risk of developing lung cancer.

Don't smoke: Tobacco use is the major cause of lung cancer in the United States. About 90% of lung cancer deaths in men and almost 80% of lung cancer deaths in women in this country are due to smoking. The most important thing a person can do to prevent lung cancer is to not start smoking, or to quit if he or she currently smokes.

Quitting smoking will lower risk of lung cancer compared to not quitting. This is true no matter how old a person is. The longer a person goes without smoking, the more his or her risk will improve compared to those who continue to smoke. However, the risk in people who have quit is still higher than the risk in people who have never smoked. For tips on quitting, visit smokefree.gov.

Centers for Disease Control and Prevention (CDC) helps support a national network of quitlines that makes free "quit smoking" support available by telephone to smokers anywhere in the United States. The toll-free number is 800-QUIT-NOW (800-784-8669); TTY 800-332-8615.

For smokers, avoiding other things that increase risk for lung cancer may help lower risk, but not as much as quitting smoking.

Avoid secondhand smoke: Make your home and car smoke-free.

Make your home and workplace safer: The EPA recommends that all homes be tested for radon. Radon detectors can be purchased or arrangements can be made for qualified testers to come into the home. Some states offer free or low-cost radon test kits.

Health and safety guidelines in the workplace can help workers avoid things that can cause cancer (carcinogens). Visit the National Institute for Occupational Safety and Health (at www.cdc.gov/niosh/topics/cancer) for more information.

Eat a healthy diet: Scientists are studying many different foods and dietary supplements to see if they can prevent lung cancer. There is much we still need to know. We do know that fruits and carotenoid-rich foods probably protect against lung cancer.

Symptoms

Different people have different symptoms for lung cancer. Some people have symptoms related to the lungs. Some people whose lung cancer has spread to other parts of the body (metastasized) have symptoms specific to that part of the body. Some people just have general symptoms of not feeling well. Most people with lung cancer don't have symptoms until the cancer is advanced. Lung cancer symptoms may include the following:

- Coughing that gets worse or doesn't go away
- Chest pain
- Shortness of breath
- Wheezing
- Coughing up blood
- Feeling very tired all the time (fatigue)
- Weight loss with no known cause

Other changes that can sometimes occur with lung cancer may include repeated bouts of pneumonia and swollen or enlarged lymph nodes (glands) inside the chest in the area between the lungs.

These symptoms can happen with other illnesses, too. People with symptoms should talk to their doctor, who can help find the cause.

Screening

Screening means testing for a disease when there are no symptoms or history of that disease. Doctors recommend a screening test to find a disease early on (early detection), when treatment may work better. Scientists have studied several types of screening tests for lung cancer.

Several tests have been studied to see if they can detect lung cancer early with the goal of decreasing deaths from lung cancer. There is little evidence that chest X-rays or sputum cytology can prevent people from dying from lung cancer. Screening for lung cancer with chest X-rays was once promoted by some experts, but researchers found out that people who were screened did not have a lower death rate than people who were not screened. Promising results have been reported recently that people who had low-dose helical CT scans did have a lower chance of dying from lung cancer than people who had chest X-rays.

Screening also has its downside. Screening tests may find spots (abnormalities) in the lungs. These spots could be cancer or not cancer (benign). More tests may be needed to find out if the spot is a cancer. These tests might include removing a small piece of lung tissue for more testing (biopsy). This means that some people might have a surgical procedure even though they don't have cancer (false positive). These procedures have risks associated with them and can cause anxiety and cost money.

Experts do not know if the benefits of screening (early detection) outweigh the potential harms (false positives), especially for people who do not smoke. For these reasons, experts do not currently recommend for or against lung cancer screening.

Diagnosis and Treatment

There are two main types of lung cancer: small cell lung cancer and non-small cell lung cancer. These categories refer to what the cancer cells look like under a microscope. Non-small cell lung cancer is more common than small cell lung cancer.

Lung cancer stage depends on the extent of disease, which includes information about how big a cancer is or how far it has spread through the lungs, lymph nodes, and the rest of the body.

Doctors use information about the type of lung cancer and stage to plan treatment and to monitor progress of treatment.

Types of Treatment

There are several ways to treat lung cancer. The treatment depends on the type of lung cancer and how far it has spread. Treatments include surgery, chemotherapy, radiation therapy, and targeted therapy. People with lung cancer often get more than one kind of treatment.

- **Surgery:** Doctors cut out and remove the cancer in an operation.

- **Chemotherapy:** Chemotherapy involves the use of drugs to shrink or kill the cancer. The drugs could be pills or medicines given through an IV (intravenous) tube.

- **Radiation therapy:** Radiation uses high-energy rays (similar to X-rays) to kill the cancer cells. The rays are aimed at the part of the body where the cancer is.

- **Targeted therapy:** Targeted therapy uses drugs to block the growth and spread of cancer cells. The drugs could be pills or medicines given through an IV tube. Bevacizumab (Avastin) and erlotinib (Tarceva) can be used to treat non-small cell lung cancer.

People with non-small cell lung cancer can be treated with surgery, chemotherapy, radiation therapy, targeted therapy, or a combination of these treatments. People with small cell lung cancer are usually treated with radiation therapy and chemotherapy.

These treatments may be provided by different doctors on your medical team. Pulmonologists are doctors who are experts in diseases of the lungs. Surgeons are doctors who perform operations. Medical oncologists are doctors who are experts in cancer and treat cancers with medicines. Radiation oncologists are doctors who treat cancers with radiation.

Survivorship

People with lung cancer may experience symptoms caused by the cancer or by cancer treatments (side effects). Common symptoms include shortness of breath, coughing, wheezing, coughing up blood, pain, fever, and weight loss. These symptoms usually can be treated. Patients with lung cancer should discuss their concerns about symptoms and side effects with their doctors. Doctors can help answer questions and make a plan for comfort care.

People with lung cancer should quit smoking if they smoke. Patients with lung cancer should ask their doctor about medical options that can aid smoking cessation such as nicotine replacement therapy, bupropion, or varenicline.

People with lung cancer should eat a healthy diet to keep up their strength. Side effects from cancer treatment such as nausea or appetite loss may make this challenging.

Regular physical activity may improve quality of life after a lung cancer diagnosis. Patients with lung cancer should discuss an exercise plan with their doctor.

Chapter 41

Skin Cancer

Skin cancer is the most common form of cancer in the United States. The two most common types of skin cancer—basal cell and squamous cell carcinomas—are highly curable. However, melanoma, the third most common skin cancer, is more dangerous. About 65%–90% of melanomas are caused by exposure to ultraviolet (UV) light.

Ultraviolet Light

UV rays are an invisible kind of radiation that comes from the sun, tanning beds, and sunlamps. UV rays can penetrate and change skin cells.

The three types of UV rays are ultraviolet A (UVA), ultraviolet B (UVB), and ultraviolet C (UVC):

- UVA is the most common kind of sunlight at the earth's surface and reaches beyond the top layer of human skin. Scientists believe that UVA rays can damage connective tissue and increase a person's risk of skin cancer.

- Most UVB rays are absorbed by the ozone layer, so they are less common at the earth's surface than UVA rays. UVB rays don't reach as far into the skin as UVA rays, but they can still be damaging.

- UVC rays are very dangerous, but they are absorbed by the ozone layer and do not reach the ground.

Excerpted from "Basic Information about Skin Cancer," Centers for Disease Control and Prevention (www.cdc.gov), 2012.

Too much exposure to UV rays can change skin texture, cause the skin to age prematurely, and can lead to skin cancer. UV rays also have been linked to eye conditions such as cataracts.

UV Index

The National Weather Service and the Environmental Protection Agency developed the UV Index (www.epa.gov/sunwise/uvindex.html) to forecast the risk of overexposure to UV rays. It lets you know how much caution you should take when working, playing, or exercising outdoors.

The UV Index predicts exposure levels on a 1–15 scale; higher levels indicate a higher risk of overexposure. Calculated on a next-day basis for dozens of cities across the United States, the UV Index takes into account clouds and other local conditions that affect the amount of UV rays reaching the ground.

Risk Factors

People with certain risk factors are more likely than others to develop skin cancer. Risk factors vary for different types of skin cancer, but some general risk factors are having the following:

- A lighter natural skin color
- Family history of skin cancer
- A personal history of skin cancer
- Exposure to the sun through work and play
- A history of sunburns early in life
- A history of indoor tanning
- Skin that burns, freckles, reddens easily, or becomes painful in the sun
- Blue or green eyes
- Blond or red hair
- Certain types and a large number of moles

Tanning and Burning

Ultraviolet rays come from the sun or from indoor tanning (using a tanning bed, booth, or sunlamp to get tan). When UV rays reach the skin's inner layer, the skin makes more melanin. Melanin is the pigment that colors the skin. It moves toward the outer layers of the skin and becomes visible as a tan.

A tan does not indicate good health. A tan is a response to injury, because skin cells signal that they have been hurt by UV rays by producing more pigment.

People burn or tan depending on their skin type, the time of year, and how long they are exposed to UV rays. The six types of skin, based on how likely it is to tan or burn, are the following:

I: Always burns, never tans, sensitive to UV exposure

II: Burns easily, tans minimally

III: Burns moderately, tans gradually to light brown

IV: Burns minimally, always tans well to moderately brown

V: Rarely burns, tans profusely to dark

VI: Never burns, deeply pigmented, least sensitive

Although everyone's skin can be damaged by UV exposure, people with skin types I and II are at the highest risk.

Prevention

Protection from UV radiation is important all year round, not just during the summer or at the beach. UV rays from the sun can reach you on cloudy and hazy days, as well as bright and sunny days. UV rays also reflect off of surfaces like water, cement, sand, and snow. Indoor tanning exposes users to UV radiation.

The hours between 10 a.m. and 4 p.m. daylight savings time (9 a.m. to 3 p.m. standard time) are the most hazardous for UV exposure outdoors in the continental United States. UV rays from sunlight are the greatest during the late spring and early summer in North America.

CDC recommends easy options for protection from UV radiation:

- Seek shade, especially during midday hours.

- Wear clothing to protect exposed skin.

- Wear a hat with a wide brim to shade the face, head, ears, and neck.

- Wear sunglasses that wrap around and block as close to 100% of both UVA and UVB rays as possible.

- Use sunscreen with sun protective factor (SPF) 15 or higher and both UVA and UVB protection.

- Avoid indoor tanning.

Shade

You can reduce your risk of skin damage and skin cancer by seeking shade under an umbrella, tree, or other shelter before you need relief from the sun. Your best bet to protect your skin is to use sunscreen or wear protective clothing when you're outside—even when you're in the shade.

Clothing

Loose-fitting long-sleeved shirts and long pants made from tightly woven fabric offer the best protection from the sun's UV rays. A wet T-shirt offers much less UV protection than a dry one. Darker colors may offer more protection than lighter colors.

If wearing this type of clothing isn't practical, at least try to wear a T-shirt or a beach cover-up. Keep in mind that a typical T-shirt has an SPF rating lower than 15, so use other types of protection as well.

Hats

For the most protection, wear a hat with a brim all the way around that shades your face, ears, and the back of your neck. A tightly woven fabric, such as canvas, works best to protect your skin from UV rays. Avoid straw hats with holes that let sunlight through. A darker hat may offer more UV protection.

If you wear a baseball cap, you should also protect your ears and the back of your neck by wearing clothing that covers those areas, using sunscreen with at least SPF 15, or by staying in the shade.

Sunglasses

Sunglasses protect your eyes from UV rays and reduce the risk of cataracts. They also protect the tender skin around your eyes from sun exposure.

Sunglasses that block both UVA and UVB rays offer the best protection. Most sunglasses sold in the United States, regardless of cost, meet this standard. Wrap-around sunglasses work best because they block UV rays from sneaking in from the side.

Sunscreen

The sun's UV rays can damage your skin in as little as 15 minutes. Put on sunscreen before you go outside, even on slightly cloudy or cool days. Don't forget to put a thick layer on all parts of exposed skin. Get help for hard-to-reach places like your back.

How sunscreen works: Most sun protection products work by absorbing, reflecting, or scattering sunlight. They contain chemicals that interact with the skin to protect it from UV rays. All products do not have the same ingredients; if your skin reacts badly to one product, try another one or call a doctor.

SPF: Sunscreens are assigned a sun protection factor (SPF) number that rates their effectiveness in blocking UV rays. Higher numbers indicate more protection. You should use a sunscreen with at least SPF 15.

Reapplication: Sunscreen wears off. Put it on again if you stay out in the sun for more than two hours and after you swim or do things that make you sweat.

Expiration date: Check the sunscreen's expiration date. Sunscreen without an expiration date has a shelf life of no more than three years, but its shelf life is shorter if it has been exposed to high temperatures.

Cosmetics: Some make-up and lip balms contain some of the same chemicals used in sunscreens. If they do not have at least SPF 15, don't use them by themselves.

Indoor Tanning

Using a tanning bed, booth, or sunlamp to get tan is called "indoor tanning." Indoor tanning has been linked with skin cancers including melanoma (the deadliest type of skin cancer), squamous cell carcinoma, and cancers of the eye (ocular melanoma).

Dangers of Indoor Tanning

Indoor tanning exposes users to both UVA and UVB rays, which damage the skin and can lead to cancer. Using a tanning bed is particularly dangerous for younger users; people who begin tanning younger than age 35 have a 75% higher risk of melanoma. Using tanning beds also increases the risk of wrinkles and eye damage and changes skin texture.

Myths about Indoor Tanning

"Tanning indoors is safer than tanning in the sun." Indoor tanning and tanning outside are both dangerous. Although tanning beds operate on a timer, the exposure to ultraviolet (UV) rays can vary based on the age and type of light bulbs. You can still get a burn from tanning indoors, and even a tan indicates damage to your skin.

"I can use a tanning bed to get a base tan, which will protect me from getting a sunburn." A tan is a response to injury: skin cells respond to damage from UV rays by producing more pigment. The best way to protect your skin from the sun is by using the tips for skin cancer prevention above.

"Indoor tanning is a safe way to get vitamin D, which prevents many health problems." Vitamin D is important for bone health, but studies showing links between vitamin D and other health conditions are inconsistent. Although it is important to get enough vitamin D, the safest way is through diet or supplements. Tanning harms your skin, and the amount of time spent tanning to get enough vitamin D varies from person to person.

Chapter 42

Thyroid Cancer

Thyroid cancer is a disease in which malignant (cancer) cells form in the tissues of the thyroid gland.

The thyroid is a gland at the base of the throat near the trachea (windpipe). It is shaped like a butterfly, with a right lobe and a left lobe. The isthmus, a thin piece of tissue, connects the two lobes. A healthy thyroid is a little larger than a quarter. It usually cannot be felt through the skin. The thyroid uses iodine, a mineral found in some foods and in iodized salt, to help make several hormones. Thyroid hormones do the following:

- Control heart rate, body temperature, and how quickly food is changed into energy (metabolism)

- Control the amount of calcium in the blood

There are four main types of thyroid cancer:

- **Papillary thyroid cancer:** The most common type of thyroid cancer

- **Follicular thyroid cancer:** Hürthle cell carcinoma, a form of follicular thyroid cancer, is treated the same way

- **Medullary thyroid cancer**

- **Anaplastic thyroid cancer**

Excerpted from PDQ Cancer Information Summary. National Cancer Institute; Bethesda, MD. Thyroid Cancer Treatment (PDQ®): Patient Version. Updated 06/2012. Available at: http://cancer.gov. Accessed March 12, 2013.

Age, gender, and exposure to radiation can affect the risk of developing thyroid cancer. Anything that increases your risk of getting a disease is called a risk factor. Having a risk factor does not mean that you will get cancer; not having risk factors doesn't mean that you will not get cancer. People who think they may be at risk should discuss this with their doctor. Risk factors for thyroid cancer include the following:

• Being between 25 and 65 years old

• Being female

• Being exposed to radiation to the head and neck as a child or being exposed to atomic bomb radiation. The cancer may occur as soon as five years after exposure

• Having a history of goiter (enlarged thyroid)

• Having a family history of thyroid disease or thyroid cancer

• Having certain genetic conditions such as familial medullary thyroid cancer (FMTC), multiple endocrine neoplasia type 2A syndrome, and multiple endocrine neoplasia type 2B syndrome

• Being Asian

Medullary thyroid cancer is sometimes caused by a change in a gene that is passed from parent to child. The genes in cells carry hereditary information from parent to child. A certain change in a gene that is passed from parent to child (inherited) may cause medullary thyroid cancer. A test has been developed that can find the changed gene before medullary thyroid cancer appears. The patient is tested first to see if he or she has the changed gene. If the patient has it, other family members may also be tested. Family members, including young children, who have the changed gene can decrease the chance of developing medullary thyroid cancer by having a thyroidectomy (surgery to remove the thyroid).

Possible signs of thyroid cancer include a swelling or lump in the neck. Thyroid cancer may not cause early symptoms. It is sometimes found during a routine physical exam. Symptoms may occur as the tumor gets bigger. Other conditions may cause the same symptoms. Check with your doctor if you have any of the following problems:

• A lump in the neck

• Trouble breathing

• Trouble swallowing

• Hoarseness

Tests that examine the thyroid, neck, and blood are used to detect (find) and diagnose thyroid cancer. The following tests and procedures may be used:

- **Physical exam and history:** An exam of the body to check general signs of health, including checking for signs of disease, such as lumps or swelling in the neck, voice box, and lymph nodes, and anything else that seems unusual. A history of the patient's health habits and past illnesses and treatments will also be taken.

- **Laryngoscopy:** A procedure in which the doctor checks the larynx (voice box) with a mirror or with a laryngoscope. A laryngoscope is a thin, tube-like instrument with a light and a lens for viewing. A thyroid tumor may press on vocal cords. The laryngoscopy is done to see if the vocal cords are moving normally.

- **Blood hormone studies:** A procedure in which a blood sample is checked to measure the amounts of certain hormones released into the blood by organs and tissues in the body. An unusual (higher or lower than normal) amount of a substance can be a sign of disease in the organ or tissue that makes it. The blood may be checked for abnormal levels of thyroid-stimulating hormone (TSH). TSH is made by the pituitary gland in the brain. It stimulates the release of thyroid hormone and controls how fast follicular thyroid cells grow. The blood may also be checked for high levels of the hormone calcitonin and antithyroid antibodies.

- **Blood chemistry studies:** A procedure in which a blood sample is checked to measure the amounts of certain substances, such as calcium, released into the blood by organs and tissues in the body. An unusual (higher or lower than normal) amount of a substance can be a sign of disease in the organ or tissue that makes it.

- **Ultrasound exam:** A procedure in which high-energy sound waves (ultrasound) are bounced off internal tissues or organs and make echoes. The echoes form a picture of body tissues called a sonogram. This procedure can show the size of a thyroid tumor and whether it is solid or a fluid-filled cyst. Ultrasound may be used to guide a fine-needle aspiration biopsy.

- **CT scan (computed tomography, or CAT scan):** A procedure that makes a series of detailed pictures of areas inside the body, taken from different angles. The pictures are made by a computer linked to an X-ray machine. A dye may be injected into a vein or swallowed to help the organs or tissues show up more clearly.

- **Fine-needle aspiration biopsy of the thyroid:** The removal of thyroid tissue using a thin needle. The needle is inserted through the skin into the thyroid. Several tissue samples are removed from different parts of the thyroid. A pathologist views the tissue samples under a microscope to look for cancer cells.

- **Surgical biopsy:** The removal of the thyroid nodule or one lobe of the thyroid during surgery so the cells and tissues can be viewed under a microscope by a pathologist to check for signs of cancer.

Certain factors affect prognosis (chance of recovery) and treatment options:

- The age of the patient
- The type of thyroid cancer
- The stage of the cancer
- The patient's general health
- Whether the patient has multiple endocrine neoplasia type 2B (MEN 2B)
- Whether the cancer has just been diagnosed or has recurred (come back)

Different types of treatment are available for patients with thyroid cancer. Some treatments are standard (the currently used treatment), and some are being tested in clinical trials. A treatment clinical trial is a research study meant to help improve current treatments or obtain information on new treatments for patients with cancer. When clinical trials show that a new treatment is better than the standard treatment, the new treatment may become the standard treatment. Patients may want to think about taking part in a clinical trial.

Five types of standard treatment are used:

Surgery: Surgery is the most common treatment of thyroid cancer. One of the following procedures may be used:

- **Lobectomy:** Removal of the lobe in which thyroid cancer is found (biopsies of lymph nodes in the area may be done to see if they contain cancer)

- **Near-total thyroidectomy:** Removal of all but a very small part of the thyroid

- **Total thyroidectomy:** Removal of the whole thyroid

- **Lymphadenectomy:** Removal of lymph nodes in the neck that contain cancer

Radiation therapy, including radioactive iodine therapy: Radiation therapy is a cancer treatment that uses high-energy X-rays or other types of radiation to kill cancer cells or keep them from growing. There are two types of radiation therapy. External radiation therapy uses a machine outside the body to send radiation toward the cancer. Internal radiation therapy uses a radioactive substance sealed in needles, seeds, wires, or catheters that are placed directly into or near the cancer. The way the radiation therapy is given depends on the type and stage of the cancer being treated.

Radiation therapy may be given after surgery to kill any thyroid cancer cells that were not removed. Follicular and papillary thyroid cancers are sometimes treated with radioactive iodine (RAI) therapy. RAI is taken by mouth and collects in any remaining thyroid tissue, including thyroid cancer cells that have spread to other places in the body. Since only thyroid tissue takes up iodine, the RAI destroys thyroid tissue and thyroid cancer cells without harming other tissue. Before a full treatment dose of RAI is given, a small test dose is given to see if the tumor takes up the iodine.

Chemotherapy: Chemotherapy is a cancer treatment that uses drugs to stop the growth of cancer cells, either by killing the cells or by stopping them from dividing. When chemotherapy is taken by mouth or injected into a vein or muscle, the drugs enter the bloodstream and can reach cancer cells throughout the body (systemic chemotherapy). When chemotherapy is placed directly into the cerebrospinal fluid, an organ, or a body cavity such as the abdomen, the drugs mainly affect cancer cells in those areas (regional chemotherapy). The way the chemotherapy is given depends on the type and stage of the cancer being treated.

Thyroid hormone therapy: Hormone therapy is a cancer treatment that removes hormones or blocks their action and stops cancer cells from growing. Hormones are substances made by glands in the body and circulated in the bloodstream. In the treatment of thyroid cancer, drugs may be given to prevent the body from making TSH, a hormone that can increase the chance that thyroid cancer will grow or recur.

Also, because thyroid cancer treatment kills thyroid cells, the thyroid is not able to make enough thyroid hormone. Patients are given thyroid hormone replacement pills.

Targeted therapy: Targeted therapy is a type of treatment that uses drugs or other substances to identify and attack specific cancer cells without harming normal cells. Tyrosine kinase inhibitor (TKI) therapy is a type of targeted therapy that blocks signals needed for tumors to grow. Vandetanib is a TKI used to treat thyroid cancer.

Follow-up tests may be needed. Some of the tests that were done to diagnose the cancer or to find out the stage of the cancer may be repeated. Some tests will be repeated in order to see how well the treatment is working. Decisions about whether to continue, change, or stop treatment may be based on the results of these tests. This is sometimes called re-staging.

Some of the tests will continue to be done from time to time after treatment has ended. The results of these tests can show if your condition has changed or if the cancer has recurred. These tests are sometimes called follow-up tests or checkups.

Part Six

Other Health Conditions with Issues of Significance to Women

Chapter 43

Alzheimer Disease

An estimated 4.5 million Americans—more than half of them women—have Alzheimer's disease in the United States. Given the aging of the baby boomers and the growing numbers of "oldest old," those 85 and above, that figure is expected to more than triple by 2050, when an estimated 13.1 million Americans will be living with the disease.

A Women's Health Concern

Although Alzheimer's affects men and women at nearly the same rates (women are slightly more likely to get Alzheimer's disease than men), Alzheimer's disease has particular relevance for women. That's because the prevalence of the disease in women, or the number of women living with the disease at any one time, is twice as high as for men simply because women live longer. Increasing age is a major risk factor for developing the disease. Thus, about half of all women over 85 will eventually be diagnosed with Alzheimer's disease.

Additionally, in the family women are the primary caregivers for those with the disease. The Family Caregiving Alliance notes that the typical caregiver is a 46-year-old woman, married and working outside the home. Overall, she spends as much as 50% more time giving care than male caregivers, providing an estimated $148 billion in unpaid care annually. And this is not a benign task. There are real health risks for the women who take on this type of caregiving. For instance, studies find that middle-aged and older women who provided care for an ill or disabled spouse are six times as likely to suffer depressive or anxious symptoms as those who had no caregiving responsibilities. Additionally, the chronic stress can weaken the caregiver's immune system, more than double her risk of cardiovascular disease, result in an increased risk of developing hypertension, and contribute to an overall increased risk of death. Studies find that the changes in a woman's immune functioning may continue for up to two years after the person they were caring for dies.

There are ways to manage the stress of caregiving so you don't get sick. Social workers suggest the following to feel more comfortable with the caregiving:

- Have everything in order for your loved ones in terms of legal, financial, and medical issues.

- Anticipate end-of-life needs.

- Take care of the family relationships so they can come together to make decisions.

- Find what it is that gives you solace and peace so you can cope.

Knowledge of the Disease

Despite the prevalence of the disease and the high-profile death of former president Ronald Reagan from complications associated with it, Americans' overall knowledge about Alzheimer's—and the progress being made in preventing, diagnosing, and treating it—is lacking. One survey found that fewer than half of all Americans know that treatments are available that can ease the symptoms and improve the quality of life.

Although researchers still don't know for sure what causes Alzheimer's disease, most believe it is related to the abnormal processing of normal brain proteins, particularly amyloid precursor protein and tau, another type of protein. For some reason, these proteins can begin to be abnormally processed and assemble themselves into lesions, called neurofibrillary tangles and senile plaques, then destroy parts of the brain.

Other theories link the disease's development to the death of cells critical for maintaining levels of certain brain chemicals required for awareness and judgment; chronic inflammation; accumulation of heavy metals in the brain; and vascular factors that affect the health of blood vessels in the brain.

There are two forms of Alzheimer's disease: familial, in which genes directly cause the disease, and sporadic, the most common, in which genes may influence one's risk of developing the disease. Most cases of familial disease, also called "early onset Alzheimer's disease," occur before a person turns 60. This form, however, affects less than 5% of those with Alzheimer's. The majority of people with the disease are diagnosed after age 65.

The disease itself is progressive. In the beginning, people may have problems with simple memory-related tasks: writing checks or taking the bus somewhere; but by the end, they "forget" most everything—how to use the toilet, eat, and even walk. People with Alzheimer's often exhibit significant personality changes as well. Victims may have mood changes, including depression, and may become agitated and/or aggressive at times.

Diagnosing Alzheimer's disease can be tricky. The average patient with Alzheimer's will deny they have a problem so it's up to the family to be proactive in receiving help from the primary care physician. In addition, the only way to get a confirmed diagnosis is through a brain autopsy after death, but doctors are getting better at using cognitive memory tests and, if necessary, brain imaging technology like MRIs or PET scans, to evaluate changes in the brain.

If you think you or someone else in your family has Alzheimer's disease, make sure you get a complete medical workup, including MRI [magnetic resonance imaging] or CT [computed tomography] scans and blood work to rule out other causes of dementia. More than 150 medical conditions—some temporary—can cause dementia. Those include depression, drug intoxication, thyroid disease, brain tumors, and stroke.

Stages of the Disease

Although Alzheimer's disease progresses differently in each individual, there are stages that appear to be common to the disease.

- During the mild stage, caregivers and others may notice that the individual is having problems planning or organizing, reading a paragraph and understanding it, or performing properly at work. They may have problems performing math in their head, such as counting backwards by sevens, and performing complex tasks, such as shopping or paying bills.

- During moderate or mid-stage Alzheimer's disease, an individual may need help choosing the right clothing, may be unable to recall important personal details like his or her birthday or address, or may get confused about where they are.

471

- By the time the disease reaches late stage, individuals lose most awareness of recent experiences and events, as well as their surroundings or the name of their spouse. They may need help getting dressed and experience disruptions in their normal sleep/wake cycle.

- By the end, they are no longer able to respond to their environment, speak, walk without help, or even smile. They have problems swallowing and their reflexes become abnormal. However, there is often quite a lot of overlap between the stages and a patient may exhibit symptoms of several stages at once.

Treatment for Alzheimer's Disease

Today, there are five FDA [U.S. Food and Drug Administration]-approved drugs to treat the disease, none of which do much more than temporarily stabilize or slow the progression. Four of the drugs are known as cholinesterase inhibitors. They work by increasing the amount of neurotransmitter acetylcholine in the brain, which helps brain cells communicate, and work best when prescribed early in the disease. The newest drug, memantine (Namenda), is the first available for those with moderate to severe Alzheimer's disease. It works on a different neurotransmitter called glutamate and is now being tested in people with earlier stages of the disease.

Other drugs in development are directed at the underlying causes of the disease to help prevent the formation of the brain-robbing plaques and tangles in the first place. Additionally, vaccines, which eliminate the plaques after they've formed, are also being developed.

Prevention of Alzheimer's Disease

One of the most intriguing discoveries about Alzheimer's in the last few years is that many of the risk factors for cardiovascular disease are also risk factors for Alzheimer's disease. Those risk factors include high blood pressure, being overweight or obese, high cholesterol levels, high levels of homocysteine (an amino acid in the blood), and a sedentary lifestyle.

Researchers have several theories behind this link. One is that having an intact vascular, or blood, system within the brain helps maximize the brain's potential. If blood flow is restricted because of buildup of plaque or clots in blood vessels, or if blood vessels become too stiff to enable the smooth flow of blood, less oxygen gets to the brain and fewer waste products leave the brain.

It appears that it's most likely there are two primary causes of dementia: an Alzheimer's disease type "pathology," represented by the neurofibrillary tangles and senile plaques of the disease, and vascular dementia, resulting from significant changes in blood vessels in the brain. Another theory suggests that cholesterol plays a role in the development of the amyloid plaques that are a hallmark of the disease. It may be that both theories are going to end up being true, so that having a healthy blood vessel structure in the brain is really a big help. Paying attention to cardiovascular risk factors may have a big impact in delaying the onset of Alzheimer's and may also influence the course of the disease once someone is diagnosed.

Some of the Major Strategies for Preventing Alzheimer's Disease

- **Regular exercise:** It turns out that regular physical activity can reduce the risk of Alzheimer's by up to 50% in all individuals, and up to 60% for women with high levels of physical activity.

- **Regular use of non-steroidal anti-inflammatory drugs (NSAIDs), like aspirin:** No one is suggesting that you begin taking a daily aspirin to prevent Alzheimer's because that link hasn't been proven yet. However, since taking a baby aspirin daily is recommended to prevent cardiovascular disease in high-risk individuals, you may want to talk to your doctor about this option. In one large Canadian study, regular use of NSAIDs was significantly related to a 35% reduction in the risk of Alzheimer's, results duplicated in several other population-based studies.

- **Stretch your mind:** Certain activities that stretch your mind, like chess or crossword puzzles, actually help rewire your brain, increasing the number of synapse, or connections between brain cells. One study found such activities could lower your risk of developing Alzheimer's or any other form of dementia by as much as 75%.

- **Eat a healthful diet:** Specifically, studies suggest that fruits and vegetables high in antioxidants (the darker the better), cold-water fish high in omega-3 fatty acids, and nuts can play a protective role. Along the same lines, limit high-fat, high-cholesterol foods to protect the health of your blood vessels.

- **Maintain a healthy weight:** If you follow all this advice, this should come easily. One major long-term study of 1,500 adults presented at the 9th International Conference on Alzheimer's

Disease and Related Disorders in 2004 found those who were obese in middle age were twice as likely to develop dementia in later life.

Chapter 44

Anemia and Bleeding Disorders

Chapter Contents

Section 44.1

Anemia

Excerpted from "Anemia Fact Sheet," U.S. Department of
Health and Human Services Office on Women's Health
(www.womenshealth.gov), May 13, 2008.

What is anemia?

Anemia occurs when you have fewer than the normal number of
red blood cells in your blood or when the red blood cells in your blood
don't have enough hemoglobin. Hemoglobin is a protein. It gives the
red color to your blood. Its main job is to carry oxygen from your lungs
to all parts of your body. If you have anemia, your blood does not carry
enough oxygen to all the parts of your body. Without oxygen, your organs and tissues cannot work as well as they should. More than three
million people in the United States have anemia. Women and people
with chronic diseases are at the greatest risk for anemia.

What are the types and causes of anemia?

Anemia happens in these situations:

- When the body loses too much blood (such as with heavy periods,
  certain diseases, and trauma)

- When the body has problems making red blood cells

- When red blood cells break down or die faster than the body can
  replace them with new ones

There are many types of anemia, all with different causes:

Iron deficiency anemia (IDA): IDA is the most common type of
anemia. IDA happens when you don't have enough iron in your body.
You need iron to make hemoglobin.

A person can have a low iron level because of blood loss. In women,
iron and red blood cells are lost when bleeding occurs from very heavy
and long periods, as well as from childbirth. Women also can lose iron
and red blood cells from uterine fibroids, which can bleed slowly. Other

ways iron and red blood cells can be lost include ulcers, colon polyps, or colon cancer; regular use of aspirin; infections; severe injury; and surgery.

Eating foods low in iron also can cause IDA. Meat, poultry, fish, eggs, dairy products, or iron-fortified foods are the best sources of iron found in food. Pregnancy can cause IDA if a woman doesn't consume enough iron for both her and her unborn baby.

Some people have enough iron in their diet but have problems absorbing it because of diseases, such as Crohn disease and celiac disease, or drugs they are taking.

Vitamin deficiency anemia (or megaloblastic anemia): Low levels of vitamin B12 or folate are the most common causes of this type of anemia.

- **Vitamin B12 deficiency anemia (or pernicious anemia):** This type of anemia happens due to a lack of vitamin B12 in the body. This type of anemia occurs most often in people whose bodies are not able to absorb vitamin B12 from food because of an autoimmune disorder. It also can happen because of intestinal problems.

- **Folate deficiency anemia:** Folate, also called folic acid, is also needed to make red blood cells. This type of anemia can occur if you don't consume enough folate or if you have problems absorbing vitamins. It also may occur during the third trimester of pregnancy, when your body needs extra folate.

Anemias caused by underlying diseases: Some diseases can hurt the body's ability to make red blood cells. For example, anemia is common in people with kidney disease.

Anemias caused by inherited blood disease: If you have a blood disease in your family, such as sickle cell anemia or thalassemia, you are at greater risk to also have this disease.

What are the signs of anemia?

Anemia takes some time to develop. In the beginning, you may not have any signs or they may be mild. But as it gets worse, you may have these symptoms:

- Fatigue (very common)
- Weakness (very common)
- Dizziness
- Headache

- Numbness or coldness in your hands and feet
- Low body temperature
- Pale skin
- Rapid or irregular heartbeat
- Shortness of breath
- Chest pain
- Irritability

How do I find out if I have anemia?

Your doctor can tell if you have anemia by a blood test called a complete blood count (CBC). Your doctor also will do a physical exam and talk to you about the food you eat, the medicines you are taking, and your family health history. If you have anemia, your doctor may want to do other tests to find out what's causing it.

What is the treatment for anemia?

The treatment your doctor prescribes for you will depend on the cause of the anemia. Treatment may include changes in foods you eat, taking dietary supplements (like vitamins or iron pills), changing the medicines you are taking, or in more severe forms of anemia, medical procedures such as blood transfusion or surgery.

Some types of anemia may be life threatening if not diagnosed and treated. Too little oxygen in the body can damage organs. With anemia, the heart must work harder to make up for the lack of red blood cells or hemoglobin. This extra work can harm the heart and even lead to heart failure.

How do I prevent anemia?

There are steps you can take to help prevent some types of anemia.

- Eat foods high in iron, like 100% iron-fortified breads and cereals, liver, lentils and beans, oysters, tofu, green leafy vegetables, red meat, fish, and dried fruits.

- Eat and drink foods that help your body absorb iron, like orange juice, strawberries, broccoli, or other fruits and vegetables with vitamin C.

- Don't drink coffee or tea with meals. These drinks make it harder for your body to absorb iron.

- Lack of calcium can hurt your absorption of iron. If you have a hard time getting enough iron, talk to your doctor about the best way to also get enough calcium.

- Make sure you consume enough folic acid and vitamin B12.

- Make balanced food choices. Food fads and dieting can lead to anemia.

- Talk to your doctor about taking iron pills (supplements). Do not take these pills without talking to your doctor first.

- If you are a nonpregnant woman of childbearing age, get tested for anemia every 5 to 10 years. This can be done during a regular health exam.

How much iron do I need every day?

Most people get enough iron by making healthy, balanced food choices and eating iron-rich foods. But some groups of women are at greater risk for low iron levels:

- Teenage girls/women of childbearing age (who have heavy bleeding during their period, who have had more than one child, or use an intrauterine device [IUD])

- Pregnant women (about half of pregnant women have iron-deficiency anemia)

- Female athletes who engage in regular, intense exercise

These groups of people should be screened at times for iron deficiency. If the tests show that the body isn't getting enough iron, iron pills (supplements) may be prescribed. Many doctors prescribe iron pills during pregnancy because many pregnant women don't get enough iron.

Since meat, poultry, and seafood are the best sources of iron found in food, some vegetarians may need to take a higher amount of iron each day.

Table 44.1. Recommended Dietary Allowances for Iron for Adult Women

Age	Women	Pregnant	Breastfeeding
14 to 18 years	15 milligrams (mg)	27 mg	10 mg
19 to 50 years	18 mg	27 mg	9 mg
51+ years	8 mg	n/a	n/a

Pregnant women need to consume twice as much iron as women who are not pregnant. But about half of all pregnant women do not get enough iron. If a pregnant woman does not get enough iron for herself or her growing baby, she has an increased chance of having preterm birth and a low-birth-weight baby. If you're pregnant, follow these tips:

- Make sure you get 27 mg of iron every day. Take an iron supplement (pill). It may be part of your prenatal vitamin.

- Get tested for anemia at your first prenatal visit.

- Ask if you need to be tested for anemia four to six weeks after delivery.

What happens if my body gets more iron than it needs?

Iron overload happens when too much iron builds up in the body over time. This condition is called hemochromatosis. The extra iron can damage the organs, mainly the liver, heart, and pancreas. Most people with hemochromatosis inherit it from their parents. It is one of the most common genetic (runs in families) diseases in the United States. Some other diseases also can lead to iron overload. It also can happen from years of taking too much iron or from repeated blood transfusions or dialysis.

Signs of early hemochromatosis may include the following:

- Fatigue
- Weakness
- Weight loss
- Abdominal pain
- Joint pain
- Fluttering in chest

As iron builds up in the body, common symptoms include these:

- Arthritis
- Impotence
- Missed periods
- Heart problems like shortness of breath, chest pain, and changes in rate or rhythm
- Early menopause
- Loss of sex drive

Signs of advanced hemochromatosis include the following:

- Arthritis
- Liver disease
- Damage to the pancreas, possibly causing diabetes
- Chronic abdominal pain

- Severe fatigue

- Weakening of the heart muscle

- Heart failure

- Changes in skin color, making it look gray, yellow, or bronze

Treatment depends on how severe the iron overload is. The first step is to get rid of the extra iron in the body. Most people undergo a process called phlebotomy, which means removing blood. It is simple and safe. A pint of blood will be taken once or twice a week for several months to a year, and sometimes longer. Once iron levels go back to normal, you will give a pint of blood every two to four months for life. People who cannot give blood can take medicine to remove extra iron. This is called iron chelation therapy. Although treatment cannot cure the problems caused by hemochromatosis, it will help most of them. Arthritis is the only problem that does not improve after excess iron is removed.

Section 44.2

Bleeding Disorders

"Bleeding Disorders in Women," Centers for Disease
Control and Prevention (www.cdc.gov), March 22, 2012.

A bleeding disorder is a condition that keeps your blood from clotting properly after a cut or injury. Women are more likely to notice the symptoms of a bleeding disorder because of heavy or abnormal bleeding during their menstrual periods and after childbirth.

Heavy bleeding is one of the most common problems women report to their doctors. It affects more than 10 million American women each year. This means that about one out of every five women has it.

Signs and Symptoms of a Bleeding Disorder

- Heavy menstrual periods that have the following symptoms:

  - Bleeding for more than seven days

- Flooding or gushing of blood that limits daily activities
- Passing clots that are bigger than a quarter
- Changing a tampon or pad, possibly even both, every hour or more often on heaviest day(s)
- Being diagnosed as "low in iron" or having received treatment for anemia
- Having experienced prolonged or heavy bleeding episodes such as might occur as a result of the following:
  - Dental surgery, other surgery, or childbirth
  - Frequent nose bleeds (longer than 10 minutes)
  - Bleeding from cuts or injury (longer than 5 minutes)
  - Easy bruising (weekly, raised, and larger than a quarter in size)
- Having any of the aforementioned bleeding symptoms and a family member with a bleeding disorder such as von Willebrand disease or a clotting factor deficiency such as hemophilia

Talk to Your Doctor

If you have **one or more** of these signs and symptoms, please talk with your doctor or other health care professional. Bleeding disorders can be dangerous if they are not treated. Women with untreated bleeding disorders face serious risks after childbirth, dental surgery, other surgery, or injury. Talking openly with your doctor is very important in making sure you are diagnosed properly and get the right treatment.

Chapter 45

Arthritis (Osteoarthritis)

Osteoarthritis is the most common form of arthritis among older people. The disease affects both men and women. Before age 45, osteoarthritis is more common in men than in women. After age 45, osteoarthritis is more common in women. Osteoarthritis is one of the most frequent causes of physical disability among older adults.

Osteoarthritis occurs when cartilage, the tissue that cushions the ends of the bones within the joints, breaks down and wears away. In some cases, all of the cartilage may wear away, leaving bones that rub up against each other.

Symptoms range from stiffness and mild pain that comes and goes to severe joint pain. Osteoarthritis affects hands, low back, neck, and weight-bearing joints such as knees, hips, and feet. Osteoarthritis affects just joints, not internal organs.

Causes and Risk Factors

Researchers suspect that osteoarthritis is caused by a combination of factors in the body and the environment. The chance of developing osteoarthritis increases with age. It is estimated that 33.6% (12.4 million) of individuals age 65 and older are affected by the disease.

Excerpted from "Osteoarthritis," National Institute on Aging (nihseniorhealth .gov), June 2011.

483

Osteoarthritis often results from years of wear and tear on joints. This wear and tear mostly affects the cartilage, the tissue that cushions the ends of bones within the joint. Osteoarthritis occurs when the cartilage begins to fray, wear away, and decay.

Putting too much stress on a joint that has been previously injured, improper alignment of joints, and excess weight all may contribute to the development of osteoarthritis.

Symptoms

Different types of arthritis have different symptoms. In general, people with most forms of arthritis have pain and stiffness in their joints.

Osteoarthritis usually develops slowly and can occur in any joint but often occurs in weight-bearing joints. Early in the disease, joints may ache after physical work or exercise. Most often, osteoarthritis occurs in the hands, hips, knees, neck, or low back.

Common signs of osteoarthritis include the following:

- Joint pain, swelling, and tenderness

- Stiffness after getting out of bed

- A crunching feeling or sound of bone rubbing on bone

Not everyone with osteoarthritis feels pain, however. In fact, only a third of people with X-ray evidence of osteoarthritis report pain or other symptoms. A patient's attitude, daily activities, and levels of anxiety or depression have a lot to do with how severe the symptoms of osteoarthritis may be.

Diagnosis

To make a diagnosis of osteoarthritis, most doctors use a combination of methods and tests including a medical history, a physical examination, X-rays, and laboratory tests.

- A medical history is the patient's description of symptoms and when and how they began. The description covers pain, stiffness, and joint function and how these have changed over time.

- A physical examination includes the doctor's examination of the joints, skin, reflexes, and muscle strength. The doctor observes the patient's ability to walk, bend, and carry out activities of daily living.

- X-rays are limited in their capacity to reveal how much joint damage may have occurred in osteoarthritis. X-rays usually don't show osteoarthritis damage until there has been a significant loss of cartilage.

Questions Your Doctor May Ask

It is important for people with joint pain to give the doctor a complete medical history. Answering these questions will help your doctor make an accurate diagnosis:

- Is the pain in one or more joints?
- When does the pain occur and how long does it last?
- When did you first notice the pain?
- Does activity make the pain better or worse?
- Have you had any illnesses or accidents that may account for the pain?
- Is there a family history of any arthritis or rheumatic diseases?
- What medicines are you taking?

Treatment

Osteoarthritis treatment plans often include ways to manage pain and improve function. Such plans can include exercise, rest and joint care, pain relief, weight control, medicines, surgery, and nontraditional treatment approaches.

Current treatments for osteoarthritis can relieve symptoms such as pain and disability, but right now there are no treatments that can cure osteoarthritis.

Exercise: Exercise is one of the best treatments for osteoarthritis. It can improve mood and outlook, decrease pain, increase flexibility, and help you maintain a healthy weight.

The amount and form of exercise will depend on which joints are involved, how stable the joints are, whether or not the joint is swollen, and whether a joint replacement has already been done. Ask your doctor or physical therapist what exercises are best for you.

Heat or cold: For temporary relief of pain from osteoarthritis, you can use warm towels, hot packs, or a warm bath or shower. In some cases, cold packs such as a bag of ice or frozen vegetables wrapped in a towel can relieve pain or numb the sore area.

A doctor or physical therapist can recommend if heat or cold is the best treatment. For osteoarthritis in the knee, wearing insoles or cushioned shoes may reduce joint stress.

Medications: Doctors consider a number of factors when choosing medicines for their patients. In particular, they look at the type of pain the patient may be having and any possible side effects from the drugs.

For pain relief, doctors usually start with acetaminophen because the side effects are minimal. If acetaminophen does not relieve pain, then nonsteroidal anti-inflammatory drugs (NSAIDs) such as ibuprofen and naproxen may be used. Some NSAIDs are available over the counter, while more than a dozen others are available only with a prescription.

Other medications, including corticosteroids, hyaluronic acid, and topical creams, are also used. Most medicines used to treat osteoarthritis have side effects, so it is important for people to learn about the medicines they take. For example, people over age 65 and those with any history of ulcers or stomach bleeding should use NSAIDs with caution.

There are measures you can take to help reduce the risk of side effects associated with NSAIDs. These include taking medications with food and avoiding stomach irritants such as alcohol, tobacco, and caffeine. In some cases, it may help to take another medication along with an NSAID to coat the stomach or block stomach acids. Although these measures may help, they are not always completely effective.

Protecting and supporting the affected joints: Protecting and supporting the affected joint or joints is important. Some people use canes and splints to protect and take pressure off the joints. Splints or braces are used to provide extra support for weakened joints.

Surgery: For some people, surgery helps relieve the pain and disability of osteoarthritis. A doctor may perform surgery to smooth out, fuse, or reposition bones, or to replace joints.

The decision to have an operation depends on several factors. Both surgeon and patient should consider the patient's level of disability, intensity of pain, lifestyle, age, and occupation.

Research

Genetic research: Researchers suspect that heredity plays a role in some osteoarthritis cases. For example, scientists have identified a mutation, or gene defect, affecting collagen—an important part of cartilage—in patients with an inherited kind of osteoarthritis that starts at an early age.

In the future, a test to determine who carries a genetic defect or defects could help people reduce their risk for osteoarthritis with lifestyle adjustments

Research on tissue engineering: Tissue engineering is an exciting area of research in osteoarthritis. This approach involves removing cells from a healthy part of the body and placing them in an area of diseased or damaged tissue. In some cases, this improves joint movement.

Research on exercise: Researchers also are studying whether exercise can treat or prevent osteoarthritis. Studies on knee osteoarthritis and exercise found that strengthening the thigh muscle, also known as the quadriceps, can relieve symptoms of knee osteoarthritis and prevent more damage.

Studies also show that people with knee osteoarthritis who exercise appropriately feel less pain and function better.

Research on acupuncture: Early research suggests that acupuncture, which is the use of fine needles inserted at specific points in the skin, may provide pain relief for some patients.

The Glucosamine and Chondroitin Arthritis Intervention Trial (GAIT)

Some people claim that the dietary supplements glucosamine and chondroitin sulfate can relieve the symptoms of osteoarthritis. GAIT tested whether or not glucosamine and/or chondroitin have a beneficial effect for people with knee osteoarthritis. The results of the four-year study indicated that these supplements did not provide significant relief from osteoarthritis pain among all participants. However, a smaller subgroup of study participants with moderate-to-severe pain showed significant relief with the combined supplements. A long-term GAIT study revealed that subjects who took the supplements (alone or in combination) had outcomes similar to those experienced by patients who took a NSAID or a placebo pill.

Chapter 46

Autoimmune and Related Diseases

Chapter Contents

Section 46.1

Autoimmune Diseases Overview

Excerpted from "Autoimmune Diseases Fact Sheet," U.S. Department of Health and Human Services Office on Women's Health (www.womenshealth.gov), April 14, 2010.

What are autoimmune diseases?

Our bodies have an immune system, which is a complex network of special cells and organs that defends the body from germs and other foreign invaders. At the core of the immune system is the ability to tell the difference between self and nonself: what's you and what's foreign. A flaw can make the body unable to tell the difference. When this happens, the body makes autoantibodies that attack normal cells by mistake. At the same time special cells called regulatory T cells fail to do their job of keeping the immune system in line. The result is a misguided attack on your own body. This causes the damage we know as autoimmune disease. The body parts that are affected depend on the type of autoimmune disease. There are more than 80 known types.

Although each disease is unique, many share hallmark symptoms, such as fatigue, dizziness, and low-grade fever. For many autoimmune diseases, symptoms come and go, or can be mild sometimes and severe at others. When symptoms go away for a while, it's called remission. Flares are the sudden and severe onset of symptoms.

How common are autoimmune diseases?

Overall, autoimmune diseases are common, affecting more than 23.5 million Americans. They are a leading cause of death and disability. Yet some autoimmune diseases are rare, while others, such as Hashimoto disease, affect many people.

Who gets autoimmune diseases?

Autoimmune diseases can affect anyone. Yet certain people are at greater risk, including the following:

- **Women of childbearing age:** More women than men have auto-immune diseases, which often start during their childbearing years.

- **People with a family history:** Some autoimmune diseases run in families, such as lupus and multiple sclerosis. It is also common for different types of autoimmune diseases to affect different members of a single family. Inheriting certain genes can make it more likely to get an autoimmune disease. But a combination of genes and other factors may trigger the disease to start.

- **People who are around certain things in the environment:** Certain events or environmental exposures may cause some autoimmune diseases or make them worse. Sunlight, chemicals called solvents, and viral and bacterial infections are linked to many autoimmune diseases.

- **People of certain races or ethnic backgrounds:** Some autoimmune diseases are more common or more severely affect certain groups of people more than others. For instance, type 1 diabetes is more common in white people. Lupus is most severe for African American and Hispanic people.

How do I find out if I have an autoimmune disease?

Getting a diagnosis can be a long and stressful process. Although each autoimmune disease is unique, many share some of the same symptoms. And many symptoms of autoimmune diseases are the same for other types of health problems. This makes it hard for doctors to find out if you really have an autoimmune disease and which one it might be. But if you are having symptoms that bother you, it's important to find the cause. Don't give up if you're not getting any answers. You can take these steps to help find out the cause of your symptoms:

- Write down a complete family health history that includes extended family and share it with your doctor.

- Record any symptoms you have, even if they seem unrelated, and share it with your doctor.

- See a specialist who has experience dealing with your most major symptom. For instance, if you have symptoms of inflammatory bowel disease, start with a gastroenterologist. Ask your regular doctor, friends, and others for suggestions.

- Get a second, third, or fourth opinion if need be. If your doctor doesn't take your symptoms seriously or tells you they are stress related or in your head, see another doctor.

What types of doctors treat autoimmune diseases?

Juggling your health care needs among many doctors and specialists can be hard. But specialists, along with your main doctor, may be helpful in managing some symptoms of your autoimmune disease. If you see a specialist, make sure you have a supportive main doctor to help you. Often, your family doctor may help you coordinate care if you need to see one or more specialists. Here are some specialists who treat autoimmune diseases:

- **Nephrologist:** A doctor who treats kidney problems, such as inflamed kidneys caused by lupus; kidneys are organs that clean the blood and produce urine

- **Rheumatologist:** A doctor who treats arthritis and other rheumatic diseases, such as scleroderma and lupus

- **Endocrinologist:** A doctor who treats gland and hormone problems, such as diabetes and thyroid disease

- **Neurologist:** A doctor who treats nerve problems, such as multiple sclerosis and myasthenia gravis

- **Hematologist:** A doctor who treats diseases that affect blood, such as some forms of anemia

- **Gastroenterologist:** A doctor who treats problems with the digestive system, such as inflammatory bowel disease

- **Dermatologist:** A doctor who treats diseases that affect the skin, hair, and nails, such as psoriasis and lupus

- **Physical therapist:** A health care worker who uses proper types of physical activity to help patients with stiffness, weakness, and restricted body movement

- **Occupational therapist:** A health care worker who can find ways to make activities of daily living easier for you, despite your pain and other health problems

- **Speech therapist:** A health care worker who can help people with speech problems from illness such as multiple sclerosis

- **Audiologist:** A health care worker who can help people with hearing problems, including inner ear damage from autoimmune diseases

- **Vocational therapist:** A health care worker who offers job training for people who cannot do their current jobs because of their illness or other health problems

- **Counselor for emotional support:** A health care worker who is specially trained to help you to find ways to cope with your illness and help you work through your feelings of anger, fear, denial, and frustration

Are there medicines to treat autoimmune diseases?

There are many types of medicines used to treat autoimmune diseases. The type of medicine you need depends on which disease you have, how severe it is, and your symptoms. Treatment can do the following:

- **Relieve symptoms:** Some people can use over-the-counter drugs for mild symptoms, like aspirin and ibuprofen for mild pain. Others with more severe symptoms may need prescription drugs to help relieve symptoms such as pain, swelling, depression, anxiety, sleep problems, fatigue, or rashes. For others, treatment may be as involved as having surgery.

- **Replace vital substances the body can no longer make on its own:** Some autoimmune diseases, like diabetes and thyroid disease, can affect the body's ability to make substances it needs to function. With diabetes, insulin injections are needed to regulate blood sugar. Thyroid hormone replacement restores thyroid hormone levels in people with underactive thyroid.

- **Suppress the immune system:** Some drugs can suppress immune system activity. These drugs can help control the disease process and preserve organ function. For instance, these drugs are used to control inflammation in affected kidneys in people with lupus to keep the kidneys working. Medicines used to suppress inflammation include chemotherapy given at lower doses than for cancer treatment and drugs used in patients who have had an organ transplant to protect against rejection. A class of drugs called anti-TNF medications blocks inflammation in some forms of autoimmune arthritis and psoriasis.

I want to have a baby. Does having an autoimmune disease affect pregnancy?

Women with autoimmune diseases can safely have children. But there could be some risks for the mother or baby, depending on the disease and how severe it is. For instance, pregnant women with lupus have a higher risk of preterm birth and stillbirth. Pregnant women with myasthenia gravis (MG) might have symptoms that lead to trouble breathing during pregnancy. For some women, symptoms tend to improve during pregnancy, while others find their symptoms tend to flare up. Also, some medicines used to treat autoimmune diseases might not be safe to use during pregnancy.

If you want to have a baby, talk to your doctor before you start trying to get pregnant. Your doctor might suggest that you wait until your disease is in remission or suggest a change in medicines before you start trying. You also might need to see a doctor who cares for women with high-risk pregnancies.

How can I manage my life now that I have an autoimmune disease?

Although most autoimmune diseases don't go away, you can treat your symptoms and learn to manage your disease so you can enjoy life! Women with autoimmune diseases lead full, active lives. It is important, though, to see a doctor who specializes in these types of diseases, follow your treatment plan, and adopt a healthy lifestyle.

If you are living with an autoimmune disease, there are things you can do each day to feel better:

- **Eat healthy, well-balanced meals:** Make sure to include fruits and vegetables, whole grains, fat-free or low-fat milk products, and lean sources of protein. Limit saturated fat, trans fat, cholesterol, salt, and added sugars. If you follow a healthy eating plan, you will get the nutrients you need from food.

- **Get regular physical activity:** But be careful not to overdo it. Talk with your doctor about what types of physical activity you can do. A gradual and gentle exercise program often works well for people with long-lasting muscle and joint pain. Some types of yoga or tai chi exercises may be helpful.

- **Get enough rest:** Rest allows your body tissues and joints the time they need to repair. If you don't get enough sleep, your stress level and your symptoms could get worse. You also can't fight off sickness as well when you sleep poorly. When you are well-rested, you can tackle your problems better and lower your risk for illness. Most people need at least seven to nine hours of sleep each day to feel well-rested.

- **Reduce stress:** Stress and anxiety can trigger symptoms to flare up with some autoimmune diseases. So finding ways to simplify your life and cope with daily stressors will help you to feel your best. Meditation, self-hypnosis, and guided imagery are simple relaxation techniques that might help you to reduce stress, lessen your pain, and deal with other aspects of living with your disease. Joining a support group or talking with a counselor might also help you to manage your stress and cope with your disease.

How can I deal with flares?

Flares are the sudden and severe onset of symptoms. You might notice that certain triggers, such as stress or being out in the sun, cause your symptoms to flare. Knowing your triggers, following your treatment plan, and seeing your doctor regularly can help you to prevent flares or keep them from becoming severe. If you suspect a flare is coming, call your doctor. Don't try a "cure" you heard about from a friend or relative.

Section 46.2

Celiac Disease

Excerpted from "Celiac Disease," National Digestive Diseases Information Clearinghouse, National Institute of Diabetes and Digestive and Kidney Diseases (digestive.niddk.nih.gov), January 27, 2012.

What is celiac disease?

Celiac disease is a digestive disease that damages the small intestine and interferes with absorption of nutrients from food. People who have celiac disease cannot tolerate gluten, a protein in wheat, rye, and barley. Gluten is found mainly in foods but may also be found in everyday products such as medicines, vitamins, and lip balms.

When people with celiac disease eat foods or use products containing gluten, their immune system responds by damaging or destroying villi—the tiny, fingerlike protrusions lining the small intestine. Villi normally allow nutrients from food to be absorbed through the walls of the small intestine into the bloodstream. Without healthy villi, a person becomes malnourished, no matter how much food one eats.

Celiac disease is both a disease of malabsorption—meaning nutrients are not absorbed properly—and an abnormal immune reaction to gluten. Celiac disease is genetic, meaning it runs in families. Sometimes the disease is triggered—or becomes active for the first time—after surgery, pregnancy, childbirth, viral infection, or severe emotional stress.

What are the symptoms of celiac disease?

Symptoms of celiac disease vary from person to person. Symptoms may occur in the digestive system or in other parts of the body. Digestive symptoms are more common in infants and young children. Adults are less likely to have digestive symptoms and may instead have one or more of the following:

- Unexplained iron-deficiency anemia
- Fatigue
- Bone or joint pain
- Arthritis
- Bone loss or osteoporosis
- Depression or anxiety
- Tingling numbness in the hands and feet
- Seizures
- Missed menstrual periods
- Infertility or recurrent miscarriage
- Canker sores inside the mouth
- An itchy skin rash called dermatitis herpetiformis

People with celiac disease may have no symptoms but can still develop complications of the disease over time. Long-term complications include malnutrition—which can lead to anemia, osteoporosis, and miscarriage, among other problems—liver diseases, and cancers of the intestine.

How common is celiac disease?

Celiac disease affects people in all parts of the world. Originally thought to be a rare childhood syndrome, celiac disease is now known to be a common genetic disorder. More than two million people in the

United States have the disease, or about 1 in 133 people. Among people who have a first-degree relative—a parent, sibling, or child—diagnosed with celiac disease, as many as 1 in 22 people may have the disease.

How is celiac disease diagnosed and treated?

Recognizing celiac disease can be difficult because some of its symptoms are similar to those of other diseases. As doctors become more aware of the many varied symptoms of the disease and reliable blood tests become more available, diagnosis rates are increasing.

The only treatment for celiac disease is a gluten-free diet. Doctors may ask a newly diagnosed person to work with a dietitian on a gluten-free diet plan. For most people, following this diet will stop symptoms, heal existing intestinal damage, and prevent further damage. Improvement begins within days of starting the diet. The small intestine usually heals in three to six months in children but may take several years in adults. A healed intestine means a person now has villi that can absorb nutrients from food into the bloodstream.

To stay well, people with celiac disease must avoid gluten for the rest of their lives. Eating even a small amount of gluten can damage the small intestine. The damage will occur in anyone with the disease, including people without noticeable symptoms.

A gluten-free diet means not eating foods that contain wheat, rye, and barley. The foods and products made from these grains should also be avoided. In other words, a person with celiac disease should not eat most grain, pasta, cereal, and many processed foods.

Some people with celiac disease show no improvement on the gluten-free diet. The most common reason for poor response to the diet is that small amounts of gluten are still being consumed. Hidden sources of gluten include additives such as modified food starch, preservatives, and stabilizers made with wheat. And because many corn and rice products are produced in factories that also manufacture wheat products, they can be contaminated with wheat gluten.

Rarely, the intestinal injury will continue despite a strictly gluten-free diet. People with this condition, known as refractory celiac disease, have severely damaged intestines that cannot heal. Because their intestines are not absorbing enough nutrients, they may need to receive nutrients directly into their bloodstream through a vein, or intravenously. Researchers are evaluating drug treatments for refractory celiac disease.

Section 46.3

Chronic Fatigue Syndrome

Excerpted from "Chronic Fatigue Syndrome Fact Sheet,"
U.S. Department of Health and Human Services Office
on Women's Health (www.womenshealth.gov), September
22, 2009.

What is chronic fatigue syndrome (CFS)?

A person with CFS feels completely worn-out and overtired. This extreme tiredness makes it hard to do the daily tasks that most of us do without thinking—like dressing, bathing, or eating. Sleep or rest does not make the tiredness go away. It can be made worse by moving, exercising, or even thinking.

CFS can happen over time or come on suddenly. People who get CFS over time get more and more tired over weeks or months. People who get CFS suddenly feel fine one day and then feel extremely tired the next.

A person with CFS may have muscle pain, trouble focusing, or insomnia (not being able to sleep). The extreme tiredness may come and go. In some cases the extreme tiredness never goes away. The extreme tiredness must go on for at least six months before a diagnosis of CFS can be made.

What causes CFS?

No one knows for sure what causes CFS. Many people with CFS say it started after an infection, such as a cold or stomach bug. It also can follow infection with the Epstein-Barr virus. This is the same virus that causes infectious mononucleosis (sometimes called "mono"). Some people with CFS say it started after a time of great stress, such as the loss of a loved one or major surgery.

It can be hard to figure out if a person has CFS because extreme tiredness is a common symptom of many illnesses. Also, some medical treatments, such as chemotherapy, can cause extreme tiredness.

What are the signs of CFS?

The signs of CFS can come and go or they can stay with a person. At first, you may feel like you have the flu. As well as extreme tiredness and weakness, main CFS symptoms include the following:

- Feeling very tired for more than a day (24 hours) after physical or mental exercise

- Forgetting things or having a hard time focusing

- Feeling tired even after sleeping

- Muscle pain or aches

- Pain or aches in joints without swelling or redness

- Headaches of a new type, pattern, or strength

- Tender lymph nodes in the neck or under the arm

- Sore throat

These symptoms are the main signs of CFS. CFS symptoms may also include the following:

- Visual disturbances (blurring, sensitivity to light, eye pain)

- Psychological symptoms (irritability, mood swings, panic attacks, anxiety)

- Chills and night sweats

- Low-grade fever or low body temperature

- Irritable bowel

- Allergies and sensitivities to foods, odors, chemicals, medications, and noise/sound

- Numbness, tingling, or burning sensations in the face, hands, or feet

- Difficulty sitting or standing straight up, dizziness, balance problems, and fainting

Symptoms of CFS vary widely from person to person and may be serious or mild. Most symptoms cannot be seen by others, which makes it hard for friends, family members, and the public to understand the challenges a person with CFS faces. If you think you may have CFS, talk to your doctor.

How common is CFS? Who gets it?

Experts think at least one million Americans have CFS. Fewer than 20% of these cases have been diagnosed, however.

Women are four times as likely as men to develop CFS. The illness occurs most often in people ages 40–59. Still, people of all ages can get CFS. CFS is less common in children than in adults. Studies suggest that CFS occurs more often in adolescents than in children under the age of 12.

CFS occurs in all ethnic groups and races and in countries around the world. People of all income levels can develop CFS, although there is evidence that it is more common in lower-income than in higher-income persons. CFS is sometimes seen in members of the same family, but there is no evidence that it is contagious. Instead, it may run in families because of a genetic link.

How would my doctor know if I have CFS?

It can be hard for your doctor to diagnose CFS because there is no lab test for it. Also, many signs of CFS are also signs of other illnesses or side effects of medical treatments. All cases are diagnosed by the 1994 Centers for Disease Control and Prevention (CDC) definition, which is also sometimes called the "Fukuda criteria" after the name of a leading researcher in the field. If you think you may have CFS, see your doctor. Your doctor will do the following:

- Ask you about your physical and mental health

- Do a physical exam

- Order urine and blood tests, which will tell your doctor if something other than CFS might be causing your symptoms

- Order more tests, if your urine and blood tests do not show a cause for your symptoms

- Classify you as having CFS if you have been extremely tired for six months or more and tests do not show a cause for your symptoms and you have four or more of the symptoms listed in this section

This process can take a long time (even years), so try to be patient with your doctor. While these tests are being done, talk to your doctor about ways to help ease your symptoms. Although CFS is not a form of depression, many patients develop depression as a result of dealing with a long-term illness.

How is CFS treated?

Right now, there is no cure for CFS. But there are things you can do to feel better. Talk to your doctor about ways to ease your symptoms and deal with your tiredness. You might also try the following:

Lifestyle changes: Try to stop or do less of the things that seem to trigger your tiredness. For a week or two write down what you do each day. Note when you feel really tired. Then, look over this list to find out which activities tend to tire you out. An occupational therapist can help you by looking at your daily habits and suggesting changes to help you save energy. Your doctor can help you find an occupational therapist near where you live.

At the end of the day, try thinking about how much energy you think you had that day and how much energy you actually used that day. If you keep these two amounts of energy similar over time, you may slowly gain more strength and energy. Think about which activities are most important to you and which activities you do not need to do as often. Make sure to tell other people in your life how much energy you can actually use each day. They can help make sure you don't do too much. It is important to remember that energy can mean mental, emotional, or physical energy.

Medications: Over-the-counter pain relievers such as Advil, Motrin, or Aleve can help with body aches, headaches, and muscle and joint pain. Nondrowsy antihistamines can help with allergy symptoms, such as runny nose and itchy eyes. Prescription medications like doxepin or amitriptyline can help improve sleep.

Some people say their CFS symptoms get better with complementary or alternative treatments, such as massage, acupuncture, chiropractic care, yoga, stretching, or self-hypnosis. Keep in mind that many alternative treatments, dietary supplements, and herbal remedies claim to cure CFS, but they might do more harm than good. Talk to your doctor before seeing someone else for treatment or before trying alternative therapies.

Also, keep in mind that your doctor may need to learn more about CFS to better help you. If you feel your doctor doesn't know a lot about CFS or has doubts about it being a "real" illness, see another doctor for a second opinion. Contact a local university medical school or research center for help finding a doctor who treats people with CFS.

What can I do to cope with CFS?

It's normal to feel cranky, sad, angry, or upset when you have an illness like CFS. Some things that might help you to feel better include the following:

- Consider talk therapy to help you learn how to deal with your feelings.

- Join a CFS support group. Sometimes it helps to talk with people who are going through the same thing.

What if I can't work because of CFS?

If you can't work because of CFS, get in touch with the Social Security Administration (www.ssa.gov, or toll free 800-772-1213) for help with disability benefits. It can be hard to get these benefits on your own. Working with a lawyer who specializes in disability benefits could make this process easier.

Section 46.4

Fibromyalgia

Excerpted from "Fibromyalgia Fact Sheet,"
U.S. Department of Health and Human Services Office on
Women's Health (www.womenshealth.gov), June 29, 2010.

What is fibromyalgia?

Fibromyalgia is a disorder that causes aches and pain all over the body. People with fibromyalgia also have "tender points" throughout their bodies. Tender points are specific places on the neck, shoulders, back, hips, arms, and legs that hurt when pressure is put on them.

What are the symptoms of fibromyalgia?

In addition to pain, people with fibromyalgia could also have the following:

- Cognitive and memory problems (sometimes called "fibro fog")
- Trouble sleeping
- Morning stiffness
- Headaches

- Irritable bowel syndrome
- Painful menstrual periods
- Numbness or tingling of hands and feet
- Restless legs syndrome
- Temperature sensitivity
- Sensitivity to loud noises or bright lights

How common is fibromyalgia? Who is mainly affected?

Fibromyalgia affects as many as five million Americans ages 18 and older. Most people with fibromyalgia are women (about 80%–90%). However, men and children also can have the disorder. Most people are diagnosed during middle age.

Fibromyalgia can occur by itself, but people with certain other diseases, such as rheumatoid arthritis, lupus, and other types of arthritis, may be more likely to have it. Individuals who have a close relative with fibromyalgia are more likely to develop it themselves.

What causes fibromyalgia?

The causes of fibromyalgia are not known. Researchers think a number of factors might be involved. Fibromyalgia can occur on its own, but has also been linked to the following:

- Having a family history of fibromyalgia
- Being exposed to stressful or traumatic events, such as the following:
  - Car accidents
  - Injuries to the body caused by performing the same action over and over again (called "repetitive" injuries)
  - Infections or illnesses
  - Being sent to war

How is fibromyalgia diagnosed?

People with fibromyalgia often see many doctors before being diagnosed. One reason for this may be that pain and fatigue, the main symptoms of fibromyalgia, also are symptoms of many other conditions. Therefore, doctors often must rule out other possible causes of these symptoms before diagnosing fibromyalgia. Fibromyalgia cannot be found by a lab test.

A doctor who knows about fibromyalgia, however, can make a diagnosis based upon two criteria:

- **A history of widespread pain lasting more than three months:** Pain must be present in both the right and left sides of the body as well as above and below the waist.

- **Presence of tender points:** The body has 18 sites that are possible tender points. For fibromyalgia diagnosis a person must have 11 or more tender points. For a point to be "tender," the patient must feel pain when pressure is put on the site. People who have fibromyalgia may feel pain at other sites, too, but those 18 sites on the body are used for diagnosis.

Your doctor may try to rule out other causes of your pain and fatigue. Testing for some of these things may make sense to you. For instance, you may find it reasonable that your doctor wants to rule out rheumatoid arthritis, since that disease also causes pain. Testing for other conditions—such as lupus, multiple sclerosis, or sleep apnea—may make less sense to you. But fibromyalgia can mimic or even overlap many other conditions. Talk with your doctor. He or she can help you understand what each test is for and how each test is part of making a final diagnosis.

How is fibromyalgia treated?

Fibromyalgia can be hard to treat. It's important to find a doctor who has treated others with fibromyalgia. Many family doctors, general internists, or rheumatologists can treat fibromyalgia. Rheumatologists are doctors who treat arthritis and other conditions that affect the joints and soft tissues.

Treatment often requires a team approach. The team may include your doctor, a physical therapist, and possibly other health care providers. A pain or rheumatology clinic can be a good place to get treatment. Treatment for fibromyalgia may include the following:

Pain management: Three medicines have been approved by the U.S. Food and Drug Administration (FDA) to treat fibromyalgia. These are pregabalin (Lyrica), duloxetine (Cymbalta), and milnacipran (Savella). Other medications are being developed and may also receive FDA approval in the future. Your doctor may also suggest non-narcotic pain relievers, low-dose antidepressants, or other classes of medications that might help improve certain symptoms.

Sleep management: Getting the right amount of sleep at night may help improve your symptoms. Here are tips for good sleep:

- Keep regular sleep habits. Try to get to bed at the same time and get up at the same time every day—even on weekends and vacations.

- Avoid caffeine and alcohol in the late afternoon and evening.

- Time your exercise. Regular daytime exercise can improve nighttime sleep. But avoid exercising within three hours of bedtime, which can be stimulating, keeping you awake.

- Avoid daytime naps. Sleeping in the afternoon can interfere with nighttime sleep. If you feel you cannot get by without a nap, set an alarm for one hour. When it goes off, get up and start moving.

- Reserve your bed for sleeping. Watching the late news, reading a suspense novel, or working on your laptop in bed can stimulate you, making it hard to sleep.

- Keep your bedroom dark, quiet, and cool.

- Avoid liquids and spicy meals before bed. Heartburn and late-night trips to the bathroom do not lead to good sleep.

- Wind down before bed. Avoid working right up to bedtime. Do relaxing activities, such as listening to soft music or taking a warm bath, that get you ready to sleep. (A warm bath also may soothe aching muscles.)

Psychological support: Living with a chronic condition can be hard on you. If you have fibromyalgia, find a support group. Counseling sessions with a trained counselor may improve your understanding of your illness.

Other treatments: Complementary therapies may help you. Talk to your physician before trying any alternative treatments. These include the following:

- Physical therapy
- Massage
- Myofascial release therapy
- Water therapy
- Light aerobics
- Applying heat or cold
- Acupuncture
- Yoga

- Relaxation or breathing exercises
- Cognitive therapy
- Biofeedback
- Herbs or nutritional supplements
- Osteopathic or chiropractic manipulation

What can I do to try to feel better?

Besides taking medicine prescribed by your doctor, there are many things you can do to lessen the impact of fibromyalgia on your life, including the following:

- **Getting enough sleep:** Getting enough sleep and the right kind of sleep can help ease the pain and fatigue of fibromyalgia. Most adults need seven to eight hours of "restorative" sleep per night. Restorative sleep leaves you feeling well-rested and ready for your day to start when you wake up. It is hard for people with fibromyalgia to get a good night's sleep. It is important to discuss any sleep problems with your doctor, who can recommend treatment for them.

- **Exercising:** Although pain and fatigue may make exercise and daily activities difficult, it is crucial to be as physically active as possible. Research has repeatedly shown that regular exercise is one of the most effective treatments for fibromyalgia. People who have too much pain or fatigue to do hard exercise should just begin to move more and become more active in routine daily activities. Then they can begin with walking (or other gentle exercise) and build their endurance and intensity slowly.

- **Making changes at work:** Most people with fibromyalgia continue to work, but they may have to make big changes to do so. For example, some people cut down the number of hours they work, switch to a less demanding job, or adapt a current job. If you face obstacles at work, your employer may make changes that will enable you to keep your job. An occupational therapist can help you design a more comfortable workstation or find more efficient and less painful ways to lift. A number of federal laws protect the rights of people with disabilities.

- **Eating well:** Although some people with fibromyalgia report feeling better when they eat or avoid certain foods, no specific diet has been proven to influence fibromyalgia. Of course, it is important to have a healthy, balanced diet. Not only will proper nutrition give you more energy and make you generally feel better, it will also help you avoid other health problems.

Will fibromyalgia get better with time?

Fibromyalgia is a chronic condition, meaning it lasts a long time—possibly a lifetime. However, it may be comforting to know that fibromyalgia is not a progressive disease. It is never fatal, and it will not cause damage to the joints, muscles, or internal organs. In many people, the condition does improve over time.

What is the difference between fibromyalgia and chronic fatigue syndrome?

CFS and fibromyalgia are alike in many ways. In fact, it is not uncommon for a person to have both fibromyalgia and CFS. Some experts believe that fibromyalgia and CFS are in fact the same disorder, but expressed in slightly different ways. Both CFS and fibromyalgia have pain and fatigue as symptoms.

The main symptom of CFS is extreme tiredness. CFS often begins after having flu-like symptoms. But people with CFS do not have the tender points that people with fibromyalgia have.

What if I can't work because of fibromyalgia?

Many experts in fibromyalgia do not suggest patients go on disability. These experts have found that if patients stop working, they do the following:

- Stop moving as much during the day
- Lose contact with co-workers
- Lose a "sense of purpose" in life

All these things can make a patient feel more alone and depressed. These three things tend to make fibromyalgia symptoms worse. However, if you cannot work because of your fibromyalgia, contact the Social Security Administration for help with disability benefits. Social Security Disability Insurance (SSDI) and Supplemental Security Insurance (SSI) are the largest federal programs providing financial assistance to people with disabilities. For information about the SSDI and SSI programs, contact the Social Security Administration (at www.ssa.gov or 800-772-1213).

Section 46.5

Lupus

Excerpted from "What Is Lupus?" National Institute
of Arthritis and Musculoskeletal and Skin Diseases
(www.niams.nih.gov), October 2009.

What is lupus?

The immune system is designed to attack foreign substances in
the body. If you have lupus, something goes wrong with your immune
system and it attacks healthy cells and tissues. This can damage many
parts of the body such as the following:

- Joints
- Kidneys
- Lungs
- Brain
- Skin
- Heart
- Blood vessels

There are many kinds of lupus. The most common type, systemic
lupus erythematosus, affects many parts of the body. Other types of
lupus are the following:

- **Discoid lupus erythematosus** causes a skin rash that doesn't
  go away.

- **Subacute cutaneous lupus erythematosus** causes skin sores
  on parts of the body exposed to sun.

- **Drug-induced lupus** can be caused by medications.

- **Neonatal lupus** is a rare type of lupus that affects newborns.

Who gets lupus?

Anyone can get lupus, but it most often affects women. Lupus is
also more common in women of African American, Hispanic, Asian,
and Native American descent than in Caucasian women.

What causes lupus?

The cause of lupus is not known. Research suggests that genes play an important role, but genes alone do not determine who gets lupus. It is likely that many factors trigger the disease.

What are the symptoms of lupus?

Symptoms of lupus vary, but some of the most common symptoms of lupus are the following:

- Pain or swelling in joints
- Muscle pain
- Fever with no known cause
- Red rashes, most often on the face
- Chest pain when taking a deep breath
- Hair loss
- Pale or purple fingers or toes
- Sensitivity to the sun
- Swelling in legs or around eyes
- Mouth ulcers
- Swollen glands
- Feeling very tired

Less common symptoms include these:

- Anemia (a decrease in red blood cells)
- Dizzy spells
- Confusion
- Headaches
- Feeling sad
- Seizures

Symptoms may come and go. The times when a person is having symptoms are called flares, which can range from mild to severe. New symptoms may appear at any time.

How is lupus diagnosed?

There is no single test to diagnose lupus. It may take months or years for a doctor to diagnose lupus. Your doctor may use many tools to make a diagnosis:

- Medical history
- Complete exam
- Blood tests
- Skin biopsy (looking at skin samples under a microscope)
- Kidney biopsy (looking at tissue from your kidney under a microscope)

How is lupus treated?

You may need special kinds of doctors to treat the many symptoms of lupus. Your health care team may include the following:

- A family doctor
- Rheumatologists, doctors who treat arthritis and other diseases that cause swelling in the joints
- Clinical immunologists, doctors who treat immune system disorders
- Nephrologists, doctors who treat kidney disease
- Hematologists, doctors who treat blood disorders
- Dermatologists, doctors who treat skin diseases
- Neurologists, doctors who treat problems with the nervous system
- Cardiologists, doctors who treat heart and blood vessel problems
- Endocrinologists, doctors who treat problems related to the glands and hormones
- Nurses
- Psychologists
- Social workers

Your doctor will develop a treatment plan to fit your needs. You and your doctor should review the plan often to be sure it is working. You should report new symptoms to your doctor right away so that treatment can be changed if needed.

The goals of the treatment plan are to accomplish the following:

- Prevent flares
- Treat flares when they occur
- Reduce organ damage and other problems

Treatments may include drugs to do the following:

- Reduce swelling and pain
- Prevent or reduce flares
- Help the immune system
- Reduce or prevent damage to joints
- Balance the hormones

In addition to medications for lupus itself, sometimes other medications are needed for problems related to lupus such as high cholesterol, high blood pressure, or infection. Alternative treatments are those that are not part of standard treatment. No research shows that this kind of treatment works for people with lupus. You should talk to your doctor about alternative treatments.

What can I do?

It is vital that you take an active role in your treatment. One key to living with lupus is to know about the disease and its impact. Being able to spot the warning signs of a flare can help you prevent the flare or make the symptoms less severe. Many people with lupus have certain symptoms just before a flare:

- Feeling more tired
- Pain
- Rash
- Fever
- Stomach ache
- Headache
- Dizziness

You should see your doctor often, even when symptoms are not severe. These visits will help you and your doctor to do the following:

- Look for changes in symptoms
- Predict and prevent flares
- Change the treatment plan as needed
- Detect side effects of treatment

It is also important to find ways to cope with the stress of having lupus. Exercising and finding ways to relax may make it easier for you to cope. A good support system can also help.

Learning more about lupus is very important. Studies have shown that patients who are informed and involved in their own care do the following:

- Have less pain

- Make fewer visits to the doctor

- Feel better about themselves

- Remain more active

What are concerns with pregnancy and contraception for women with lupus?

Women with lupus can and do have healthy babies. There are a few things to keep in mind if you are pregnant or thinking about becoming pregnant:

- Pregnancy in women with lupus is considered high risk, but most women with lupus carry their babies safely.

- Pregnant women with lupus should see their doctors often.

- Lupus can flare during pregnancy.

- Pregnancy counseling and planning before pregnancy are important.

Women with lupus who do not wish to become pregnant or who are taking medicine that could be harmful to an unborn baby may want reliable birth control. Recent studies have shown that oral contraceptives (birth control pills) are safe for women with lupus.

Section 46.6

Rheumatoid Arthritis

Excerpted from "Rheumatoid Arthritis,"
National Institutes of Health (nihseniorhealth.gov),
May 2012.

Rheumatoid arthritis is an inflammatory disease that causes pain, swelling, stiffness, and loss of function in the joints. It can cause mild to severe symptoms. Rheumatoid arthritis not only affects the joints, but may also attack tissue in the skin, lungs, eyes, and blood vessels. People with rheumatoid arthritis may feel sick, tired, and sometimes feverish.

Rheumatoid arthritis is classified as an autoimmune disease. An autoimmune disease occurs when the immune system turns against parts of the body it is designed to protect.

Rheumatoid arthritis generally occurs in a symmetrical pattern. This means that if one knee or hand is involved, the other one is, too. It can occur at any age, but usually begins during a person's most productive years.

Rheumatoid arthritis occurs much more frequently in women than in men. About two to three times as many women as men have the disease.

Causes and Risk Factors

Scientists believe that rheumatoid arthritis may result from the interaction of many factors such as genetics, hormones, and the environment. Although rheumatoid arthritis sometimes runs in families, the actual cause of rheumatoid arthritis is still unknown.

Research suggests that a person's genetic makeup is an important part of the picture, but not the whole story. Some evidence shows that infectious agents, such as viruses and bacteria, may trigger rheumatoid arthritis in people with an inherited tendency to develop the disease. However, a specific agent or agents are not yet known.

It is important to note that rheumatoid arthritis is not contagious. A person cannot catch it from someone else.

Symptoms and Diagnosis

Different types of arthritis have different symptoms. In general, people with most forms of arthritis have pain and stiffness in their joints. Rheumatoid arthritis is characterized by inflammation of the joint lining. This inflammation causes warmth, redness, swelling, and pain around the joints. A person also feels sick, tired, and sometimes feverish. Rheumatoid arthritis generally occurs in a symmetrical pattern. If one knee or hand is affected, the other one is also likely to be affected.

Diagnostic Tests

Rheumatoid arthritis can be difficult to diagnose in its early stages for several reasons. First, there is no single test for the disease. In addition, symptoms differ from person to person and can be more severe in some people than in others.

Common tests for rheumatoid arthritis include the following:

- **The rheumatoid factor test:** Rheumatoid factor is an antibody that is present eventually in the blood of most people with rheumatoid arthritis However, not all people with rheumatoid arthritis test positive for rheumatoid factor, especially early in the disease. Also, some people who do test positive never develop the disease.

- **The citrulline antibody test:** This blood test detects antibodies to cyclic citrullinated peptide (anti-CCP). This test is positive in most people with rheumatoid arthritis and can even be positive years before rheumatoid arthritis symptoms develop. When used with the rheumatoid factor test, the citrulline antibody test results are very useful in confirming a rheumatoid arthritis diagnosis.

Other common tests for rheumatoid arthritis include the following:

- The erythrocyte sedimentation rate, which indicates the presence of inflammation in the body

- A test for white blood cell count

- A blood test for anemia

Symptoms of rheumatoid arthritis can be similar to those of other types of arthritis and joint conditions, and it may take some time to rule out other conditions. Finally, the full range of symptoms develops over time, and only a few symptoms may be present in the early stages.

Treatment

Treatments for rheumatoid arthritis can help relieve your pain, reduce swelling, slow down or help prevent joint damage, increase your ability to function, and improve your sense of well-being.

Exercise, medication, and, in some cases, surgery are common treatments for rheumatoid arthritis. People with rheumatoid arthritis need a good balance between rest and exercise; they should rest more when the disease is active and exercise more when it is not.

Reducing stress also is important. Doing relaxation exercises and taking part in support groups are two ways to help reduce stress. For more information on exercise classes, you may want to contact the Arthritis Foundation at 800-283-7800.

Medications

Most people who have rheumatoid arthritis take medications. Some drugs only provide relief for pain; others reduce inflammation. Still others, called disease-modifying anti-rheumatic drugs, or DMARDs, can often slow the course of the disease.

- DMARDs include methotrexate, leflunomide, sulfasalazine, and cyclosporine.

- Steroids, which are also called corticosteroids, are another type of drug used to reduce inflammation for people with rheumatoid arthritis. Cortisone, hydrocortisone, and prednisone are some commonly used steroids.

- New types of drugs called biologic response modifiers also can help reduce joint damage. These drugs include etanercept, infliximab, anakinra, golimumab, adalimumab, rituximab, and abatacept.

Early treatment with powerful drugs and drug combinations instead of single drugs may help prevent the disease from progressing and greatly reduce joint damage.

Surgery

In some cases, a doctor will recommend surgery to restore function or relieve pain in a damaged joint. Surgery may also improve a person's ability to perform daily activities. Joint replacement and tendon reconstruction are two types of surgery available to patients with severe joint damage.

Diet

Special diets, vitamin supplements, and other alternative approaches have been suggested for treating rheumatoid arthritis. Although such approaches may not be harmful, scientific studies have not yet shown any benefits.

An overall nutritious diet with the right amount of calories, protein, and calcium is important. Some people need to be careful about drinking alcoholic beverages because of the medications they take for rheumatoid arthritis.

Scientists are making rapid progress in understanding the complexities of rheumatoid arthritis. They are learning more about how and why it develops and why some people have more severe symptoms than others.

Research

Research efforts are focused on developing drugs that can reduce inflammation and slow or stop the disease with few side effects.

Some evidence shows that infectious agents, such as viruses and bacteria, may contribute to triggering rheumatoid arthritis in people with an inherited tendency to develop the disease. Investigators are trying to identify the infectious agents and understand how they work. This knowledge could lead to new therapies.

Why More Women Than Men

Researchers are also exploring why so many more women than men develop rheumatoid arthritis. In the hope of finding clues, they are studying complex relationships between the hormonal, nervous, and immune systems in rheumatoid arthritis.

For example, they are exploring whether and how the normal changes in the levels of steroid hormones such as estrogen and testosterone during a person's lifetime may be related to the development, improvement, or flares of the disease. Scientists are also examining why rheumatoid arthritis often improves during pregnancy.

Chapter 47

Cardiovascular Disorders

Chapter Contents

Section 47.1

Heart Disease in Women

Excerpted from "Heart Disease Fact Sheet," U.S. Department
of Health and Human Services Office on Women's Health
(www.womenshealth.gov), February 2, 2009.

What is heart disease?

Heart disease includes a number of problems affecting the heart
and the blood vessels in the heart. Types of heart disease include the
following:

- **Coronary artery disease (CAD)** is the most common type and
  is the leading cause of heart attacks. When you have CAD, your
  arteries become hard and narrow. Blood has a hard time getting
  to the heart, so the heart does not get all the blood it needs. CAD
  can lead to the following:

  - **Angina** is chest pain or discomfort that happens when the
    heart does not get enough blood. It may feel like a pressing or
    squeezing pain, often in the chest, but sometimes the pain is in
    the shoulders, arms, neck, jaw, or back. It can also feel like indi-
    gestion (upset stomach). Angina is not a heart attack, but hav-
    ing angina means you are more likely to have a heart attack.

  - A **heart attack** occurs when an artery is severely or com-
    pletely blocked, and the heart does not get the blood it needs
    for more than 20 minutes.

- **Heart failure** occurs when the heart is not able to pump blood
  through the body as well as it should. This means that other organs, which normally get blood from the heart, do not get enough
  blood. It does not mean that the heart stops. Signs of heart failure include the following:

  - Shortness of breath

  - Swelling in feet, ankles, and legs

  - Extreme tiredness

- **Heart arrhythmias** are changes in the beat of the heart. Most people have felt dizzy, faint, out of breath or had chest pains at one time. These changes in heartbeat are harmless for most people. As you get older, you are more likely to have arrhythmias. Don't panic if you have a few flutters or if your heart races once in a while. If you have flutters and other symptoms such as dizziness or shortness of breath, call 911 right away.

Do women need to worry about heart disease?

Yes. Among all U.S. women who die each year, one in four dies of heart disease. In 2004, nearly 60% more women died of cardiovascular disease (both heart disease and stroke) than from all cancers combined. The older a woman gets, the more likely she is to get heart disease. But women of all ages should be concerned about heart disease.

Both men and women have heart attacks, but more women who have heart attacks die from them. Treatments can limit heart damage, but they must be given as soon as possible after a heart attack starts. Ideally, treatment should start within one hour of the first symptoms.

If you think you're having a heart attack, call 911 right away. Tell the operator your symptoms and that you think you're having a heart attack.

African American and Hispanic American/Latina women should be concerned about getting heart disease because they tend to have more risk factors than white women. These risk factors include obesity, lack of physical activity, high blood pressure, and diabetes.

What can I do to prevent heart disease?

You can reduce your chances of getting heart disease by taking these steps:

- **Know your blood pressure:** People with high blood pressure often have no symptoms, so have your blood pressure checked every one to two years and get treatment if you need it.

- **Don't smoke:** If you're having trouble quitting, there are products and programs that can help.

- **Get tested for diabetes:** People with diabetes have high blood glucose (often called blood sugar). People with high blood glucose often have no symptoms, so have your blood glucose checked regularly.

- **Get your cholesterol and triglyceride levels tested:** High blood cholesterol can clog your arteries and keep your heart from getting the blood it needs. This can cause a heart attack. Triglycerides are a form of fat in your blood stream. High levels of triglycerides are linked to heart disease in some people. People with high blood cholesterol or high blood triglycerides often have no symptoms, so have both levels checked regularly.

- **Maintain a healthy weight:** Being overweight raises your risk for heart disease. Healthy food choices and physical activity are important to staying at a healthy weight:

  - Start by adding more fruits, vegetables, and whole grains to your diet.

  - Each week, aim to get at least 2 hours and 30 minutes of moderate physical activity, 1 hour and 15 minutes of vigorous physical activity, or a combination of moderate and vigorous activity.

- **If you drink alcohol, limit it to no more than** one drink (one 12-ounce beer, one 5-ounce glass of wine, or one 1 1/2-ounce shot of hard liquor) a day.

- **Find healthy ways to cope with stress:** Lower your stress level by talking to your friends, exercising, or writing in a journal.

What does high blood pressure have to do with heart disease?

Blood pressure is the force your blood makes against the walls of your arteries. The pressure is highest when your heart pumps blood into your arteries—when it beats. It is lowest between heart beats, when your heart relaxes. A doctor or nurse will write down your blood pressure as the higher number over the lower number. A blood pressure reading below 120/80 is usually considered normal. Very low blood pressure (lower than 90/60) can sometimes be a cause of concern and should be checked out by a doctor.

High blood pressure, or hypertension, is a blood pressure reading of 140/90 or higher. Years of high blood pressure can damage artery walls, causing them to become stiff and narrow. As a result, your heart cannot get the blood it needs to work well. This can cause a heart attack.

A blood pressure reading of 120/80 to 139/89 is considered prehypertension. This means that you don't have high blood pressure now but are likely to develop it in the future.

If you have hypertension or prehypertension, you may be able to lower your blood pressure by following the advice to prevent heart disease. If lifestyle changes do not lower your blood pressure, your doctor may prescribe medicine.

What does high cholesterol have to do with heart disease?

Cholesterol is a waxy substance found in cells in all parts of the body. When there is too much cholesterol in your blood, cholesterol can build up on the walls of your arteries and cause blood clots. Cholesterol can clog your arteries and keep your heart from getting the blood it needs. This can cause a heart attack.

There are two types of cholesterol:

- Low-density lipoprotein (LDL) is often called the "bad" type of cholesterol because it can clog the arteries that carry blood to your heart. For LDL, lower numbers are better. Less than 100 mg/dL (milligrams per deciliter) is best.

- High-density lipoprotein (HDL) is known as "good" cholesterol because it takes the bad cholesterol out of your blood and keeps it from building up in your arteries. For HDL, higher numbers are better. More than 60 mg/dL is best.

All women age 20 and older should have their blood cholesterol and triglyceride levels checked at least once every five years. For total cholesterol level, less than 200 mg/dL is best. For triglyceride levels, less than 150mg/dL is best.

How can I lower my cholesterol?

You can lower your cholesterol by taking these steps:

- **Maintain a healthy weight:** If you are overweight, losing weight can help lower your total cholesterol and LDL ("bad cholesterol") levels.

- **Eat better:** Eat foods low in saturated fats, trans fats, and cholesterol.

- **Eat more** of the following:

  - Fish, poultry chicken, turkey, and lean meats (round, sirloin, tenderloin), skin removed before eating (broil, bake, roast, or poach foods)

- Skim (fat-free) or low-fat (1%) milk and cheeses, and low-fat or nonfat yogurt

- Fruits and vegetables (try for five a day)

- Cereals, breads, rice, and pasta made from whole grains

- **Eat less** of the following:

  - Organ meats (liver, kidney, brains)

  - Egg yolks

  - Fats (butter, lard) and oils

  - Packaged and processed foods

- **Get moving:** Exercise can help lower LDL and raise HDL.

- **Take your medicine:** If your doctor has prescribed medicine to lower your cholesterol, take it exactly as you have been told to.

How do I know if I have heart disease?

Heart disease often has no symptoms. But there are some signs to watch for. Chest or arm pain or discomfort can be a symptom of heart disease and a warning sign of a heart attack. Shortness of breath, dizziness, nausea, abnormal heartbeats, or feeling very tired also are signs. Talk with your doctor if you're having any of these symptoms. Your doctor will take a medical history, do a physical exam, and may order tests.

What are the signs of a heart attack?

For both women and men, the most common sign of a heart attack is pain or discomfort in the center of the chest. The pain or discomfort can be mild or strong. It can last more than a few minutes, or it can go away and come back.

Other common signs of a heart attack include the following:

- Pain or discomfort in one or both arms, back, neck, jaw, or stomach

- Shortness of breath (often occurs before or along with the chest pain or discomfort)

- Nausea or vomiting

- Feeling faint or woozy

- Breaking out in a cold sweat

Women are more likely than men to have these other common signs of a heart attack, particularly shortness of breath, nausea or vomiting, and pain in the back, neck, or jaw. Women are also more likely to have less common signs of a heart attack, including the following:

- Heartburn
- Feeling tired or weak
- Heart flutters
- Loss of appetite
- Coughing

Sometimes the signs of a heart attack happen suddenly, but they can also develop slowly, over hours, days, and even weeks before a heart attack occurs.

The more heart attack signs that you have, the more likely it is that you are having a heart attack. Also, if you've already had a heart attack, your symptoms may not be the same for another one. Even if you're not sure you're having a heart attack, you should still have it checked out.

If you think you, or someone else, may be having a heart attack, wait no more than a few minutes—five at most—before calling 911.

One of my family members had a heart attack. Does that mean I'll have one too?

If your dad or brother had a heart attack before age 55, or if your mom or sister had one before age 65, you're more likely to develop heart disease. This does not mean you will have a heart attack. It means you should take extra good care of your heart to keep it healthy.

Sometimes my heart beats really fast and other times it feels like my heart skips a beat. Am I having a heart attack?

Most people have changes in their heartbeat from time to time. These changes in heartbeat are, for most people, harmless. As you get older, you're more likely to have heartbeats that feel different. Don't panic if you have a few flutters or if your heart races once in a while. If you have flutters and other symptoms such as dizziness or shortness of breath (feeling like you can't get enough air), call 911.

Should I take a daily aspirin to prevent heart attack or stroke?

Aspirin may be helpful for women at high risk, such as women who have already had a heart attack. Aspirin can have serious side effects and may be harmful when mixed with certain medicines. If you're thinking about taking aspirin, talk to your doctor first. If your doctor thinks aspirin is a good choice for you, be sure to take it exactly as your doctor tells you to.

Does taking birth control pills or the patch increase my risk for heart disease?

Taking birth control pills is generally safe for young, healthy women if they do not smoke. But birth control pills can pose heart disease risks for some women, especially women older than 35; women with high blood pressure, diabetes, or high cholesterol; and women who smoke. Talk with your doctor if you have questions about the pill.

Recent studies show that women who use the patch may be exposed to more estrogen than women who use the birth control pill. Research is underway to see if the risk for blood clots is higher in patch users. Talk with your doctor if you have questions about the patch.

If you're using one of the birth control methods, watch for the following signs of trouble. If you have any of these symptoms, call 911:

- Eye problems such as blurred or double vision
- Pain in the upper body or arm
- Bad headaches
- Problems breathing
- Spitting up blood
- Swelling or pain in the leg
- Yellowing of the skin or eyes
- Breast lumps
- Unusual (not normal) heavy bleeding from your vagina

Does menopausal hormone therapy (MHT) increase a woman's risk for heart disease?

Menopausal hormone therapy can help with some symptoms of menopause, including hot flashes, vaginal dryness, mood swings, and bone loss, but there are risks, too. For some women, taking hormones can increase their chances of having a heart attack or stroke. If you decide to use hormones, use them at the lowest dose that helps for the shortest time needed. Talk with your doctor if you have questions about MHT.

Section 47.2

Stroke in Women

Excerpted from "Stroke Fact Sheet," U.S. Department of
Health and Human Services Office on Women's Health
(www.womenshealth.gov), January 28, 2009.

What is a stroke?

A stroke is sometimes called a "brain attack." A stroke can injure
the brain like a heart attack can injure the heart. A stroke occurs when
part of the brain doesn't get the blood it needs.

There are two types of stroke:

- **Ischemic stroke (most common type):** This type of stroke
  happens when blood is blocked from getting to the brain. This
  often happens because the artery is clogged with fatty deposits
  (atherosclerosis) or a blood clot.

- **Hemorrhagic stroke:** This type of stroke happens when a
  blood vessel in the brain bursts and blood bleeds into the brain.
  This type of stroke can be caused by an aneurysm—a thin or
  weak spot in an artery that balloons out and can burst.

Both types of stroke can cause brain cells to die. This may cause a
person to lose control of their speech, movement, and memory. If you
think you are having a stroke, call 911.

What is a "mini-stroke"?

A "mini-stroke," also called a transient ischemic attack or TIA,
happens when, for a short time, less blood than normal gets to the
brain. You may have some signs of stroke or you may not notice any
signs.

A "mini-stroke" lasts from a few minutes up to a day. Many people
do not even know they have had a stroke. A "mini-stroke" can be a
sign of a full stroke to come. If you think you are having a "mini-
stroke," call 911.

What are the signs of a stroke?

A stroke happens fast. Most people have two or more of these signs. If you have any of these signs, call 911:

- Sudden numbness or weakness of face, arm, or leg (mainly on one side of the body)
- Sudden trouble seeing in one or both eyes
- Sudden trouble walking, dizziness, or loss of balance
- Sudden confusion or trouble talking or understanding speech
- Sudden bad headache with no known cause

Women may have unique symptoms:
- Sudden face and arm or leg pain
- Sudden hiccups
- Sudden nausea
- Sudden tiredness
- Sudden chest pain
- Sudden shortness of breath
- Sudden pounding or racing heartbeat

How is stroke diagnosed?

The doctor will usually start by asking the patient what happened and when the symptoms began. Then the doctor will ask the patient some questions to see if she or he is thinking clearly. The doctor also will test the patient's reflexes to see if she or he may have had any physical damage. The doctor may order one or more of the following tests:

- Imaging tests that give a picture of the brain, including CT (computed tomography) scanning and MRI (magnetic resonance imaging) scanning, which are useful for finding out if a stroke is caused by a blockage or by bleeding in the brain
- Electrical tests, such as EEG (electroencephalogram) and an evoked response test, to record the electrical impulses and sensory processes of the brain
- Blood flow tests, such as Doppler ultrasound tests, to show any changes in the blood flow to the brain

What are the effects of stroke?

It depends on the type of stroke, the area of the brain where the stroke occurs, and the extent of brain injury. A mild stroke can cause little or no brain damage. A major stroke can cause severe brain damage and even death.

The brain is divided into four main parts: the right hemisphere (or half), the left hemisphere (or half), the cerebellum, and the brain stem.

A stroke in the right half of the brain can cause the following:

- **Problems judging distances:** The stroke survivor may misjudge distances and fall or be unable to guide her hands to pick something up.

- **Impaired judgment and behavior:** The stroke survivor may try to do things that she should not do, such as driving a car.

- **Short-term memory loss:** The stroke survivor may be able to remember events from 30 years ago, but not what she ate for breakfast that morning.

A stroke in the left half of the brain can cause these symptoms:

- **Speech and language problems:** The stroke survivor may have trouble speaking or understanding others.

- **Slow and cautious behavior:** The stroke survivor may need a lot of help to complete tasks.

- **Memory problems:** The stroke survivor may not remember what she did 10 minutes ago or she may have a hard time learning new things.

A stroke in the cerebellum, or the part of the brain that controls balance and coordination, can cause the following:

- Abnormal reflexes of the head and upper body

- Balance problems

- Dizziness, nausea, and vomiting

Strokes in the brain stem are very harmful because the brain stem controls all our body's functions that we don't have to think about, such as eye movements, breathing, hearing, speech, and swallowing. Since impulses that start in the brain must travel through the brain stem on their way to the arms and legs, patients with a brain stem stroke may also develop paralysis, or may not be able to move or feel on one or both sides of the body.

In many cases, a stroke weakens the muscles, making it hard to walk, eat, or dress without help. Some symptoms may improve with time and rehabilitation or therapy.

Who is at risk for stroke?

It is a myth that stroke occurs only in older adults. A person of any age can have a stroke. But stroke risk does increase with age. For every 10 years after the age of 55, the risk of stroke doubles, and two-thirds of all strokes occur in people over 65 years old. Stroke also seems to run in some families. Stroke risk doubles for a woman if someone in her immediate family (mom, dad, sister, or brother) has had a stroke.

Compared to white women, African American women have more strokes and have a higher risk of disability and death from stroke. This is partly because more African American women have high blood pressure, a major stroke risk factor. Women who smoke or who have high blood pressure, atrial fibrillation (a kind of irregular heart beat), heart disease, or diabetes are more likely to have a stroke. Hormonal changes with pregnancy, childbirth, and menopause are also linked to an increased risk of stroke.

How do I prevent a stroke?

Experts think that up to 80% of strokes can be prevented. Some stroke risk factors cannot be controlled. But you can reduce your chances of having a stroke by taking these steps:

- **Know your blood pressure:** Your heart moves blood through your body. If it is hard for your heart to do this, your heart works harder, and your blood pressure will rise. People with high blood pressure often have no symptoms, so have your blood pressure checked every one to two years. If you have high blood pressure, your doctor may suggest you make some lifestyle changes, such as eating less salt and exercising more. Your doctor may also prescribe medicine to help lower your blood pressure.

- **Don't smoke:** If you are having trouble quitting, there are products and programs that can help.

- **Get tested for diabetes:** People with diabetes have high blood glucose (often called blood sugar). People with high blood sugar often have no symptoms, so have your blood sugar checked regularly. Having diabetes raises your chances of having a stroke. If you have diabetes, your doctor will decide if you need diabetes pills or insulin shots. Your doctor can also help you make a healthy eating and exercise plan.

- **Get your cholesterol and triglyceride levels tested:** Cholesterol is a waxy substance found in all parts of your body. Cholesterol can clog your arteries and keep your brain from getting the blood it needs. This can cause a stroke. Triglycerides are a form of fat in your blood stream. High levels of triglycerides are linked to stroke in some people. People with high blood cholesterol or high blood triglycerides often have no symptoms, so have your blood cholesterol and triglyceride levels checked regularly.

- **Maintain a healthy weight:** Being overweight raises your risk for stroke. Make healthy food choices and get plenty of exercise. Each week, aim for at least 2 hours and 30 minutes of moderate-intensity aerobic physical activity, 1 hour and 15 minutes of vigorous-intensity aerobic physical activity, or a combination of moderate and vigorous activity.

- **If you drink alcohol, limit it to no more than one drink** (one 12-ounce beer, one 5-ounce glass of wine, or one 1 1/2-ounce shot of hard liquor) a day.

- **Find healthy ways to cope with stress:** Lower your stress level by talking to your friends, exercising, or writing in a journal.

How is stroke treated?

Strokes caused by blood clots can be treated with clot-busting drugs such as TPA, or tissue plasminogen activator. TPA must be given within three hours of the start of a stroke to work, and tests must be done first. This is why it is so important for a person having a stroke to get to a hospital fast.

Other medicines are used to treat and to prevent stroke. Anticoagulants, such as warfarin, and antiplatelet agents, such as aspirin, block the blood's ability to clot and can help prevent a stroke in patients with high risk, such as a person who has atrial fibrillation (a kind of irregular heartbeat).

Surgery is sometimes used to treat or prevent stroke. Carotid endarterectomy is a surgery to remove fatty deposits clogging the carotid artery in the neck, which could lead to a stroke. For hemorrhagic stroke, a doctor may perform surgery to place a metal clip at the base of an aneurysm (a thin or weak spot in an artery that balloons out and can burst) or remove abnormal blood vessels.

529

What about rehabilitation?

Rehabilitation is a very important part of recovery for many stroke survivors. The effects of stroke may mean that you must change, re-learn, or redefine how you live. Stroke rehabilitation is designed to help you return to independent living.

Rehabilitation does not reverse the effects of a stroke. Its goals are to build your strength, capability, and confidence so you can continue your daily activities despite the effects of your stroke. Rehabilitation services may include the following:

- Physical therapy to restore movement, balance, and coordination

- Occupational therapy to relearn basic skills such as bathing and dressing

- Speech therapy to relearn how to talk

Section 47.3

Varicose and Spider Veins

Excerpted from "Varicose Veins and Spider Veins Fact Sheet,"
U.S. Department of Health and Human Services Office on Women's
Health (www.womenshealth.gov), June 2, 2010.

What are varicose veins and spider veins?

Varicose veins are enlarged veins that can be blue, red, or flesh colored. They often look like cords and appear twisted and bulging. They can be swollen and raised above the surface of the skin. Varicose veins are often found on the thighs, backs of the calves, or the inside of the leg.

Spider veins are like varicose veins but smaller. They also are closer to the surface of the skin than varicose veins. Often, they are red or blue. They can look like tree branches or spider webs. They can be found on the legs and face and can cover either a very small or very large area.

What causes varicose veins and spider veins?

Varicose veins can be caused by weak or damaged valves in the veins. Veins have valves that act as one-way flaps to prevent blood from flowing backward as it moves up your legs. If the valves become weak, blood can leak back into the veins and collect there. (This problem is called venous insufficiency.) When backed-up blood makes the veins bigger, they can become varicose.

Spider veins can be caused by the backup of blood. They can also be caused by hormone changes, exposure to the sun, and injuries.

How common are abnormal leg veins?

About 50% to 55% of women and 40% to 45% of men in the United States suffer from some type of vein problem. Varicose veins affect half of people 50 years and older.

What factors increase my risk of varicose veins and spider veins?

Many factors increase a person's chances of developing varicose or spider veins:

- **Increasing age:** As you get older, the valves in your veins may weaken and not work as well.

- **Medical history:** Being born with weak vein valves or having family members with vein problems also increases your risk.

- **Hormonal changes:** These occur during puberty, pregnancy, and menopause or by taking birth control pills and other medicines containing estrogen and progesterone.

- **Pregnancy:** During pregnancy, there is a huge increase in the amount of blood in the body. This can cause veins to enlarge.

- **Obesity:** Being overweight or obese can put extra pressure on your veins.

- **Lack of movement:** Sitting or standing for a long time may force your veins to work harder, especially if you sit with your legs bent or crossed.

- **Sun exposure:** This can cause spider veins on the cheeks or nose of a fair-skinned person.

Why do varicose veins and spider veins usually appear in the legs?

Most varicose and spider veins appear in the legs due to the pressure of body weight, force of gravity, and task of carrying blood from the bottom of the body up to the heart.

Compared with other veins in the body, leg veins have the toughest job of carrying blood back to the heart. They endure the most pressure. This pressure can be stronger than the one-way valves in the veins.

What are the signs of varicose veins?

Varicose veins can often be seen on the skin. Some other common symptoms of varicose veins in the legs include the following:

- Aching pain that may get worse after sitting or standing for a long time

- Throbbing or cramping

- Heaviness

- Swelling

- Rash that's itchy or irritated

- Darkening of the skin (in severe cases)

- Restless legs

Are varicose veins and spider veins dangerous?

Spider veins rarely are a serious health problem, but they can cause uncomfortable feelings in the legs. If there are symptoms from spider veins, most often they will be itching or burning. Less often, spider veins can be a sign of blood backup deeper inside that you can't see on the skin.

Varicose veins may not cause any problems, or they may cause aching pain, throbbing, and discomfort. In some cases, varicose veins can lead to more serious health problems. These include the following:

- Sores or skin ulcers due to chronic (long-term) backing up of blood

- Bleeding

- Superficial thrombophlebitis, a blood clot that forms in a vein just below the skin

- Deep vein thrombosis, which is a blood clot in a deeper vein; it can cause a "pulling" feeling in the calf, pain, warmth, redness, and swelling

Should I see a doctor about varicose veins?

You should see a doctor about varicose veins if you have any of the following:

- The vein has become swollen, red, or very tender or warm to the touch
- There are sores or a rash on the leg or near the ankle
- The skin on the ankle and calf becomes thick and changes color
- One of the varicose veins begins to bleed
- Your leg symptoms are interfering with daily activities
- The appearance of the veins is causing you distress
- You're having pain, even if it's just a dull ache

How are varicose veins diagnosed?

Your doctor may diagnose your varicose veins based on a physical exam. Your doctor will look at your legs while you're standing or sitting with your legs dangling. He or she may ask you about your symptoms. Sometimes, you may have other tests to find out the extent of the problem and to rule out other disorders.

You might have an ultrasound, which is used to see the veins' structure, check the blood flow in your veins, and look for blood clots. Although less likely, you might have a venogram. This test can be used to get a more detailed look at blood flow through your veins.

How are varicose and spider veins treated?

Your doctor may recommend lifestyle changes if your varicose veins don't cause many symptoms. If symptoms are more severe, your doctor may recommend medical treatments. Some treatment options include the following:

Compression stockings: Compression stockings put helpful pressure on your veins. There are three kinds of compression stockings:

- Support pantyhose offer the least amount of pressure. They provide pressure all over instead of where it is needed most.

- Over-the-counter gradient compression hose give a little more pressure. They are sold in medical supply stores and drugstores.

- Prescription-strength gradient compression hose offer the greatest amount of pressure. They are sold in medical supply stores and drugstores. You need to be fitted for them.

Sclerotherapy: Sclerotherapy is the most common treatment for both spider veins and varicose veins. The doctor uses a needle to inject a liquid chemical into the vein. The chemical causes the vein walls to swell, stick together, and seal shut. This stops the flow of blood, and the vein turns into scar tissue. In a few weeks, the vein should fade. This treatment does not require anesthesia and can be done in your doctor's office.

The same vein may need to be treated more than once. Treatments are usually done every four to six weeks. You may be asked to wear gradient compression stockings after sclerotherapy to help with healing and decrease swelling.

Ultrasound-guided sclerotherapy (or echo-sclerotherapy) uses ultrasound imaging to guide the needle. It can be useful in treating veins that cannot be seen on the skin's surface.

Surface laser treatments: In some cases, laser treatments can effectively treat spider veins and smaller varicose veins. This technique sends very strong bursts of light through the skin onto the vein. This makes the vein slowly fade and disappear. Not all skin types and colors can be safely treated with lasers.

No needles or incisions are used, but the heat from the laser can be quite painful. Cooling helps reduce the pain. Laser treatments last for 15 to 20 minutes. Generally, two to five treatments are needed to remove spider veins in the legs. Laser therapy usually isn't effective for varicose veins larger than three millimeters (about a tenth of an inch).

Endovenous techniques (radiofrequency and laser): These methods for treating the deeper veins of the legs, called the saphenous veins, have replaced surgery for most patients with severe varicose veins. These techniques can be done in a doctor's office.

The doctor puts a very small tube, called a catheter, into the vein. A small probe is placed through the tube. The device can use radiofrequency or laser energy to seal the vein. The procedure can be done using just local anesthesia. You might have slight bruising after treatment.

Healthy veins around the closed vein take over the normal flow of blood. The symptoms from the varicose vein improve.

Surgery: Surgery is used mostly to treat very large varicose veins. Types of surgery for varicose veins include the following:

- **Surgical ligation and stripping:** Problem veins are tied shut and completely removed from the leg through small cuts in the skin. Removing the veins does not affect the circulation of blood in the leg. This surgery requires general anesthesia and must be done in an operating room. It takes between one and four weeks to recover from the surgery. This surgery is generally safe. Pain in the leg is the most common side effect, although there are other less common side effects.

- **PIN stripping:** An instrument called a PIN stripper is inserted into a vein. The tip of the PIN stripper is sewn to the end of the vein, and when it is removed, the vein is pulled out. This procedure can be done in an operating room or an outpatient center. General or local anesthesia can be used.

- **Ambulatory phlebectomy:** Tiny cuts are made in the skin, and hooks are used to pull the vein out of the leg. Only the parts of your leg that are being pricked will be numbed with anesthesia. The vein is usually removed in one treatment. Very large varicose veins can be removed with this treatment while leaving only very small scars. Patients can return to normal activity the day after treatment. Possible side effects of the treatment include slight bruising and temporary numbness.

How can I prevent varicose veins and spider veins?

Not all varicose and spider veins can be prevented. But there are some steps you can take to reduce your chances of getting new varicose and spider veins and ease discomfort from the ones you already have:

- Wear sunscreen to protect your skin from the sun and to limit spider veins on the face.

- Exercise regularly to improve your leg strength, circulation, and vein strength. Focus on exercises that work your legs, such as walking or running.

- Control your weight to avoid placing too much pressure on your legs.

- Don't cross your legs for long times when sitting. It's possible to injure your legs that way, and even a minor injury can increase the risk of varicose veins.

- Elevate your legs when resting as much as possible.

- Don't stand or sit for long periods of time. If you must stand for a long time, shift your weight from one leg to the other every few minutes. If you must sit for long periods of time, stand up and move around or take a short walk every 30 minutes.

- Wear elastic support stockings and avoid tight clothing that constricts your waist, groin, or legs.

- Avoid wearing high heels for long periods of time.

- Eat a low-salt diet rich in high-fiber foods. Eating fiber reduces the chances of constipation, which can contribute to varicose veins. Eating less salt can help with the swelling that comes with varicose veins.

Can varicose and spider veins return even after treatment?

Current treatments for varicose veins and spider veins have very high success rates compared to traditional surgical treatments. Over a period of years, however, more abnormal veins can develop because there is no cure for weak vein valves. Ultrasound can be used to keep track of how badly the valves are leaking. Ongoing treatment can help keep this problem under control.

The single most important thing you can do to slow down the development of new varicose veins is to wear gradient compression support stockings as much as possible during the day.

Chapter 48

Carpal Tunnel Syndrome in Women

What is carpal tunnel syndrome (CTS)?

Carpal tunnel syndrome is the name for a group of problems that includes swelling, pain, tingling, and loss of strength in your wrist and hand. Your wrist is made of small bones that form a narrow groove or carpal tunnel. Tendons and a nerve called the median nerve must pass through this tunnel from your forearm into your hand. The median nerve controls the feelings and sensations in the palm side of your thumb and fingers. Sometimes swelling and irritation of the tendons can put pressure on the wrist nerve causing the symptoms of CTS. A person's dominant hand is the one that is usually affected. However, nearly half of CTS sufferers have symptoms in both hands.

CTS has become more common in the United States and is quite costly in terms of time lost from work and expensive medical treatment. The U.S. Department of Labor reported that in 2003 the average number of missed days of work due to CTS was 23 days, costing over $2 billion a year. It is thought that about 3.7% of the general public in this country suffer from CTS.

What are the symptoms of CTS?

Typically, CTS begins slowly with feelings of burning, tingling, and numbness in the wrist and hand. The areas most affected are the thumb,

Excerpted from "Carpal Tunnel Syndrome Fact Sheet," U.S. Department of Health and Human Services Office on Women's Health (www.womenshealth.gov), June 1, 2009.

index, and middle fingers. At first, symptoms may happen more often at night. Many CTS sufferers do not make the connection between a daytime activity that might be causing the CTS and the delayed symptoms. Also, many people sleep with their wrist bent, which may cause more pain and symptoms at night. As CTS gets worse, the tingling may be felt during the daytime too, along with pain moving from the wrist to your arm or down to your fingers. Pain is usually felt more on the palm side of the hand.

Another symptom of CTS is weakness of the hands that gets worse over time. Some people with CTS find it difficult to grasp an object, make a fist, or hold onto something small. The fingers may even feel like they are swollen even though they are not. Over time, this feeling will usually happen more often.

If left untreated, those with CTS can have a loss of feeling in some fingers and permanent weakness of the thumb. Thumb muscles can actually waste away over time. Eventually, CTS sufferers may have trouble telling the difference between hot and cold temperatures by touch.

What causes CTS and who is more likely to develop it?

Women are three times more likely to have CTS than men. Although there is limited research on why this is the case, scientists have several ideas. It may be that the wrist bones are naturally smaller in most women, creating a tighter space through which the nerves and tendons must pass. Other researchers are looking at genetic links that make it more likely for women to have musculoskeletal injuries such as CTS. Women also deal with strong hormonal changes during pregnancy and menopause that make them more likely to suffer from CTS. Generally, women are at higher risk of CTS between the ages of 45 and 54. Then, the risk increases for both men and women as they age.

There are other factors that can cause CTS, including certain health problems and, in some cases, the cause is unknown.

These are some of the things that might raise your chances of developing CTS:

- **Genetic predisposition:** The carpal tunnel is smaller in some people than others.

- **Repetitive movements:** People who do the same movements with their wrists and hands over and over may be more likely to develop CTS. People with certain types of jobs are more likely to have CTS, including manufacturing and assembly line workers, grocery store checkers, violinists, and carpenters. Some hobbies and sports that use repetitive hand movements can also cause CTS, such as golfing, knitting, and gardening. Whether or not long-term typing or computer use causes CTS is still being debated.

- **Injury or trauma:** A sprain or a fracture of the wrist can cause swelling and pressure on the nerve, increasing the risk of CTS. Forceful and stressful movements of the hand and wrist can also cause trauma, such as strong vibrations caused by heavy machinery or power tools.

- **Pregnancy:** Pregnant women at greater risk of getting CTS, especially during the last few months. Most doctors treat CTS in pregnant women with wrist splits or rest, rather than surgery, as CTS almost always goes away following childbirth.

- **Menopause:** Hormonal changes during menopause can put women at greater risk of getting CTS. Also, in some postmenopausal women, the wrist structures become enlarged and can press on the wrist nerve.

- **Breast cancer:** Some women who have a mastectomy get lymphedema, the build-up of fluids that go beyond the lymph system's ability to drain it. In mastectomy patients, this causes pain and swelling of the arm. Although rare, some of these women will get CTS due to pressure on the nerve from this swelling.

- **Medical conditions:** People who have diabetes, hypothyroidism, lupus, obesity, and rheumatoid arthritis are more likely to get CTS. In some of these patients, the normal structures in the wrist can become enlarged and lead to CTS.

Also, smokers with CTS usually have worse symptoms and recover more slowly than nonsmokers.

How is CTS treated?

It is important to be treated by a doctor in order to avoid permanent damage to the wrist nerve and muscles of the hand and thumb. Underlying causes such as diabetes or a thyroid problem should be addressed first. Left untreated, CTS can cause nerve damage that leads to loss of feeling and less hand strength. Over time, the muscles of the thumb can become weak and damaged. You can even lose the ability to feel hot and cold by touch. Permanent injury occurs in about 1% of those with CTS.

CTS is much easier to treat early on. Most CTS patients get better after first-step treatments and the following tips for protecting the wrist. Treatments for CTS include the following:

- **Wrist splint:** A splint can be worn to support and brace your wrist in a neutral position so that the nerves and tendons can recover. A splint can be worn 24 hours a day or only at night. Splinting works best when done within three months of having any symptoms of CTS.

- **Rest:** For people with mild CTS, stopping or doing less of a repetitive movement may be all that is needed.

- **Medication:** The short-term use of nonsteroidal anti-inflammatory drugs (NSAIDs) may be helpful to control CTS pain. NSAIDs include aspirin, ibuprofen, and other nonprescription pain relievers. In severe cases, an injection of cortisone may help to reduce swelling. Your doctor may also give you corticosteroids in a pill form. But these treatments only relieve symptoms temporarily.

- **Physical therapy:** A physical therapist can help you do special exercises to make your wrist and hand stronger. There are also many different kinds of treatments that can make CTS better and help relieve symptoms. Massage, yoga, ultrasound, chiropractic manipulation, and acupuncture are just a few such options that have been found to be helpful. You should talk with your doctor before trying these alternative treatments.

- **Surgery:** CTS surgery is one of the most common surgeries done in the United States. Generally, surgery is only an option for severe cases of CTS and/or after other treatments have failed for a period of at least six months. Open release surgery is a common approach to CTS surgery and involves making a small incision in the wrist or palm and cutting the ligament to enlarge the carpal tunnel. This surgery is done under a local anesthetic to numb the wrist and hand area and is an outpatient procedure.

What is the best way to prevent CTS?

The following steps can help to prevent CTS:

- **Prevent workplace musculoskeletal injury:** Make sure that your workspace and equipment are at the right height and distance for your hands and wrist to work with less strain. If you are working on a computer, the keyboard should be at a height that allows your wrist to rest comfortably without having to bend at an angle. Desk or table workspace should be about 27 to 29 inches above the floor for most people. It also helps to keep your elbows close to your sides as you type to reduce the strain on your forearm. Keeping good posture and wrist position can lower your risk of getting CTS.

- **Take breaks:** Allowing your hand and wrist to rest and recover every so often will lower your risk of swelling. Experts believe that taking a 10- to 15-minute break every hour is a good way to prevent CTS.

- **Vary tasks:** Avoid repetitive movements without changing up your routine. Try to do tasks that use different muscle movements during each hour. Break up tasks that require repetitive wrist and hand motion with those that do not.

- **Relax your grip:** Sometimes, people get into a habit of tensing muscles without needing to. Practice doing hand and wrist motion tasks more gently and less tightly.

- **Do exercises:** After doing repetitive movements for a while, you can sometimes cancel out the effects of those movements by flexing and bending your wrists and hands in the opposite direction. For example, after typing with your wrist and hand extended, it is helpful to make a tight fist and hold it for a second, then stretch out the fingers and hold for a few seconds.

- **Stay warm:** Muscles that are warm are less likely to get hurt, and the risk of getting CTS is greater in a cold environment. It is important to keep your hands warm while you work, even if you must wear fingerless gloves.

Chapter 49

Chronic Pain

Chapter Contents

Section 49.1

Chronic Pain in Women

"Halt the Hurt! Dealing with Chronic Pain," National Institutes of Health *News in Health* (newsinhealth.nih.gov), March 2012, and excerpts from "Pain: Hope through Research," National Institute of Neurological Disorders and Stroke (www.ninds.nih.gov), September 19, 2012.

Halt the Hurt! Dealing with Chronic Pain

Pain—it's something we've all experienced. From our first skinned knee to the headaches, back pain, and creaky joints as we age, pain is something we encounter many times. Most pain is acute and goes away quickly. But in some cases, when pain develops slowly or persists for months or even years, then it's called chronic pain, and it can be tricky to treat.

Chronic pain is a huge problem. Over 115 million people nationwide—about one in three Americans—suffer from some kind of long-term pain. It's the leading reason that people miss work.

Chronic pain differs in many ways from acute pain. Acute pain is part of the body's response to an injury or short-term illness. Acute pain can help prevent more serious injury. For instance, it can make you quickly pull your finger away from a hot stove or keep your weight off a broken ankle. The causes of acute pain can usually be diagnosed and treated, and the pain eventually ends.

But the causes of chronic pain aren't always clear. "It's a complex problem that involves more than just the physical aspects of where the hurt seems to be," says Dr. John Killen, deputy director of National Institute of Health (NIH)'s National Center for Complementary and Alternative Medicine. "There's a lot of accumulating scientific evidence that chronic pain is partly a problem of how the brain processes pain."

Chronic pain can come in many forms, and it accompanies several conditions including low-back pain, arthritis, cancer, migraine, fibromyalgia, endometriosis, and inflammatory bowel disease. These persistent pains can severely limit your ability to move around and perform day-to-day tasks. Chronic pain can lead to depression and anxiety. It's hard to look on the bright side when pain just won't go away. Some experts say that chronic pain is a disease itself.

The complexities of chronic pain can make it difficult to treat. Many of today's medications for chronic pain target inflammation. These drugs include aspirin, ibuprofen and COX-2 inhibitors. But if taken at high doses for a long time, these drugs can irritate your stomach and digestive system and possibly harm your kidneys. And they don't work for everyone.

"With hard-to-treat pain, the opioids are also used, sometimes in combination with the other drugs," says Dr. Raymond Dionne, who oversees some of NIH's clinical pain research. Opioids include prescription painkillers such as codeine and morphine and brand-name drugs such as Vicodin, Oxycontin, and Percocet. Opioids affect the processes by which the brain perceives pain. If used improperly, though, opioids can be addictive, and increasingly high doses may be needed to keep pain in check.

"As with all drugs, you have to find a balance between effectiveness and side effects," says Dionne. He and other researchers have studied potential new pain medications to learn more about how they work in the body. But for the most part, pain medications are similar to those used five or more decades ago. That's why some researchers are looking for approaches beyond medications.

"One thing we know is that currently available drug therapies don't provide all the answers. Many people find that medications don't fully relieve their chronic pain, and they can experience unpleasant side effects," Killen says. "Evidence on a number of fronts, for several conditions, suggests that mind and body approaches can be helpful additions to conventional medicine for managing chronic pain."

Research has shown that patients with chronic low-back pain might benefit from acupuncture, massage therapy, yoga, or cognitive-behavioral therapy (a type of talk therapy).

NIH-funded scientists have also found that people with fibromyalgia pain might find relief through tai chi. This mind-body technique combines meditation, slow movements, deep breathing, and relaxation.

But how much these approaches truly help is still an open question. Studies of pain relief can be difficult to interpret. Researchers must rely on patients to complete questionnaires and rate their own levels of pain.

One puzzler is that the exposure to the exact same pain-causing thing, or stimulus, can lead to completely different responses in different people. For example, when an identical heat stimulus is applied to different people's arms, one may report feeling uncomfortable, while another might say that the pain is extreme.

"How do we account for these differences? We've now learned that genes play a role," says Dr. Sean Mackey, who heads Stanford University's neuroscience and pain lab. "Some differences involve our personality and mood states, including anxiety."

Mackey and his team are using brain scans to gain insights into how we process and feel pain. One study found that a painful stimulus can activate different brain regions in people who are anxious than in those who are fearful of pain.

In another study, volunteers were taught strategies that could turn on specific brain regions. One technique involved mentally changing the meaning of the pain and thinking about it in a nonthreatening way.

"We found that with repeated training, people can learn how to build up this brain area, almost like a muscle, and make its activity much stronger," says Mackey. "That led to a significant improvement overall in their pain perception." The researchers also found that different types of mental strategies, such as distraction, engaged different brain regions.

Another study found that intense feelings of passionate love can provide surprisingly effective pain relief. "It turns out that the areas of the brain activated by intense love are the same areas that drugs use to reduce pain," says Mackay.

"We can't write a prescription for patients to go home and have a passionate love affair," says Mackey. "But we can suggest that you go out and do things that are rewarding, that are emotionally meaningful. Go for a walk on a moonlit beach. Go listen to some music you never listened to before. Do something that's novel and exciting."

That's a prescription that should be painless to try.

Pain: Hope through Research: Gender and Pain

It is now widely believed that pain affects men and women differently. While the sex hormones estrogen and testosterone certainly play a role in this phenomenon, psychology and culture, too, may account at least in part for differences in how men and women receive pain signals. For example, young children may learn to respond to pain based on how they are treated when they experience pain. Some children may be cuddled and comforted, while others may be encouraged to tough it out and to dismiss their pain.

Many investigators are turning their attention to the study of gender differences and pain. Women, many experts now agree, recover more quickly from pain, seek help more quickly for their pain, and are less likely to allow pain to control their lives. They also are more likely to marshal a variety of resources—coping skills, support, and distraction—with which to deal with their pain.

Research in this area is yielding fascinating results. For example, male experimental animals injected with estrogen, a female sex hormone, appear to have a lower tolerance for pain—that is, the addition of estrogen appears to lower the pain threshold. Similarly, the presence of testosterone, a male hormone, appears to elevate tolerance for pain in female mice: the animals are simply able to withstand pain better. Female mice deprived of estrogen during experiments react to stress similarly to male animals. Estrogen, therefore, may act as a sort of pain switch, turning on the ability to recognize pain.

Investigators know that males and females both have strong natural pain-killing systems, but these systems operate differently. For example, a class of painkillers called kappa-opioids is named after one of several opioid receptors to which they bind, the kappa-opioid receptor, and they include the compounds nalbuphine (Nubain) and butorphanol (Stadol). Research suggests that kappa-opioids provide better pain relief in women.

Though not prescribed widely, kappa-opioids are currently used for relief of labor pain and in general work best for short-term pain. Investigators are not certain why kappa-opioids work better in women than men. Is it because a woman's estrogen makes them work, or because a man's testosterone prevents them from working? Or is there another explanation, such as differences between men and women in their perception of pain? Continued research may result in a better understanding of how pain affects women differently from men, enabling new and better pain medications to be designed with gender in mind.

Section 49.2

Chronic Pain and Emotion

"Why Chronic Pain Is All In Your Head" by Marla Paul, July 2, 2012. Reprinted with permission from *Northwestern News*, www.northwestern.edu/ newscenter. © 2012 Northwestern University. All rights reserved.

When people have similar injuries, why do some end up with chronic pain while others recover and are pain free? The first longitudinal brain imaging study to track participants with a new back injury has found the chronic pain is all in their heads—quite literally.

A new Northwestern Medicine study shows for the first time that chronic pain develops the more two sections of the brain—related to emotional and motivational behavior—talk to each other. The more they communicate, the greater the chance a patient will develop chronic pain.

The finding provides a new direction for developing therapies to treat intractable pain, which affects 30 to 40 million adults in the United States.

Researchers were able to predict, with 85% accuracy at the beginning of the study, which participants would go on to develop chronic pain based on the level of interaction between the frontal cortex and the nucleus accumbens.

The study is published in the journal *Nature Neuroscience*.

"For the first time we can explain why people who may have the exact same initial pain either go on to recover or develop chronic pain," said A. Vania Apkarian, senior author of the paper and professor of physiology at Northwestern University Feinberg School of Medicine.

"The injury by itself is not enough to explain the ongoing pain. It has to do with the injury combined with the state of the brain. This finding is the culmination of 10 years of our research."

The more emotionally the brain reacts to the initial injury, the more likely the pain will persist after the injury has healed. "It may be that these sections of the brain are more excited to begin with in certain individuals, or there may be genetic and environmental influences that predispose these brain regions to interact at an excitable level," Apkarian said.

The nucleus accumbens is an important center for teaching the rest of the brain how to evaluate and react to the outside world, Apkarian noted, and this brain region may use the pain signal to teach the rest of the brain to develop chronic pain.

"Now we hope to develop new therapies for treatment based on this finding," Apkarian added.

Chronic pain participants in the study also lost gray matter density, which is likely linked to fewer synaptic connections or neuronal and glial shrinkage, Apkarian said. Brain synapses are essential for communication between neurons.

"Chronic pain is one of the most expensive health care conditions in the U.S. yet there still is not a scientifically validated therapy for this condition," Apkarian said. Chronic pain costs an estimated $600 billion a year, according to a 2011 National Academy of Sciences report. Back pain is the most prevalent chronic pain condition.

A total of 40 participants who had an episode of back pain that lasted 4 to 16 weeks—but with no prior history of back pain—were studied. All subjects were diagnosed with back pain by a clinician. Brain scans were conducted on each participant at study entry and for three more visits during one year.

Other Northwestern authors on the paper include lead author Marwan N. Baliki, Bogdan Petre, Souraya Torbey, Kristina M. Herrmann, Lejian Huang, and Thomas J. Schnitzer.

The study was funded by the National Institute of Neurological Disorders and Stroke of the National Institutes of Health grant NS35115.

Chapter 50

Diabetes in Women

What is diabetes?

Diabetes means that your blood glucose (sugar) is too high. Your blood always has some glucose in it because the body uses glucose for energy; it's the fuel that keeps you going. But too much glucose in the blood is not good for your health.

Your body changes most of the food you eat into glucose. Your blood takes the glucose to the cells throughout your body. The glucose needs insulin to get into the body's cells. Insulin is a hormone made in the pancreas, an organ near the stomach. Insulin helps the glucose from food get into body cells. If your body does not make enough insulin or the insulin does not work right, the glucose can't get into the cells, so it stays in the blood. This makes your blood glucose level high, causing you to have diabetes.

If not controlled, diabetes can lead to blindness, heart disease, stroke, kidney failure, amputations (having a toe or foot removed, for example), and nerve damage. In women, diabetes can cause problems during pregnancy and make it more likely that your baby will be born with birth defects.

What is prediabetes?

Prediabetes means your blood glucose is higher than normal but lower than the diabetes range. It also means you are at risk of getting type 2

Excerpted from "Diabetes Fact Sheet," U.S. Department of Health and Human Services Office on Women's Health (www.womenshealth.gov), February 18, 2010.

diabetes and heart disease. There is good news though: You can reduce the risk of getting diabetes and even return to normal blood glucose levels with modest weight loss and moderate physical activity. If you are told you have prediabetes, have your blood glucose checked again in one to two years.

What are the different types of diabetes?

There are three main types of diabetes:

- Type 1 diabetes is commonly diagnosed in children and young adults, but it's a lifelong condition. If you have this type of diabetes, your body does not make insulin, so you must take insulin every day. Treatment for type 1 diabetes includes taking insulin shots or using an insulin pump, making healthy food choices, getting regular physical activity, taking aspirin daily (for many people), and controlling blood pressure and cholesterol levels.

- Type 2 diabetes is the most common type of diabetes—about 9 out of 10 people with diabetes have type 2 diabetes. You can get type 2 diabetes at any age, even during childhood. In type 2 diabetes, your body makes insulin, but the insulin can't do its job, so glucose is not getting into the cells. Treatment includes taking medicine, making healthy food choices, getting regular physical activity, taking aspirin daily (for many people), and controlling blood pressure and cholesterol levels. If you have type 2 diabetes, your body generally produces less and less insulin over time. This means that you may need to increase your medications or start using insulin in order to keep your diabetes in good control.

- Gestational diabetes occurs during pregnancy. This type of diabetes occurs in about 1 in 20 pregnancies. During pregnancy your body makes hormones that keep insulin from doing its job. To make up for this, your body makes extra insulin. But in some women this extra insulin is not enough, so they get gestational diabetes. Gestational diabetes usually goes away when the pregnancy is over. Women who have had gestational diabetes are very likely to develop type 2 diabetes later in life.

Who gets diabetes?

About 24 million Americans have diabetes, about half of whom are women. As many as one quarter do not know they have diabetes.

Type 1 diabetes occurs at about the same rate in men and women, but it is more common in Caucasians than in other ethnic groups.

Type 2 diabetes is more common in older people, mainly in people who are overweight. It is more common in African Americans, Hispanic Americans/Latinos, and American Indians.

What causes diabetes?

Type 1 and type 2 diabetes: The exact causes of both types of diabetes are still not known. For both types, genetic factors make it possible for diabetes to develop. But something in the person's environment is also needed to trigger the onset of diabetes. With type 1 diabetes, those environmental triggers are unknown. With type 2 diabetes, the exact cause is also unknown, but it is clear that excess weight helps trigger the disease. Most people who get type 2 diabetes are overweight.

Gestational diabetes: Changing hormones and weight gain are part of a healthy pregnancy, but these changes make it hard for your body to keep up with its need for insulin. When that happens, your body doesn't get the energy it needs from the foods you eat.

Am I at risk for diabetes?

The risk factors for type 1 diabetes are unknown. Things that can put you at risk for type 2 diabetes include the following:

- Age—being older than 45
- Overweight or obesity
- Family history—having a mother, father, brother, or sister with diabetes
- Race/ethnicity—your family background is African American, American Indian/Alaska Native, Hispanic American/Latino, Asian American/Pacific Islander and Native Hawaiian
- Having a baby with a birth weight more than nine pounds
- Having diabetes during pregnancy (gestational diabetes)
- High blood pressure—140/90 mmHg (millimeters of mercury) or higher
- High cholesterol—total cholesterol over 240 mg/dL (milligrams/deciliter)
- Inactivity—exercising fewer than three times a week
- Abnormal results in a prior diabetes test
- Having other health conditions that are linked to problems using insulin, like polycystic ovarian syndrome (PCOS)

- Having a history of heart disease or stroke

Should I be tested for diabetes?

If you're at least 45 years old, you should get tested for diabetes, and then you should be tested again every three years. If you're 45 or older and overweight, you may want to get tested more often. If you're younger than 45, overweight, and have one or more diabetes risk factors, you should get tested now.

What are the signs of diabetes?

- Being very thirsty
- Urinating a lot
- Feeling very hungry
- Feeling very tired
- Losing weight without trying
- Having sores that are slow to heal
- Having dry, itchy skin
- Losing feeling in or having tingling in the hands or feet
- Having blurry vision
- Having more infections than usual

If you have one or more of these signs, see your doctor.

How can I take care of myself if I have diabetes?

Many people with diabetes live healthy and full lives. By following your doctor's instructions and eating right, you can too. Here are the things you'll need to do to keep your diabetes in check:

- **Follow your meal plan:** Eat lots of whole grain foods, fruits, and vegetables.
- **Get moving:** Health benefits are gained by doing the following each week:
  - 2 hours and 30 minutes of moderate intensity aerobic physical activity **or**
  - 1 hour and 15 minutes of vigorous-intensity aerobic physical activity **or**

- A combination of moderate and vigorous-intensity aerobic physical activity and muscle-strengthening activities on three days

- **Test your blood glucose:** Keep track of your blood glucose levels and talk to your doctor about ways to keep your levels on target. Many women report that their blood glucose levels go up or down around their period. If you're going through menopause, you might also notice your blood glucose levels going up and down.

- **Take your diabetes medicine** exactly as your doctor tells you.

Talk to your doctor about other things you can do to take good care of yourself. Taking care of your diabetes can help prevent serious problems in your eyes, kidneys, nerves, gums and teeth, and blood vessels.

How can I take care of myself if I have gestational diabetes?

Taking care of yourself when you have gestational diabetes is very much like taking care of yourself when you have other types of diabetes. But it can be a little scary when you're pregnant and you also have a new condition to take care of. Don't worry. Many women who've had gestational diabetes have gone on to have healthy babies. Here are the things you'll need to do:

- **Follow your meal plan:** You will meet with a dietitian or diabetes educator who will help you design a meal plan full of healthy foods for you and your baby. You will be advised to do the following:
  - Limit sweets.
  - Eat often—three small meals and one to three snacks every day.
  - Be careful about the carbohydrates you eat. Your meal plan will tell you when to eat carbohydrates and how much to eat at each meal and snack
  - Eat lots of whole grain foods, fruits, and vegetables.

- **Get moving:** Try to be active for at least 2 hours and 30 minutes each week. If you're already active, your doctor can help you make an exercise plan for your pregnancy. If you haven't been active in the past, talk to your doctor. Your doctor can suggest activities, such as swimming or walking, to help keep your blood glucose on track.

- **Test your blood glucose:** Your doctor may ask you to use a small device called a blood glucose meter to check your blood glucose levels. Your diabetes team will tell you what your target blood glucose range is, how often you need to check your blood glucose, and what to do if it is not where it should be.

  - Each time you check your blood glucose, write down the results in a record book. Take the book with you when you visit your health care team.

  - Take your diabetes medicine exactly as your doctor tells you. You may need to take insulin to keep your blood glucose at the right level. Insulin will not harm your baby—it cannot move from your bloodstream to your baby's.

Is there a cure for diabetes?

There is no cure for diabetes at this time, but there is a great deal of research going on in hopes of finding cures for both type 1 and type 2 diabetes. Many different approaches to curing diabetes are being studied, and researchers are making progress.

Is there anything I can do to prevent diabetes?

Yes. The best way to prevent diabetes is to make some lifestyle changes:

- **Maintain a healthy weight:** If you're overweight, start making small changes to your eating habits by adding more whole grain foods, fruits, and vegetables. Start exercising more, even if taking a short walk is all you can do for now. If you're not sure where to start, talk to your doctor. Even a relatively small amount of weight loss—10 to 15 pounds—has been proven to delay or even prevent the onset of type 2 diabetes.

- **Eat healthy:**
  - Eat lots of whole grains, fruits, and vegetables.
  - Choose foods low in fat and cholesterol.
  - If you drink alcohol, limit it to no more than one or two drinks (one 12-ounce beer, one 5-ounce glass of wine, or one 1½-ounce shot of hard liquor) a day.

- **Get moving:** Follow the physical activity guidelines listed in this chapter to gain health benefits.

Chapter 51

Female Athlete Triad

What Is Female Athlete Triad?

Sports and exercise are part of a balanced, healthy lifestyle. People who play sports are healthier; get better grades; are less likely to experience depression; and use alcohol, cigarettes, and drugs less frequently than people who aren't athletes. But for some women, not balancing the needs of their bodies and their sports can have major consequences.

Some women who play sports or exercise intensely are at risk for a problem called female athlete triad. Female athlete triad is a combination of three conditions: disordered eating, amenorrhea, and osteoporosis. A female athlete can have one, two, or all three parts of the triad.

Triad Factor #1: Disordered Eating

Most women with female athlete triad try to lose weight as a way to improve their athletic performance. The disordered eating that accompanies female athlete triad can range from avoiding certain types of food the athlete thinks are "bad" (such as foods containing fat) to serious eating disorders like anorexia nervosa or bulimia nervosa.

Triad Factor #2: Amenorrhea

Exercising intensely and not eating enough calories can lead to decreases in estrogen, the hormone that helps to regulate the menstrual cycle. As a result, a woman's periods may become irregular or stop altogether. Of course, it's normal for teens to occasionally miss periods, especially in the first year. A missed period does not automatically mean female athlete triad. It could mean something else is going on, like pregnancy or a medical condition. If you are having sex and miss your period, talk to your doctor.

Some women who participate intensively in sports may never even get their first period because they've been training so hard. Others may have had periods, but once they increase their training and change their eating habits, their periods may stop.

Triad Factor #3: Osteoporosis

Low estrogen levels and poor nutrition, especially low calcium intake, can lead to osteoporosis, the third aspect of the triad. Osteoporosis is a weakening of the bones due to the loss of bone density and improper bone formation. This condition can ruin a female athlete's career because it may lead to stress fractures and other injuries.

Usually, the teen years are a time when girls should be building up their bone mass to their highest levels—called peak bone mass. Not getting enough calcium then can also have a lasting effect on how strong a woman's bones are later in life.

Who Gets Female Athlete Triad?

Many women have concerns about the size and shape of their bodies. But being a highly competitive athlete and participating in a sport that requires you to train extra hard can increase that worry.

Women with female athlete triad often care so much about their sports that they would do almost anything to improve their performance. Martial arts and rowing are examples of sports that classify athletes by weight class, so focusing on weight becomes an important part of the training program and can put a woman at risk for disordered eating.

Participation in sports where a thin appearance is valued can also put a woman at risk for female athlete triad. Sports such as gymnastics, figure skating, diving, and ballet are examples of sports that value a thin, lean body shape. Some athletes may even be told by coaches or judges that losing weight would improve their scores.

Even in sports where body size and shape aren't as important, such as distance running and cross-country skiing, women may be pressured by teammates, parents, partners, and coaches who mistakenly believe that "losing just a few pounds" could improve their performance.

The truth is, losing those few pounds generally doesn't improve performance at all. People who are fit and active enough to compete in sports generally have more muscle than fat, so it's the muscle that gets starved when a woman cuts back on food. Plus, if a woman loses weight when she doesn't need to, it interferes with healthy body processes such as menstruation and bone development.

In addition, for some competitive female athletes, problems such as low self-esteem, a tendency toward perfectionism, and family stress place them at risk for disordered eating.

What Are the Signs and Symptoms?

If a woman has risk factors for female athlete triad, she may already be experiencing some symptoms and signs of the disorder, such as:

- weight loss;
- no periods or irregular periods;
- fatigue and decreased ability to concentrate;
- stress fractures (fractures that occur even if a person hasn't had a significant injury);
- muscle injuries.

Women with female athlete triad often have signs and symptoms of eating disorders, such as:

- continued dieting in spite of weight loss;
- preoccupation with food and weight;
- frequent trips to the bathroom during and after meals;
- using laxatives;
- brittle hair or nails;
- dental cavities because in women with bulimia tooth enamel is worn away by frequent vomiting;
- sensitivity to cold;
- low heart rate and blood pressure;
- heart irregularities and chest pain.

How Doctors Help

An extensive physical examination is a crucial part of diagnosing female athlete triad. A doctor who thinks a woman has female athlete triad will probably ask questions about her periods, her nutrition and exercise habits, any medications she takes, and her feelings about her body. This is called the medical history.

Poor nutrition can also affect the body in many ways, so a doctor might order blood tests to check for anemia and other problems associated with the triad. The doctor also will check for medical reasons why a woman may be losing weight and missing her periods. Because osteoporosis can put someone at higher risk for bone fractures, the doctor may also request tests to measure bone density.

Doctors don't work alone to help a woman with female athlete triad. Coaches, parents, physical therapists, pediatricians and adolescent medicine specialists, nutritionists and dietitians, and mental health specialists can all work together to treat the physical and emotional problems that a woman with female athlete triad faces.

It might be tempting to shrug off several months of missed periods, but getting help right away is important. In the short term, female athlete triad may lead to muscle weakness, stress fractures, and reduced physical performance. Over the long term, it can cause bone weakness, long-term effects on the reproductive system, and heart problems.

A woman who is recovering from female athlete triad might work with a dietitian to help reach and maintain a healthy weight while eating enough calories and nutrients for health and good athletic performance. Depending on how much the woman is exercising, she may have to reduce the length of her workouts. Talking to a psychologist or therapist can help her deal with depression, pressure from coaches or family members, or low self-esteem and can help her find ways to deal with her problems other than restricting food intake or exercising excessively.

Some women may need to take hormones to supply their bodies with estrogen to help prevent further bone loss. Calcium and vitamin D supplementation can also help when someone has bone loss as the result of female athlete triad.

What If I Think Someone I Know Has It?

It's tempting to ignore female athlete triad and hope it goes away. But it requires help from a doctor and other health professionals. If a friend, sister, or teammate has signs and symptoms of female athlete triad, discuss your concerns with her and encourage her to seek treatment. If she refuses, you may need to mention your concern to a parent, coach, teacher, or school nurse.

You might worry about seeming nosy when you ask questions about a friend's health, but you're not: Your concern is a sign that you're a caring friend. Lending an ear may be just what your friend needs.

Tips for Female Athletes

Here are a few tips to help female athletes stay on top of their physical condition:

- **Keep track of your periods:** It's easy to forget when you had your last visit from Aunt Flo, so keep a calendar in your gym bag and mark down when your period starts and stops and if the bleeding is particularly heavy or light. That way, if you start missing periods, you'll know right away and you'll have accurate information to give to your doctor.

- **Don't skip meals or snacks:** If you're constantly on the go between school, practice, and competitions you may be tempted to skip meals and snacks to save time. But eating now will improve performance later, so stock your locker or bag with quick and easy favorites such as bagels, string cheese, unsalted nuts and seeds, raw vegetables, granola bars, and fruit.

- **Visit a dietitian or nutritionist who works with athletes:** He or she can help you get your dietary game plan into gear and find out if you're getting enough key nutrients such as iron, calcium, and protein. And if you need supplements, a nutritionist can recommend the best choices.

- **Do it for you:** Pressure from teammates, parents, or coaches can turn a fun activity into a nightmare. If you're not enjoying your sport, make a change. Remember: It's your body and your life. You—not your coach or teammates—will have to live with any damage you do to your body now.

Chapter 52

Gastrointestinal and Digestive Disorders Common in Women

Chapter Contents

Section 52.1

Irritable Bowel Syndrome (IBS)

Excerpted from "Irritable Bowel Syndrome (IBS) Fact Sheet,"
U.S. Department of Health and Human Services Office on Women's
Health (www.womenshealth.gov), April 14, 2010.

What is irritable bowel syndrome (IBS)?

Irritable bowel syndrome is a collection of symptoms such as cramping, abdominal pain, bloating, diarrhea, and constipation. People with IBS have some of these symptoms—such as cramping and diarrhea or bloating and constipation—for at least three months.

IBS can be uncomfortable. But it does not lead to serious disease, such as cancer. It also does not permanently harm the large intestine (colon).

Most people with IBS can ease symptoms with changes in diet, medicine, and stress relief. For some people, IBS symptoms are more severe. They may get in the way of going to work or traveling, even traveling short distances.

What causes IBS?

The cause of IBS is not known. There is also no cure for IBS, but there are ways to treat the symptoms.

Who gets IBS?

IBS is one of the most common disorders diagnosed by doctors. Up to 20% of U.S. adults have IBS symptoms.

Some people are more likely to have IBS:

- Women

- People younger than 50 (IBS usually begins before age 35)

- People with a family member who has IBS

What are the symptoms of IBS?

IBS is defined as abdominal pain or discomfort, along with a changed bowel habit (such as diarrhea or constipation), for three months or more.

The symptoms may be different from person to person and can include the following:

- Cramps or pain in the stomach area

- Constipation—infrequent stools that may be hard and dry

- Feeling like you haven't finished a bowel movement

- Diarrhea—frequent loose stools

- Alternating between diarrhea and constipation

- Mucus in the stool

- Swollen or bloated stomach area

- Gas

- Discomfort in the upper stomach area or feeling uncomfortably full or nauseous after eating a normal size meal

Women with IBS may have more symptoms during their menstrual periods.

How is IBS diagnosed?

See your doctor if you think you may have IBS. Your doctor will ask you questions about your health and examine you. He or she may even perform a rectal exam. There are no tests that can show for sure that you have IBS.

Your doctor may also perform medical tests to rule out other diseases if you have "red flag" symptoms such as these:

- Rectal bleeding

- Weight loss

- Anemia (iron deficiency)

- Nighttime symptoms, like diarrhea that awakens you

- Family history of colorectal cancer, inflammatory bowel disease, or celiac disease

Medical tests include a colonoscopy. The doctor looks inside the large intestine by inserting a scope with a tiny camera to spot inflamed tissue, abnormal growths, and ulcers. People over age 50 with IBS symptoms should also have a colonoscopy to screen for colorectal cancer, even if they don't have any "red flag" symptoms.

A doctor may also perform a blood test to check for celiac disease if you have certain types of IBS. These types are IBS-D (mostly diarrhea) or IBS-M (mixed type with diarrhea and constipation). A doctor may also check for celiac disease if you have bloating or pass a lot of gas.

Lactose intolerance may also be a concern for some people and can be checked with a breath test.

What is the treatment for IBS?

There is no cure for IBS, but there are things you can do to feel better.

Changing your diet: Foods do not cause IBS, but eating certain food may start some IBS symptoms. You can ease the symptoms of IBS by changing some eating habits.

Find out which foods make your symptoms worse by writing in a journal:

- What you eat during the day

- What symptoms you have

- When symptoms occur

You will want to limit or avoid these foods. Problem foods may be these types:

- Milk and milk products like cheese or ice cream

- Caffeinated drinks like coffee

- Carbonated drinks like soda, especially those that contain artificial sweeteners (like sorbitol) or high-fructose corn syrup

- Alcohol

- Some fruits and vegetables

Other ways to ease symptoms are the following:

- Eat a healthy, balanced diet.

- Eat more high-fiber foods such as whole grains, fruits, and vegetables (especially for people with constipation). Add foods with fiber to your diet a little at a time to let your body get used to them.

- Drink six to eight glasses of water a day (especially for people with diarrhea).

- Avoid large meals, which can cause cramping and diarrhea in people with IBS. Try eating four or five small meals a day. Or, eat less at each of your usual three meals.

Taking medicine: Your doctor may give you medicine to help with symptoms:

- Fiber supplements such as psyllium (Metamucil) to help control constipation

- Antidiarrheal medications, such as loperamide (Imodium)

- Antispasmodic agents such as peppermint oil or dicyclomine to slow contractions in the bowel, which may help with diarrhea and pain

- Antidepressant medications such as a tricyclic antidepressant or a selective serotonin reuptake inhibitor (SSRI) if symptoms include pain or depression

- An IBS medication known as lubiprostone approved by the FDA for women with severe constipation

Take your medicine exactly as your doctor tells you to. All drugs have side effects and may affect people differently. Tell your doctor about any over-the-counter medicines you take.

Counseling and stress relief: Many people who seek care for IBS also have anxiety, panic, or depression. Stress is also an issue for people with IBS because it can make the symptoms worse. Research shows that psychological therapy can help ease IBS symptoms. Therapies that can help reduce feelings of stress and anxiety include the following:

- Cognitive behavioral therapy (CBT), a short-term treatment that mixes different types of therapies and behavioral strategies, may focus on managing life stress or on changing how a person responds to anxiety about IBS symptoms.

- Dynamic psychotherapy, an intensive, short-term form of talk therapy, may focus on in-depth discussions about the link between symptoms and emotions or help people identify and resolve interpersonal conflicts.

- Hypnotherapy, where people enter an altered state of consciousness, can involve visual suggestions to imagine pain going away, for example.

General stress relief is also important. Exercising regularly is a good way to relieve stress. It also helps the bowel function better and improves overall health. Meditation, yoga, and massage may also help.

Section 52.2

Inflammatory Bowel Disease

Excerpted from "Inflammatory Bowel Disease Fact Sheet," U.S. Department of Health and Human Services Office on Women's Health (www.womenshealth.gov), August 17, 2009.

What is inflammatory bowel disease (IBD)?

Inflammatory bowel disease is the name of a group of disorders in which the intestines (small and large intestines or bowels) become inflamed (red and swollen). This inflammation causes symptoms such as the following:

- Severe or chronic (almost all of the time) pain in the abdomen
- Diarrhea—may be bloody
- Unexplained weight loss
- Loss of appetite
- Bleeding from the rectum
- Joint pain
- Skin problems
- Fever

Symptoms can range from mild to severe. Also, symptoms can come and go, sometimes going away for months or even years at a time. When people with IBD start to have symptoms again, they are said to be having a relapse or flare-up. When they are not having symptoms, the disease is said to have gone into remission.

The most common forms of IBD are ulcerative colitis and Crohn disease. The diseases are very similar. In fact, doctors sometimes have a hard time figuring out which type of IBD a person has. The main difference between the two diseases is the parts of the digestive tract they affect.

Ulcerative colitis affects the top layer of the large intestine, next to where the stool is. The disease causes swelling and tiny open sores, or ulcers, to form on the surface of the lining. The ulcers can bleed and produce pus. In severe cases of ulcerative colitis, ulcers may weaken the intestinal wall so much that a hole develops. Then the contents of the large intestine, including bacteria, spill into the abdominal cavity or leak into the blood. This causes a serious infection and requires emergency surgery.

Crohn disease can affect all layers of the intestinal wall. Areas of the intestines most often affected are the last part of the small intestine, called the ileum, and the first part of the large intestine. But Crohn disease can affect any part of the digestive tract, from the mouth to the anus. Inflammation in Crohn disease often occurs in patches, with normal areas on either side of a diseased area.

In Crohn disease, swelling and scar tissue can thicken the intestinal wall. This narrows the passageway for food that is being digested. The area of the intestine that has narrowed is called a stricture. Also, deep ulcers may turn into tunnels, called fistulas, that connect different parts of the intestine. They may also connect to nearby organs, such as the bladder or vagina, or the skin. And as with ulcerative colitis, ulcers may cause a hole to develop in the wall of the intestine.

IBD is not the same as irritable bowel syndrome (IBS), although the symptoms can be similar. Unlike inflammatory bowel disease, IBS does not cause inflammation or damage in the intestines.

In many people with IBD, medicines can control symptoms. But for people with severe IBD, surgery is sometimes needed. With treatment, most people with IBD lead full and active lives.

What causes inflammatory bowel disease?

No one knows for sure what causes IBD. Experts think that abnormal action of a person's immune system may trigger IBD. The immune system is made up of various cells and proteins. Normally, the immune system protects the body from infections caused by viruses or bacteria. Once the infection has cleared up, the immune system "shuts off."

But in people with IBD, the immune system seems to overreact to normal bacteria in the digestive tract. And once it starts working, the immune system fails to "shut off." This causes the inflammation, which damages the digestive tract and causes symptoms.

IBD runs in families. This suggests that inherited factors called genes play a role in causing IBD. Experts think that certain genes may cause the immune system to overreact in IBD.

Stress and eating certain foods do not cause IBD. But both can make IBD symptoms worse.

Can inflammatory bowel disease cause health problems in parts of the body other than the digestive tract?

Yes. Inflammatory bowel disease can cause a number of problems outside of the digestive tract.

One common problem that occurs because of loss of blood from the digestive tract is anemia. Anemia means that the amount of healthy red blood cells, which carry oxygen to organs, is below normal. This can make a person feel very tired.

Other health problems include the following:

- Arthritis and joint pain

- Weak bones and bone breaks

- Inflammation in the eye and other eye problems

- Liver inflammation

- Gallstones

- Red bumps or ulcers on the skin

- Kidney stones

- Delayed puberty and growth problems (in children and teens)

- In rare cases, lung problems

Some of these problems are caused by poor absorption of nutrients. Others are due to inflammation in parts of the body other than the digestive tract.

Some of these problems get better when the IBD is treated. Others must be treated separately.

How does a healthy digestive system work?

A normal digestive system breaks down food into nutrients. Nutrients include proteins, carbohydrates, fats, vitamins, and minerals. The body needs nutrients for energy and to stay healthy.

The digestive tract runs from the mouth to the anus. When you eat food, it goes from your mouth, down your esophagus, and into your stomach. From there, it goes into your small intestine, where the nutrients are absorbed into your blood. Leftover water and solid waste then move down into your large intestine, where most of the water is absorbed back into the blood. Solid waste leaves the body out of the anus as a bowel movement.

How does inflammatory bowel disease interfere with digestion?

When the small intestine becomes inflamed, as in Crohn disease, it is less able to absorb nutrients from food. These nutrients leave the body in the bowel movement. This is one reason why people with Crohn disease don't get enough nutrients, along with not having much appetite. Also, the undigested food that goes into the large intestine makes water absorption harder. This causes a watery bowel movement, or diarrhea.

In ulcerative colitis, the small intestine absorbs nutrients as it should. But inflammation in the large intestine keeps it from absorbing water, causing diarrhea.

Who gets inflammatory bowel disease?

Although IBD can occur in any group of people, it is more common among the following:

- People who have a family member with IBD
- Jewish people of European descent
- White people
- People who live in cities
- People who live in developed countries

Smoking also seems to affect a person's risk of getting IBD. People who smoke are more likely to develop Crohn disease but less likely to develop ulcerative colitis.

Experts think that as many as one million people in the United States have IBD. Most people with IBD begin to have symptoms between the ages of 15 and 30.

How is inflammatory bowel disease diagnosed?

If you think you have IBD, talk to your doctor. She or he will use your health history, a physical exam, and different tests to figure out if you have IBD and, if so, which type.

Tests used to diagnose IBD include the following:

- **Blood tests:** A sample of blood is studied in a lab to find signs of inflammation and anemia.
- **Stool sample:** A sample of a bowel movement is tested for blood. It is also tested for signs of an infection that can trigger a flare-up of IBD.

- **Colonoscopy or sigmoidoscopy:** For both of these tests, a long, thin tube with a lighted camera inside the tip is inserted into the anus. The image appears on a television screen. A sigmoidoscopy allows the doctor to see the lining of the lower part of the large intestine. A colonoscopy allows the doctor to see the lining of the entire large intestine and often the last part of the small intestines.

- **X-rays with barium:** In this procedure, a thick, chalky liquid called barium is used to coat the lining of the digestive tract. Areas coated with barium show up white on X-ray film.

- **Computerized axial tomography (CT or CAT scan):** A CT scan takes X-rays from several different angles around the body.

- **Capsule endoscopy:** Doctors can examine the small intestine through a capsule endoscopy. A capsule endoscopy is a small, pill-shaped camera. You swallow the pill, which then travels through your digestive system. It records video of the small intestine.

It often takes awhile for doctors to diagnose IBD. This is because IBD symptoms vary and are similar to those of many other problems.

Can I do anything to avoid getting inflammatory bowel disease?

Since doctors don't know what causes inflammatory bowel disease, there is no proven way to prevent it.

How is inflammatory bowel disease treated?

Treatments for IBD may include the following:

- Medicines
- Surgery
- Changes in the foods you eat—some people find following specific diets helps ease their symptoms.
- Nutritional supplements
- Reducing stress and getting enough rest

If you have IBD, your treatment will depend on these factors:

- Your symptoms and how severe they are
- Which part of your digestive tract is affected
- If you have health problems outside the digestive tract

Most people with IBD take medicine to control their symptoms. If medicines cannot control their disease, some people will need surgery.

What medicines are used to treat inflammatory bowel disease?

Medicines for treating IBD reduce the inflammation, relieve symptoms, and prevent flare-ups. Every patient is different. You may need to try several different medicines before you find one or more that work best for you. You should keep track of how well the drugs are working and any side effects and report all details to your doctor. The following kinds of medicines are used to treat IBD:

Aminosalicylates: Most people with mild to moderate cases of IBD are first treated with medicines called aminosalicylates. Possible side effects include nausea, vomiting, heartburn, diarrhea, and headache.

Corticosteroids: Corticosteroids are powerful and fast-acting drugs that suppress the immune system. They are given for short periods of time to treat IBD flare-ups. They are not given long-term because of possible serious side effects. Side effects may include increased risk of infection, bone loss, diabetes, and high blood pressure.

Immunomodulators: Like corticosteroids, immunomodulators suppress the immune system. They can take a long time to work (as much as six months for full effect). But, unlike corticosteroids, they can be taken long-term to prevent relapse. They are often given along with corticosteroids. As the disease is brought under control and the immunomodulator starts working, the corticosteroid dose is slowly reduced. Like corticosteroids, these medicines may raise the risk of infection. Other side effects are uncommon but may include nausea, vomiting, and headache.

Biologic therapies: Biologic therapies are proteins that block substances in the body that help cause inflammation. Biologics used to treat IBD block a substance called tumor necrosis factor alpha (TNF-alpha). Anti-TNF-alpha therapies have been used for years to treat Crohn disease and are now being used for ulcerative colitis. Blocking TNF-alpha can reduce inflammation, which can improve the symptoms of IBD.

These therapies may lower your body's ability to fight diseases. This can raise your chances of having a serious, or even life-threatening, infection. Other side effects may include stomach pain, rash, and nausea.

Antibiotics: Antibiotics are used to treat people with Crohn disease but are usually not given to people with ulcerative colitis. Antibiotics can reduce bacterial growth in the small intestine caused by stricture, fistulas, or surgery. Experts think that antibiotics may also help by suppressing the immune system.

Side effects may include nausea, vomiting, and diarrhea. Long-term use of one type of antibiotic can cause tingling of the hands and feet. If you develop this side effect, tell your doctor right away.

Other treatments: Drugs that relieve diarrhea and pain are sometimes used to treat IBD symptoms. But it is important to talk with your doctor before taking any over-the-counter drugs. Some can make your symptoms worse.

Patients who are dehydrated because of diarrhea may be treated with fluids and minerals. People with Crohn disease are sometimes given nutritional supplements.

What types of surgery are used to treat inflammatory bowel disease?

Sometimes severe IBD does not get better with medicine. In these cases, doctors may suggest surgery to fix or remove damaged parts of the intestine. Surgery can give lasting relief from symptoms and may reduce or even get rid of the need for medicine. Not every type of surgery is right for every person. People faced with the decision to have surgery should get as much information as they can from their doctors, nurses, and other patients.

Surgery for ulcerative colitis: About 25% to 40% of people with ulcerative colitis need surgery at some point in their lives. Surgery that removes the entire large intestine can completely cure ulcerative colitis. After the large intestine is removed, surgeons perform one of two types of operations to allow the body to get rid of food waste:

- In one procedure, a small opening is made in the front of the abdominal wall. Then the end of the ileum is brought through the hole. This allows waste to drain out of the body. An external pouch is worn over the opening to collect the waste, and the patient empties the pouch several times a day.

- In another procedure, the surgeon attaches the ileum to the inside of the anus where the rectum was, creating an internal pouch. Waste is stored in the pouch and passes out of the anus in the usual manner.

Surgery for Crohn disease: About 65% to 75% of people with Crohn disease need surgery at some point in their lives. Surgery can relieve symptoms and correct problems like strictures, fistulae, or bleeding in the intestine. But, since Crohn disease occurs in patches, surgery cannot cure the disease. If a part of the small or large intestine is removed, the inflammation may then affect the part next to the section that was removed.

Types of surgery for Crohn disease include the following:

- **Strictureplasty:** In this surgery, the doctor widens the strictured, or narrowed, area without removing any part of the small intestine.

- **Bowel resection:** In this surgery, the damaged part of the small or large intestine is removed and the two healthy ends are sewn back together.

- **Removal of the large intestine:** This procedure is the same as that done for ulcerative colitis. But people with Crohn can't have an internal pouch for waste because it can become inflamed. Instead, surgeons use the external pouch procedure.

Can changing the foods I eat help control inflammatory bowel disease?

No special eating plan has been proven effective for treating IBD. But for some people, changing the foods they eat may help control the symptoms of IBD.

There are no blanket food rules. Changes that help one person with IBD may not relieve symptoms in another. Talk to your doctor and maybe a dietitian about which foods you should and should not be eating. Their suggestions will depend on the part of your intestine that is affected and which disease you have.

Your doctor may suggest some of the following changes:

- Taking specific nutritional supplements, including possibly vitamin and mineral supplements

- Avoiding greasy or fried foods

- Avoiding cream sauces and meat products

- Avoiding spicy foods

- Avoiding foods high in fiber, such as nuts and raw fruits and vegetables

- Eating smaller, more frequent meals

Even though you may have to limit certain foods, you should still aim to eat meals that give you all the nutrients you need.

Can stress make inflammatory bowel disease worse?

Although stress does not cause IBD, some people find that stress can bring on a flare-up in their disease. If you think this is happening to you, try using relaxation techniques, such as slow breathing. Also, be sure to get enough sleep.

What new treatments for inflammatory bowel disease are being studied?

Researchers are studying many new treatments for IBD. These include new medicines, such as new biologic therapies. Researchers are also studying whether fish or flaxseed oils can help fight the inflammation in IBD. Some evidence supports using probiotics to treat some types of diarrhea and a form of IBD called pouchitis. Probiotics are "good" bacteria that may improve the balance of bacteria in your digestive system. Some researchers are hoping to develop new therapies by studying probiotics.

With inflammatory bowel disease, do I have a higher chance of getting colon cancer?

Yes. IBD can increase your chances of getting cancer of the colon, or large intestine. Even so, more than 90% of people with IBD do *not* get colon cancer.

What we know about colon cancer and IBD comes mostly from studying people with ulcerative colitis. Less is known about the link between Crohn disease and cancer. But research suggests that Crohn's patients have an increased risk as well. For both diseases, the risk of colon cancer depends on how long you have had IBD and how much of your colon is affected.

Also, people who have family members with colon cancer may have an even higher chance of getting the cancer.

For people with ulcerative colitis, the risk of colon cancer does not start to increase until they have had the disease for 8 to 10 years. People whose disease affects the entire colon have the highest risk of colon cancer. People whose disease affects only the rectum have the lowest risk.

People with IBD should talk to their doctors about when to begin checking for colon cancer, what tests to get, and how often to have them. Your doctor's suggestions will depend on how long you have had IBD and how severe it is.

In people who have had IBD for 8 to 10 years, most doctors recommend a colonoscopy with biopsies every one to two years. When cancer is found early, it is easier to cure and treat.

Can my inflammatory bowel disease make it harder for me to get pregnant?

If you have ulcerative colitis, you can get pregnant as easily as other women. The same is true of Crohn disease, if your disease is in remission. But if you are having a flare-up of Crohn disease, you may have trouble getting pregnant.

I have inflammatory bowel disease. Is pregnancy safe for me?

You should talk with your doctor before getting pregnant. If you think you might be pregnant, call your doctor right away. Some of the medicines used to treat IBD can harm the growing fetus.

If possible, your disease should be in remission for six months before becoming pregnant. It is also best if you have not started a new treatment or are taking corticosteroids. If you are already pregnant, you should continue taking your medicines as your doctor has told you to take them. If you stop taking your medicines and your disease flares, it may be hard to get it back under control.

In some cases, IBD gets better during pregnancy. This is because of changes in the immune system and hormone levels that occur during pregnancy.

If you have ulcerative colitis, your chances of having a normal delivery and a healthy baby are the same as for women who do not have inflammatory bowel disease. If you have a flare-up of Crohn disease during pregnancy, you have a slightly higher risk of miscarriage, preterm birth, and stillbirth.

Can inflammatory bowel disease affect my monthly period?

Yes. Some women with IBD feel worse right before and during their menstrual periods than at other times. Diarrhea, abdominal pain, and other symptoms can be more severe during these times. Women with IBD and their doctors should keep track of these monthly changes in symptoms. This will prevent overtreating the disease.

If you have not been eating well and have lost a lot of weight, your menstrual cycles can become irregular or even stop entirely.

Can inflammatory bowel disease affect my sex life?

Inflammatory bowel disease, as well as the surgery and medicines used to treat it, can all affect your sex life. Sometimes, you may just feel too tired to have sex. You may also have emotional issues related to the disease. For instance, you may not feel as confident about your body as you did before you got the disease. Even though it may be embarrassing, it is important to talk to your doctor if you are having sexual problems. She or he may have treatments that can help. For instance, if you are having pain during sex, your doctor may prescribe a hormonal cream or suppository for your vagina.

If you have an external pouch, here are some tips:

- Empty the pouch before sex.

- Use deodorizers—one in the pouch and perhaps a pill or liquid you take by mouth (ask your doctor about them).

- Make sure the pouch is secure.

- If the pouch is in the way or causes pain during sex, experiment with different positions.

- Cover up your pouch with a pouch cover or by wearing a short slip or nightie.

Talking with your partner about how having inflammatory bowel disease is affecting your sex life can help build intimacy and clear up misunderstandings. Talking with a counselor or therapist may also help you find ways to deal with your emotional issues.

Section 52.3

Gallstones

Excerpted from "Gallstones," National Digestive Diseases Information Clearinghouse, National Institute of Diabetes and Digestive and Kidney Diseases (digestive.niddk.nih.gov), February 23, 2010.

What are gallstones?

Gallstones are small, pebble-like substances that develop in the gallbladder. The gallbladder is a small, pear-shaped sac located below your liver in the right upper abdomen. Gallstones form when liquid stored in the gallbladder hardens into pieces of stone-like material. The liquid—called bile—helps the body digest fats.

Bile contains water, cholesterol, fats, bile salts, proteins, and bilirubin—a waste product. Bile salts break up fat, and bilirubin gives bile and stool a yellowish-brown color. If the liquid bile contains too much cholesterol, bile salts, or bilirubin, it can harden into gallstones.

The two types of gallstones are cholesterol stones and pigment stones. Cholesterol stones are usually yellow-green and are made primarily of hardened cholesterol. They account for about 80% of gallstones. Pigment stones are small, dark stones made of bilirubin. Gallstones can be as small as a grain of sand or as large as a golf ball. The gallbladder can develop just one large stone, hundreds of tiny stones, or a combination of the two.

Gallstones can block the normal flow of bile if they move from the gallbladder and lodge in any of the ducts that carry bile from the liver to the small intestine. Bile trapped in these ducts can cause inflammation in the gallbladder, the ducts, or, in rare cases, the liver. Sometimes gallstones passing through the common bile duct provoke inflammation in the pancreas—called gallstone pancreatitis—an extremely painful and potentially dangerous condition.

If any of the bile ducts remain blocked for a significant period of time, severe damage or infection can occur in the gallbladder, liver, or pancreas. Left untreated, the condition can be fatal. Warning signs of a serious problem are fever, jaundice, and persistent pain.

What causes gallstones?

Scientists believe cholesterol stones form when bile contains too much cholesterol, too much bilirubin, or not enough bile salts, or when the gallbladder does not empty completely or often enough. The reason these imbalances occur is not known.

The cause of pigment stones is not fully understood. The stones tend to develop in people who have liver cirrhosis, biliary tract infections, or hereditary blood disorders—such as sickle cell anemia—in which the liver makes too much bilirubin.

The mere presence of gallstones may cause more gallstones to develop. Other factors that contribute to the formation of gallstones, particularly cholesterol stones, include the following:

- **Gender:** Women are twice as likely as men to develop gallstones. Excess estrogen from pregnancy, hormone replacement therapy, and birth control pills appears to increase cholesterol levels in bile and decrease gallbladder movement, which can lead to gallstones.

- **Family history:** Gallstones often run in families, pointing to a possible genetic link.

- **Weight:** Being even moderately overweight increases the risk for developing gallstones. The most likely reason is that the amount of bile salts in bile is reduced, resulting in more cholesterol. Increased cholesterol reduces gallbladder emptying.

- **Diet:** Diets high in fat and cholesterol and low in fiber increase the risk of gallstones due to increased cholesterol in the bile and reduced gallbladder emptying.

- **Rapid weight loss:** As the body metabolizes fat during prolonged fasting and rapid weight loss—such as "crash diets"—the liver secretes extra cholesterol into bile, which can cause gallstones. In addition, the gallbladder does not empty properly.

- **Age:** People older than age 60 are more likely to develop gallstones than younger people. As people age, the body tends to secrete more cholesterol into bile.

- **Ethnicity:** American Indians have a genetic predisposition to secrete high levels of cholesterol in bile. In fact, they have the highest rate of gallstones in the United States.

- **Cholesterol-lowering drugs:** Drugs that lower cholesterol levels in the blood actually increase the amount of cholesterol secreted into bile.

- **Diabetes:** People with diabetes generally have high levels of fatty acids called triglycerides. These fatty acids may increase the risk of gallstones.

What are the symptoms of gallstones?

As gallstones move into the bile ducts and create blockage, pressure increases in the gallbladder. Symptoms of blocked bile ducts are often called a gallbladder "attack" because they occur suddenly. Gallbladder attacks often follow fatty meals, and they may occur during the night. A typical attack can cause the following:

- Steady pain in the right upper abdomen that increases rapidly and lasts from 30 minutes to several hours

- Pain in the back between the shoulder blades

- Pain under the right shoulder

Notify your doctor if you think you have experienced a gallbladder attack. Although these attacks often pass as gallstones move, your gallbladder can become infected and rupture if a blockage remains.

People with any of the following symptoms should see a doctor immediately:

- Prolonged pain—more than five hours
- Nausea and vomiting
- Fever—even low-grade—or chills
- Yellowish color of the skin or whites of the eyes
- Clay-colored stools

Many people with gallstones have no symptoms; these gallstones are called "silent stones." They do not interfere with gallbladder, liver, or pancreas function and do not need treatment.

How are gallstones diagnosed?

Frequently, gallstones are discovered during tests for other health conditions. When gallstones are suspected to be the cause of symptoms, the doctor is likely to do an ultrasound exam—the most sensitive and specific test for gallstones. The ultrasound sound waves bounce off any gallstones and show their location. Other tests may also be performed.

- **Computerized tomography (CT) scan:** The CT scan is a non-invasive X-ray that produces cross-section images of the body.

- **Cholescintigraphy (HIDA scan):** The patient is injected with a small amount of nonharmful radioactive material; the test is used to diagnose abnormal contraction of the gallbladder or obstruction of the bile ducts.

- **Endoscopic retrograde cholangiopancreatography (ERCP):** ERCP is used to locate and remove stones in the bile ducts. The doctor inserts an endoscope—a long, flexible, lighted tube with a camera—down the throat and through the stomach and into the small intestine. The endoscope helps the doctor locate the affected bile duct and the gallstone. The stone is captured in a tiny basket and removed with the endoscope.

- **Blood tests:** Blood tests may be performed to look for signs of infection, obstruction, pancreatitis, or jaundice.

How are gallstones treated?

Surgery: If you are having frequent gallbladder attacks, your doctor will likely recommend you have your gallbladder removed—an operation called a cholecystectomy. Surgery to remove the gallbladder—a nonessential organ—is one of the most common surgeries performed on adults in the United States.

Nearly all cholecystectomies are performed with laparoscopy. After giving you medication to sedate you, the surgeon makes several tiny incisions in the abdomen and inserts a laparoscope and a miniature video camera. Then the surgeon cuts the cystic duct and removes the gallbladder through one of the small incisions. Recovery after laparoscopic surgery usually involves only one night in the hospital, and normal activity can be resumed after a few days at home.

If tests show the gallbladder has severe inflammation, infection, or scarring from other operations, the surgeon may perform open surgery to remove the gallbladder. In some cases, open surgery is planned; however, sometimes these problems are discovered during the laparoscopy and the surgeon must make a larger incision. Recovery from open surgery usually requires three to five days in the hospital and several weeks at home.

The most common complication in gallbladder surgery is injury to the bile ducts. An injured common bile duct can leak bile and cause a painful and potentially dangerous infection.

If gallstones are present in the bile ducts, the physician—usually a gastroenterologist—may use ERCP to locate and remove them before or during gallbladder surgery.

Nonsurgical treatment: Nonsurgical approaches are used only in special situations—such as when a patient has a serious medical condition preventing surgery—and only for cholesterol stones. Stones commonly recur within five years in patients treated nonsurgically.

- **Oral dissolution therapy:** Drugs made from bile acid are used to dissolve gallstones. Months or years of treatment may be necessary before all the stones dissolve.

- **Contact dissolution therapy:** This experimental procedure involves injecting a drug directly into the gallbladder to dissolve cholesterol stones.

Do people need their gallbladder?

Fortunately, the gallbladder is an organ people can live without. Your liver produces enough bile to digest a normal diet. Once the gallbladder is removed, bile flows out of the liver through the hepatic ducts into the common bile duct and directly into the small intestine, instead of being store in the gallbladder. Because now the bile flows into the small intestine more often, softer and more frequent stools can occur in about 1% of people. These changes are usually temporary, but talk with your health care provider if they persist.

Chapter 53

Lung Disease in Women

What is lung disease?

Lung disease refers to disorders that affect the lungs. Breathing problems caused by lung disease may prevent the body from getting enough oxygen.

Lung disease is a major concern for women. The number of U.S. women diagnosed with lung disease is on the rise. More women are also dying from lung disease. Three of the most common lung diseases in women are asthma, chronic obstructive pulmonary disease (COPD), and lung cancer.

Asthma: Asthma is a chronic (ongoing) disease of the airways in the lungs called bronchial tubes. Bronchial tubes carry air into and out of the lungs. In people with asthma, the walls of these airways become inflamed (swollen) and oversensitive. The airways overreact to things like smoke, air pollution, mold, and many chemical sprays. They also can be irritated by allergens (like pollen and dust mites) and by respiratory infections (like a cold). When the airways overreact, they get narrower. This limits the flow of air into and out of the lungs and causes trouble breathing. Asthma symptoms include wheezing, coughing, and tightness in the chest.

Women are more likely than men to have asthma and are more likely to die from it. The percentage of women, especially young women, with asthma is rising in the United States.

Excerpted from "Lung Disease Fact Sheet," U.S. Department of Health and Human Services Office on Women's Health (www.womenshealth.gov), November 29, 2010.

Chronic obstructive pulmonary disease: COPD refers to chronic obstructive bronchitis and emphysema. These conditions often occur together. Both diseases limit airflow into and out of the lungs and make breathing difficult. COPD usually gets worse with time.

A person with COPD has ongoing inflammation of the bronchial tubes, which carry air into and out of the lungs. This irritation causes the growth of cells that make mucus. The extra mucus leads to a lot of coughing. Over time, the irritation causes the walls of the airways to thicken and develop scars. The airways may become thickened enough to limit airflow to and from the lungs. If that happens, the condition is called chronic obstructive bronchitis.

In emphysema, the lung tissue gets weak, and the walls of the air sacs (alveoli) break down. Less oxygen can pass into the blood. This causes shortness of breath, coughing, and wheezing.

More than twice as many women as men are now diagnosed with chronic bronchitis. The rate of emphysema among women has increased by 5% in recent years but has decreased among men. And more women have died from COPD than men every year since 2000.

Lung cancer: Lung cancer is a disease in which abnormal (malignant) lung cells multiply and grow without control. These cancerous cells can invade nearby tissues, spread to other parts of the body, or both. In the United States, more women now die from lung cancer than from any other type of cancer. Tobacco use is the major cause of lung cancer.

Other lung diseases: Less common lung problems that affect women include the following:

- **Pulmonary emboli:** These are blood clots that travel to the lungs from other parts of the body and plug up blood vessels in the lungs. Some factors that increase your risk include being pregnant, having recently given birth, and taking birth control pills or menopausal hormone therapy.

- **Pulmonary hypertension:** This is high blood pressure in the arteries that bring blood to the lungs. It can affect blood flow in the lungs and can reduce oxygen flow into the blood.

- **Sarcoidosis and pulmonary fibrosis:** These inflammatory diseases cause stiffening and scarring in the lungs.

- **LAM (lymphangioleiomyomatosis):** This is a rare lung disease that mostly affects women in their mid-thirties and forties. Muscle-like cells grow out of control in certain organs, including the lungs.

- **Influenza (the flu) and pneumonia:** Flu is a respiratory infection that is caused by a virus and can damage the lungs. Usually, people recover well from the flu, but it can be dangerous and even deadly for some people. Pneumonia is a severe inflammation of the lungs that can be caused by bacteria, viruses, and fungi. Fluid builds up in the lungs and may lower the amount of oxygen that the blood can get from air that's breathed in. Vaccines are the best protection against flu and pneumonia.

What causes lung disease?

Experts don't know the causes of all types of lung disease, but they do know the causes of some:

- **Smoking:** Smoke from cigarettes, cigars, and pipes is the number one cause of lung disease.

- **Radon:** This colorless, odorless gas is present in many homes and is a recognized cause of lung cancer. You can check for radon with a kit bought at many hardware stores.

- **Asbestos:** This is natural mineral fiber that is used in insulation, fireproofing materials, car brakes, and other products. Asbestos can give off small fibers that are too small to be seen and can be inhaled.

- **Air pollution:** Recent studies suggest that some air pollutants like car exhaust may contribute to lung diseases.

- **Germs:** Some diseases that affect the lungs, like the flu, are caused by bacteria, viruses, and fungi.

How would I know if I have a lung disease?

Early signs of lung disease are easy to overlook. Often, an early sign of lung disease is not having your usual level of energy. Other signs and symptoms can differ by the type of lung disease. Common signs are the following:

- Trouble breathing
- Shortness of breath
- Feeling like you're not getting enough air
- Decreased ability to exercise
- A cough that won't go away
- Coughing up blood or mucus

- Pain or discomfort when breathing in or out

How can I find out if I have asthma?

Asthma can be hard to diagnose. The signs of asthma can seem like the signs of COPD, pneumonia, bronchitis, pulmonary embolism, anxiety, and heart disease.

Common symptoms of asthma are these:

- Coughing
- Wheezing
- Chest tightness
- Shortness of breath

To diagnose asthma, the doctor asks about your symptoms and what seems to trigger them, reviews your health history, and does a physical exam.

To confirm the diagnosis, the doctor may do other tests, such as the following:

- **Spirometry:** This test measures how much air you can breathe in and out. It also measures how fast you can blow air out.

- **Bronchoprovocation:** Lung function is tested using spirometry while more stress is put on the lungs.

- **Chest X-ray or EKG (electrocardiogram):** These tests can sometimes find out if another disease or a foreign object may be causing your symptoms.

How is asthma treated?

Asthma is a chronic disease. Medicines can be used to treat asthma, but they cannot cure it. You can help control your symptoms by working with your doctor to set up and then follow a personal asthma action plan. The plan will include possible medications and ways to avoid things that trigger your asthma.

Taking medicines: Asthma medicines work by opening the lung airways. The medicines used to treat asthma fall into two groups: long-term control and quick relief.

- Long-term control medicines are to be taken every day, usually over a long period of time. They help prevent symptoms from starting. Once symptoms occur, they do not give quick relief.

584

- Quick-relief medicines are used only when needed and often relieve symptoms in minutes. They do this by quickly relaxing tightened muscles around the airways. They are taken when symptoms worsen to prevent a full-blown asthma attack and to stop attacks once they have started.

Avoiding asthma triggers: Avoid things that make your asthma worse. Common asthma triggers are tobacco smoke, animal dander, dust mites, air pollution, mold, and pollens. You can try "fragrance-free" products if your asthma is triggered by fragrances. Talk to your doctor about allergy shots if your asthma symptoms are linked to allergens that you cannot avoid. The shots may lessen or prevent the symptoms but will not cure the asthma. You can reduce your exposure to air pollution by limiting your outdoor activities on days when the air quality in your neighborhood is poor.

What about pregnancy and asthma?

If you have asthma and may become pregnant, talk to your doctor. Only in very severe cases might asthma be a reason to avoid becoming pregnant.

If you have asthma and become pregnant, you and your doctor can discuss the safety of your medicines. Changes in the medicines can sometimes make good sense. It is very important to manage your asthma symptoms when you are pregnant. Asthma that gets out of control can harm your baby.

How do I find out if I have COPD?

People with COPD have symptoms that develop very slowly over many years. As a result, many people ignore these symptoms until their disease has reached an advanced stage. COPD can be easily diagnosed and can be managed.

The symptoms of COPD include the following:

- An ongoing cough that often produces large amounts of mucus
- Shortness of breath, especially during physical activity
- Wheezing
- Chest tightness

To find out if you have COPD, the doctor will ask about your symptoms, your medical history, and your history of exposure to things that can cause COPD and will do a physical exam.

The main test to check for COPD is spirometry. For this test, you will be asked to take a deep breath and blow as hard as you can into a tube that is connected to a spirometer. This machine measures how much air you breathe out and how fast.

Other tests can include the following:

- **Chest X-ray or chest computed tomography (CT) scan:** These tests create pictures of the heart and lungs. The pictures can show signs of COPD.

- **Arterial blood gas test:** This blood test measures the oxygen and carbon dioxide levels in your blood. It can help determine how severe the COPD is and whether oxygen therapy is needed.

How is COPD treated?

Damage to the lungs cannot be repaired. The disease can be slowed by avoiding certain exposures, though. For smokers, the best approach is to stop smoking. You should also limit your exposure to smoke, dust, fumes, and irritating vapors at home and work. Also limit outdoor activities during air pollution alerts. Treatment can relieve symptoms. Common medicines are the following:

- Bronchodilators to open up air passages in the lungs

- Inhaled steroids to relieve symptoms by reducing inflammation

- Antibiotics to clear up infections in the lungs

For patients with COPD, doctors may also recommend the following:

- Flu shots

- Pneumonia shots

- Pulmonary rehabilitation

- Oxygen therapy

- Surgery (Lung transplant surgery is becoming more common for people with severe emphysema; another procedure called lung volume reduction surgery is also used to treat some patients with severe COPD of the emphysema type)

How do I find out if I have lung cancer?

Usually there are no warning signs of early lung cancer. By the time most people with lung cancer have symptoms, the cancer has become more serious.

Symptoms of lung cancer may include these:

- A cough that doesn't go away or gets worse
- Breathing trouble, like shortness of breath
- Coughing up blood
- Chest pain
- Hoarseness or wheezing
- Pneumonia that doesn't go away or that goes away and comes back

In addition, you may feel very tired or have a loss of appetite or unexplained weight loss. If you have symptoms of lung cancer, it's important to talk to your doctor. The doctor will ask about your health history, smoking history, and exposure to harmful substances. He or she will also do a physical exam and may suggest some tests.

Common tests for diagnosis of lung cancer include the following:

- **Chest X-rays:** X-rays allow doctors to see abnormal growths on the lungs.
- **CT scans:** The images can show subtle signs of cancer that don't show up on X-rays.
- **Sputum cytology:** A sample of mucus that you cough up is studied to see if it has cancer cells in it.
- **Bronchoscopy:** Doctors pass a special tube called a bronchoscope through the nose or mouth and down into the lungs. They can see into the lungs and remove small bits of tissue to test.
- **Fine-needle aspiration:** Doctors pass a needle through the chest wall into the lung to remove a small amount of tissue or fluid.
- **Thoracotomy:** Doctors cut open the chest and remove tissue from the lungs.

If I smoke, should I get tested for lung cancer?

Testing for cancer before a person has any symptoms is called screening. Screening may help find cancers early, when they may be easier to treat.

Many studies show that screening smokers with X-rays or sputum cytology does not save lives. But recently a major study showed that CT scans of older people who smoke a lot (or used to smoke a lot) can save lives.

If you're concerned about your lung cancer risk, talk to your doctor about whether screening is right for you. Of course, the best way to reduce your risk of lung cancer is not to smoke.

How is lung cancer treated?

Sometimes lung cancer treatments are used to try to cure the cancer. Other times, treatments are used to stop the cancer from spreading and to relieve symptoms. Your doctor may recommend one treatment or a combination of treatments.

Surgery is used to remove the lung tissue that has the cancerous tumor. When the cancer has not spread, surgery can cure the patient.

Radiation therapy uses a machine to aim high-energy X-rays at the tumor.

Chemotherapy uses medicine to kill cancer cells.

Targeted therapy uses medicine to block the growth and spread of cancer cells.

Can I lower my risk for lung disease?

Things you can do to reduce your risk of lung diseases include the following:

- Stop smoking.
- Avoid secondhand smoke.
- Test for radon. Find out if there are high levels of the gas radon in your home or workplace.
- Avoid asbestos. Asbestos can be a particular concern for those whose jobs put them in contact with it. This includes people who maintain buildings that have insulation or other materials that contain asbestos and people who repair car brakes or clutches.
- Protect yourself from dust and chemical fumes. Working in dusty conditions and with chemicals can increase your risk of lung disease. Many products used at home, like paints and solvents, can cause or aggravate lung disease.
- Eat a healthy diet. The National Cancer Institute notes that studies show that eating a lot of fruits or vegetables may help lower the risk of lung cancer.
- Ask your doctor if you should have a spirometry test.
- Ask your doctor about protecting yourself from flu and pneumonia with vaccinations.

Chapter 54

Mental Health Concerns among Women

Chapter Contents

Section 54.1

Anxiety Disorders

Excerpted from "Anxiety Disorders,"
U.S. Department of Health and Human Services Office on
Women's Health (www.womenshealth.gov), March 29, 2010.

Anxiety is a normal reaction to stress. It can help you cope with a
hard situation. But when anxiety becomes an extreme, irrational dread
of everyday situations, it can be disabling.

Generalized Anxiety Disorder

People with generalized anxiety disorder (GAD) go through the day
filled with worry and tension, even though there is little or nothing
to cause it. They anticipate disaster and are overly concerned about
health issues, money, family problems, or difficulties at work. Sometimes just the thought of getting through the day produces anxiety.
GAD is diagnosed when a person worries excessively about a variety of
everyday problems for at least six months. It affects about 6.8 million
adult Americans and about twice as many women as men.

Symptoms of GAD include the following:

- Unable to relax
- Startle easily
- Difficulty concentrating
- Trouble falling asleep or staying asleep
- Fatigue
- Headaches
- Muscle tension
- Muscle aches
- Difficulty swallowing
- Trembling
- Twitching

- Irritability

- Sweating

- Nausea

- Lightheadedness

- Having to go to the bathroom frequently

- Feeling out of breath

- Hot flashes

If you think you have an anxiety disorder such as GAD, the first person you should see is your family doctor. A physician can determine whether the symptoms that alarm you are due to an anxiety disorder, another medical condition, or both.

Early treatment can help keep the disease from progressing to its later stages, and people can learn effective ways to live with this disorder. Treatment options include the following:

- Medications

- Cognitive therapy (to change or get rid of destructive thought patterns)

- Behavioral therapy (to change a person's behavior)

- A combination of these treatments

Obsessive Compulsive Disorder

People with obsessive compulsive disorder (OCD) have thoughts (obsessions) or rituals (compulsions) that happen over and over again. Rituals—such as hand washing, counting, checking on a specific item (like whether the oven was left on), or cleaning—often are done in hope of stopping the thoughts. Doing these rituals, though, gives only short-term relief. Ignoring the urge to do the ritual greatly increases anxiety. Left untreated, obsessions and the need to perform rituals can take over a person's life. OCD is often a chronic, relapsing illness.

People with OCD sometimes have other mental health disorders, such as depression, eating disorders, substance abuse, attention deficit hyperactivity disorder, or other anxiety disorders. When a person also has other disorders, OCD is often harder to diagnose and treat. A person can have symptoms of OCD at the same time as, or that are part of, other brain disorders, such as Tourette syndrome. Getting the

591

right diagnosis and treatment of other disorders is important to successful treatment of OCD.

If you think you have obsessive compulsive disorder, the first person you should see is your family doctor. A physician can determine whether the symptoms that alarm you are due to an anxiety disorder, another medical condition, or both.

Research shows that people with OCD have patterns of brain activity that differ from people with other mental illnesses or people with no mental illness at all. There is also proof that both behavioral therapy and medication can help people with OCD. A type of behavioral therapy known as "exposure and response prevention" is very useful for treating OCD. In this approach, a person is exposed to whatever triggers the obsessive thoughts, and then is taught ways to avoid doing the compulsive rituals and how to deal with the anxiety.

Panic Disorder

Panic disorder is a type of anxiety disorder. Panic disorder affects women twice as often as men. Panic attacks are the most common symptom of this disorder. A person is having a panic attack when they feel the following:

- A sense of terror that strikes suddenly and repeatedly with no warning
- Chest pain
- Difficulty breathing
- Flushes or chills
- Fear of losing control
- Fear of dying

Because these attacks are so unpredictable, many women may have intense anxiety between panic attacks. While most attacks last a few minutes on average, sometimes they can last as long as 10 minutes. In rare cases, they may last an hour or more.

If you think you have an anxiety disorder such as panic disorder, the first person you should see is your family doctor. A physician can determine whether the symptoms that alarm you are due to an anxiety disorder, another medical condition, or both.

Early treatment can help keep the disease from getting worse, and people can learn effective ways to live with this disorder. Treatment options include the following:

- Medications
- Cognitive therapy (to change or get rid of destructive thought patterns)
- Behavioral therapy (to change a person's behavior)
- A combination of these treatments

Social Phobia (or Social Anxiety Disorder)

Social phobia is diagnosed when people become overwhelmingly anxious and very self-conscious in everyday social situations. People with social phobia have a strong fear of being watched and judged by others and of doing things that will embarrass them. They can worry for days or weeks before a dreaded situation. This fear may become so severe that it interferes with work, school, and other ordinary activities, and can make it hard to make and keep friends.

Physical symptoms that often accompany social phobia include the following:

- Blushing
- Sweating
- Trembling
- Nausea
- Difficulty talking

Social phobia affects about 15 million American adults and affects women and men in equal numbers. People with social phobia often have other anxiety disorders and/or depression as well. Substance abuse can develop if a person with social phobia uses alcohol or drugs to soothe their anxiety.

If you think you have an anxiety disorder such as social phobia, the first person you should see is your family doctor. A physician can determine whether the symptoms that alarm you are due to an anxiety disorder, another medical condition, or both.

Treatment options include the following:

- Medications
- Cognitive therapy (to change or get rid of destructive thought patterns)
- Behavioral therapy (to change a person's behavior)
- A combination of these treatments

Specific Phobias

A specific phobia is a strong, irrational fear of something that poses little or no actual danger. Some of the more common specific phobias are the following:

- Closed-in places
- Heights
- Escalators
- Tunnels
- Highway driving
- Water
- Flying
- Dogs
- Injuries involving blood

Such phobias aren't just extreme fear; they are irrational fear of a particular thing. You may be able to ski the world's tallest mountains with ease but be unable to go above the fifth floor of an office building. While adults with phobias realize that these fears are irrational, they often find that facing, or even thinking about facing, the feared object or situation brings on a panic attack or severe anxiety.

Specific phobias affect an estimated 19.2 million adult Americans and are twice as common in women as men. They usually appear in childhood or adolescence and tend to persist into adulthood. The causes of specific phobias are not well understood, but there is some evidence that the tendency to develop them may run in families.

If the feared situation or feared object is easy to avoid, people with specific phobias may not seek help. Treatment is needed if the phobia hurts a person's career or personal life.

If you think you have an anxiety disorder such as specific phobia, the first person you should see is your family doctor. Specific phobias respond very well to carefully targeted psychotherapy.

Section 54.2

Depression in Women

Excerpted from "Depression Fact Sheet,"
U.S. Department of Health and Human Services Office on
Women's Health (www.womenshealth.gov), March 17, 2010.

Depression affects both men and women, but more women than men are likely to be diagnosed with depression in any given year. That being said, depression is not a "normal part of being a woman," nor is it a "female weakness." Many women with depression never seek treatment. But most women, even those with the most severe depression, can get better with treatment.

What is depression?

Life is full of ups and downs. But when the down times last for weeks or months at a time or keep you from your regular activities, you may be suffering from depression. Depression is a medical illness that involves the body, mood, and thoughts. It affects the way you eat and sleep, the way you feel about yourself, and the way you think about things.

It is different from feeling "blue" or down for a few hours or a couple of days. It is not a condition that can be willed or wished away.

What are the different types of depression?

Different kinds of depression include the following:

- **Major depressive disorder:** Also called major depression, this is a combination of symptoms that hurt a person's ability to work, sleep, study, eat, and enjoy hobbies.

- **Dysthymic disorder:** Also called dysthymia, this kind of depression lasts for a long time (two years or longer). The symptoms are less severe than major depression but can prevent you from living normally or feeling well.

595

Some kinds of depression show slightly different symptoms than those described earlier. Some may start after a particular event. However, not all scientists agree on how to label and define these forms of depression:

- **Psychotic depression**, which occurs when a severe depressive illness happens with some form of psychosis, such as a break with reality, hallucinations, and delusions

- **Postpartum depression**, which is diagnosed if a new mother has a major depressive episode within one month after delivery

- **Seasonal affective disorder (SAD)**, which is a depression during the winter months, when there is less natural sunlight

What causes depression?

There are many reasons why a woman may become depressed:

- **Genetics (family history):** If a woman has a family history of depression, she may be more at risk of developing it herself.

- **Chemical imbalance:** The brains of people with depression look different than those who don't have depression. Also, the parts of the brain that manage your mood, thoughts, sleep, appetite, and behavior don't have the right balance of chemicals.

- **Hormonal factors:** Menstrual cycle changes, pregnancy, miscarriage, postpartum period, perimenopause, and menopause may all cause a woman to develop depression.

- **Stress:** Stressful life events such as trauma, loss of a loved one, a bad relationship, work responsibilities, caring for children and aging parents, abuse, and poverty may trigger depression in some people.

- **Medical illness:** Dealing with serious medical illnesses like stroke, heart attack, or cancer can lead to depression.

What are the signs of depression?

Not all people with depression have the same symptoms. Some people might only have a few, and others a lot. How often symptoms occur, and how long they last, is different for each person. Symptoms of depression include these:

- Feeling sad, anxious, or "empty"

- Feeling hopeless
- Loss of interest in hobbies and activities that you once enjoyed
- Decreased energy
- Difficulty staying focused, remembering, making decisions
- Sleeplessness, early morning awakening, or oversleeping and not wanting to get up
- No desire to eat and weight loss or eating to "feel better" and weight gain
- Thoughts of hurting yourself
- Thoughts of death or suicide
- Easily annoyed, bothered, or angered
- Constant physical symptoms that do not get better with treatment, such as headaches, upset stomach, and pain that doesn't go away

I think I may have depression. How can I get help?

Here are some people and places that can help you get treatment.

- Family doctor
- Counselors or social workers
- Family services, social service agencies, or clergy person
- Employee assistance programs (EAPs)
- Psychologists and psychiatrists

If you are unsure where to go for help, check the Yellow Pages under mental health, health, social services, suicide prevention, crisis intervention services, hotlines, hospitals, or physicians.

What if I have thoughts of hurting myself?

Depression can make you think about hurting yourself or suicide. Yet hurting yourself does just that—it hurts you. If you are thinking about hurting or even killing yourself, please ask for help! Call 911, 800-273-TALK (8255) or 800-SUICIDE, or check in your phone book for the number of a suicide crisis center. These hotlines can also tell you where to go for more help in person. You also can talk with a family member you trust, a clergy person, or a doctor. There is nothing wrong with asking for help—everyone needs help sometimes.

You might feel like your pain is too overwhelming to cope with, but those times don't last forever. People do make it through suicidal thoughts. If you can't find someone to talk with, write down your thoughts. Try to remember and write down the things you are grateful for. List the people who are your friends and family and care for you. Write about your hopes for the future. Read what you have written when you need to remind yourself that your life is IMPORTANT!

How is depression found and treated?

Most people with depression get better when they get treatment. The first step to getting the right treatment is to see a doctor. Certain medicines, and some medical conditions (such as viruses or a thyroid disorder), can cause the same symptoms as depression. Also, it is important to rule out depression that is associated with another mental illness called bipolar disorder. A doctor can rule out these possibilities with a physical exam, asking questions, and/or lab tests, depending on the medical condition.

Once identified, depression almost always can be treated. Some people with milder forms of depression do well with therapy alone. Others with moderate to severe depression might benefit from antidepressants. It may take a few weeks or months before you begin to feel a change in your mood. Some people do best with both treatments—therapy and antidepressants.

Do the following before taking medication:

- Ask your doctor to tell you about the effects and side effects of the drug.

- Tell your doctor about any alternative therapies or over-the-counter medications you are using.

- Ask your doctor when and how the medication should be stopped.

- Work with your doctor to determine which medication is right for you and what dosage is best.

- Be aware that some medications are effective only if they are taken regularly and that symptoms may come back if the medication is stopped.

Should I stop taking my antidepressant while I am pregnant?

The decision whether or not to stay on medications is a hard one. You should talk with your doctor. Medication taken during pregnancy does reach the fetus. In rare cases, some antidepressants have been associated with breathing and heart problems in newborns, as well as jitteriness, difficulty feeding, and low blood sugar after delivery. However, moms who stop medications can be at high risk of their depression coming back. In some cases, a woman and her doctor may decide to slowly lower her antidepressant dose during the last month of pregnancy. Doing so can help the newborn suffer from fewer withdrawal symptoms. After delivery, a woman can return to a full dose. This can help her feel better during the postpartum period, when risk of depression can be greater.

Should I stop taking my antidepressant while breastfeeding?

If you stopped taking your medication during pregnancy, you may need to begin taking it again after the baby is born. Be aware that because your medication can be passed into your breast milk, breast-feeding may pose some risk for a nursing infant.

However, a number of research studies show that certain antidepressants, such as some SSRIs (selective serotonin reuptake inhibitors), have been used relatively safely during breastfeeding. You should discuss with your doctor whether breastfeeding is an option or whether you should plan to feed your baby formula. Although breastfeeding has some advantages for your baby, most importantly, as a mother, you need to stay healthy so you can take care of your baby.

Is it safe for young adults to take antidepressants?

It may be safe for young people to be treated with antidepressants. However, drug companies who make antidepressants are required to post a "black box" warning label on the medication, which is the most serious type of warning on prescription drugs.

It may be possible that antidepressants make children, adolescents, and young adults more likely to think about suicide or commit suicide. In 2007, the U.S. Food and Drug Administration (FDA) said that makers of all antidepressant medications should extend the warning to include young adults up through age 24.

The warning says that patients of all ages taking antidepressants should be watched closely, especially during the first weeks of treatment. Possible side effects to look for are worsening depression, suicidal thinking or behavior, or any unusual changes in behavior such as sleeplessness, agitation, or withdrawal from normal social situations.

Can I take St. John's wort to treat depression?

St. John's wort is a plant with yellow flowers that has been used for centuries for health purposes. However, research studies from the National Institutes of Health found that St. John's wort was not effective in treating major depression.

Other research shows that St. John's wort can make some medicines not work or that it can cause dangerous side effects. The herb appears to interfere with certain drugs used to treat heart disease, HIV, depression, seizures, certain cancers, and organ transplant rejection. The herb may also make birth control pills not work as well.

How can I help myself if I am depressed?

You may feel exhausted, helpless, and hopeless. But it is important to realize that these feelings are part of the depression and do not reflect real life. As you understand your depression and begin treatment, negative thinking will fade. Do the following in the meantime:

- Engage in mild activity or exercise. Go to a movie, a ballgame, or another event or activity that you once enjoyed. Participate in religious, social, or other activities.

- Set realistic goals for yourself.

- Break up large tasks into small ones, set some priorities, and do what you can as you can.

- Try to spend time with other people and confide in a trusted friend or relative. Try not to isolate yourself.

- Expect your mood to improve gradually, not immediately. Do not expect to suddenly "snap out of" your depression.

- Postpone important decisions, such as getting married or divorced or changing jobs, until you feel better. Discuss decisions with others who know you well and have a more objective view of your situation.

- Be confident that positive thinking will replace negative thoughts as your depression responds to treatment.

Section 54.3

Eating Disorders

Excerpted from "Eating Disorders," U.S. Department of
Health and Human Services Office on Women's Health
(www.womenshealth.gov), March 29, 2010.

A woman with an eating disorder eats too much, too little, or causes
herself to throw up food. There are different types of eating disorders.

Anorexia Nervosa

Anorexia nervosa, or anorexia, is a type of eating disorder that
mainly affects adolescent girls and young women. A person with this
disease has an intense fear of gaining weight and limits the food she
eats, as well as shows the following symptoms:

- Has a low body weight
- Refuses to keep a normal body weight
- Is extremely afraid of becoming fat
- Believes she is fat even when she's very thin
- Misses three (menstrual) periods in a row (for girls/women who
  have started having their periods)

Anorexia affects your health because it can damage many parts of
your body. A person with anorexia will have many of these signs:

- Loses a lot of weight
- Talks about weight and food all the time
- Moves food around the plate; doesn't eat it
- Weighs food and counts calories
- Follows a strict diet
- Fears gaining weight
- Won't eat in front of others

- Ignores/denies hunger
- Uses extreme measures to lose weight (self-induced vomiting, laxative abuse, diuretic abuse, diet pills, fasting, and excessive exercise)
- Thinks she's fat when she's too thin
- Gets sick a lot
- Weighs self several times a day
- Acts moody
- Feels depressed
- Feels irritable
- Doesn't socialize
- Wears baggy clothes to hide appearance

Treatment

A health care team of doctors, nutritionists, and therapists will help the patient get better. They will do the following:

- Help bring the person back to a normal weight
- Treat any psychological issues related to anorexia
- Help the person get rid of any actions or thoughts that cause the eating disorder

These three steps will prevent "relapse" (relapse means to get sick again, after feeling well for a while).

Some research suggests that the use of medicines—such as antidepressants, antipsychotics, or mood stabilizers—may sometimes work for anorexic patients. It is thought that these medicines help the mood and anxiety symptoms that often coexist with anorexia. Other recent studies, however, suggest that antidepressants may not stop some patients with anorexia from relapsing. Also, no medicine has shown to work 100% of the time during the important first step of restoring a patient to healthy weight.

Some forms of psychotherapy can help make the psychological reasons for anorexia better. Psychotherapy is sometimes known as "talk therapy." It uses different ways of communicating to change a patient's thoughts or behavior. Individual counseling can help someone with anorexia. If the patient is young, counseling may involve the whole family. Support groups may also be a part of treatment.

Bulimia Nervosa

Bulimia nervosa, or bulimia, is a type of eating disorder. Someone with bulimia eats a lot of food in a short amount of time (bingeing) and then tries to get rid of the calories by purging. Purging might be done in these ways:

- Making oneself throw up
- Taking laxatives (pills or liquids that increase how fast food moves through your body and leads to a bowel movement)

A person with bulimia may also use these ways to prevent weight gain:

- Exercising a lot (more than normal)
- Restricting her eating or not eating at all (like going without food for a day)
- Taking diuretics (pills that make you urinate)

Bulimia is more than just a problem with food. It's a way of using food to feel in control of other feelings that may seem overwhelming.

Unlike anorexia, when people are severely underweight, people with bulimia may be underweight, overweight, or have a normal weight. However, someone with bulimia may have these signs:

- Thinks about food a lot
- Binges (normally in secret)
- Throws up after bingeing
- Uses laxatives, diet pills, or diuretics to control weight
- Is depressed
- Is unhappy and/or thinks a lot about her body shape and weight
- Eats large amounts of food quickly
- Goes to the bathroom all the time after she eats (to throw up)
- Exercises a lot, even during bad weather, fatigue, illness, or injury
- Unusual swelling of the cheeks or jaw area

- Cuts and calluses on the back of the hands and knuckles from making herself throw up
- White enamel of teeth wears away making teeth look clear
- Doesn't see friends or participate in activities as much
- Has rules about food—has "good" foods and "bad" foods

Treatment

Someone with bulimia can get better. A health care team of doctors, nutritionists, and therapists will help the patient learn healthy eating patterns and how to cope with their thoughts and feelings.

To stop a person from binging and purging, a doctor may recommend the patient do the following:

- **Receive nutritional advice and psychotherapy, especially cognitive behavioral therapy (CBT):** CBT is a form of psychotherapy that focuses on the important role of thinking in how we feel and what we do. CBT that has been tailored to treat bulimia has shown to be effective in changing binging and purging behavior, and eating attitudes.

- **Be prescribed medicine:** Some antidepressants, such as fluoxetine (Prozac), which is the only medication approved by the FDA for treating bulimia, may help patients who also have depression and/or anxiety. It also appears to help reduce binge-eating and purging behavior, reduces the chance of relapse, and improves eating attitudes.

Binge Eating Disorder

People with binge eating disorder often eat an unusually large amount of food and feel out of control during the binges. Unlike bulimia or anorexia, binge eaters do not throw up their food, exercise a lot, or eat only small amounts of only certain foods. Because of this, binge eaters are often overweight or obese. People with binge eating disorder also may do the following:

- Eat more quickly than usual during binge episodes
- Eat until they are uncomfortably full
- Eat when they are not hungry
- Eat alone because of embarrassment
- Feel disgusted, depressed, or guilty after overeating

About 2% of all adults in the United States (as many as four million Americans) have binge eating disorder. Binge eating disorder affects women slightly more often than men.

Treatment

People with binge eating disorder should get help from a health care professional, such as a psychiatrist, psychologist, or clinical social worker. As with bulimia, there are different ways to treat binge eating disorder that may be helpful for some people.

- Nutritional advice and psychotherapy, especially cognitive behavioral therapy (CBT), a form of psychotherapy that focuses on the important role of thinking in how we feel and what we do

- Drug therapy, such as antidepressants like fluoxetine (Prozac) or appetite suppressants prescribed by a doctor

Section 54.4

Seasonal Affective Disorder

Excerpted from "Seasonal Affective Disorder," U.S. Department of Veterans Affairs (www.mentalhealth.va.gov), January 25, 2011.

While it may be just a temporary case of "winter blues" for most people, for others the long cold days of winter can be a serious psychological problem.

It's called seasonal affective disorder—and never has an acronym been more apropos: SAD.

According to Dr. Joseph V. Pace, chief of psychiatry at the Alaska VA Medical Center, SAD is defined as "recurring depression with seasonal onset and remission."

Two seasonal patterns of SAD have been described: the fall-onset SAD and the summer-onset SAD. The fall-onset type, also known as "winter depression," is most recognized. In this subtype, major depressive episodes begin in late fall to early winter and decrease during summer months.

Dr. Pace adds that some of the symptoms of SAD include increased appetite, weight gain, sleep loss, decreased energy, and lack of motivation.

He notes that, "Usually, we do not see pure seasonal depression, but seasonal worsening of pre-existing depression..."

One of the treatments he also recommends is aerobic exercise, "which can sometimes help."

The cause of SAD is not well understood. It is believed that the decreasing daylight available in fall and winter triggers a depressive episode in people predisposed to develop the disorder. However, no studies have established a causal relationship between decreasing daylight and the development of winter SAD.

One of the most effective remedies for dealing with the condition is light therapy. Light therapy has proven effective in a limited number of small, placebo-controlled studies.

The usual dose is 10,000 lux (the intensity of light that hits or passes through a surface) beginning with one 10- to 15-minute session per day, usually in the morning, gradually increasing to 30 to 45 minutes per day, depending upon response.

It may take four to six weeks to see a response, although some patients improve within days. Therapy is continued until sufficient daily light exposure is available through other sources, typically from springtime sun.

Light therapy is considered first-line therapy in patients who are not severely suicidal, have medical reasons to avoid antidepressant drugs, have a history of a positive response to light therapy, or if the patient specifically requests it.

Medication is also an option in some cases. Drugs may be a better option in patients with significant functional impairment or who are at high suicide risk, for patients with a history of moderate to severe recurrent depression, and for patients who have had a prior positive response to antidepressants or mood stabilizers or who have failed other therapies.

Dr. Pace recommends that anyone experiencing unusual depression during the winter months should see their doctor as soon as possible.

Chapter 55

Migraine Headaches in Women

What is migraine?

A migraine headache is usually an intense, throbbing pain on one, or sometimes both, sides of the head. Most people with migraine headache feel the pain in the temples or behind one eye or ear, although any part of the head can be involved. Besides pain, migraine also can cause nausea and vomiting and sensitivity to light and sound. Some people also may see spots or flashing lights or have a temporary loss of vision.

Migraine can occur any time of the day, though it often starts in the morning. The pain can last a few hours or up to one or two days. Some people get migraines once or twice a week. Others, only once or twice a year. Most of the time, migraines are not a threat to your overall health. But migraine attacks can interfere with your day-to-day life.

We don't know what causes migraine, but some things are more common in people who have them:

- Most often, migraine affects people between the ages of 15 and 55.

- Most people have a family history of migraine or of disabling headache.

- They are more common in women.

- Migraine often becomes less severe and less frequent with age.

Excerpted from "Migraine Fact Sheet," U.S. Department of Health and Human Services Office on Women's Health (www.womenshealth.gov), May 1, 2008.

607

What causes migraines?

The exact cause of migraine is not fully understood. Most researchers think that migraine is due to abnormal changes in levels of substances that are naturally produced in the brain. When the levels of these substances increase, they can cause inflammation, which causes blood vessels in the brain to swell and press on nearby nerves, causing pain.

Genes also have been linked to migraine. People who get migraines may have abnormal genes that control the functions of certain brain cells.

Experts do know that people with migraines react to a variety of factors and events, called triggers. These triggers can vary from person to person and don't always lead to migraine. A combination of triggers is more likely to set off an attack. Many women with migraine tend to have attacks triggered by the following:

- Lack of or too much sleep

- Skipped meals

- Bright lights, loud noises, or strong odors

- Hormone changes during the menstrual cycle

- Stress and anxiety, or relaxation after stress

- Weather changes

- Alcohol (often red wine)

- Caffeine (too much or withdrawal)

- Foods that contain nitrates, such as hot dogs and lunch meats

- Foods that contain MSG (monosodium glutamate), a flavor enhancer found in fast foods, broths, seasonings, and spices

- Foods that contain tyramine, such as aged cheeses, soy products, fava beans, hard sausages, smoked fish, and Chianti wine

- Aspartame (NutraSweet and Equal)

Talk with your doctor about what sets off your headaches to help find the right treatment for you.

Are there different kinds of migraine?

Yes, there are many forms of migraine. The two forms seen most often are migraine with aura and migraine without aura.

Migraine with aura (previously called classical migraine):
With a migraine with aura, a person might have these sensory symptoms (the so-called "aura") 10 to 30 minutes before an attack:

- Seeing flashing lights, zigzag lines, or blind spots
- Numbness or tingling in the face or hands
- Disturbed sense of smell, taste, or touch
- Feeling mentally "fuzzy"

Only one in five people who get migraine experience an aura. Women have this form of migraine less often than men.

Migraine without aura (previously called common migraine):
With this form of migraine, a person does not have an aura but has all the other features of an attack.

How can I tell if I have a migraine or just a bad tension-type headache?

Compared with migraine, tension-type headache is generally less severe and rarely disabling. Although fatigue and stress can bring on both tension and migraine headaches, migraines can be triggered by certain foods, changes in the body's hormone levels, and even changes in the weather.

There also are differences in how types of headaches respond to treatment with medicines. Although some over-the-counter drugs used to treat tension-type headaches sometimes help migraine headaches, the drugs used to treat migraine attacks do not work for tension-type headaches for most people.

You can't tell the difference between a migraine and a tension-type headache by how often they occur. Both can occur at irregular intervals.

How can I tell if I have a migraine or a sinus headache?

Many people confuse a sinus headache with a migraine because pain and pressure in the sinuses, nasal congestion, and watery eyes often occur with migraine. To find out if your headache is sinus or migraine, ask yourself if you have these symptoms in addition to sinus symptoms:

- Moderate-to-severe headache
- Nausea
- Sensitivity to light

If you answer yes to two or three of these questions, then most likely you have migraine with sinus symptoms. A true sinus headache is rare and usually occurs due to sinus infection. In a sinus infection, you would also likely have a fever and thick nasal secretions that are yellow, green, or blood-tinged. A sinus headache should go away with treatment of the sinus infection.

When should I seek help for my headaches?

Sometimes, headache can signal a more serious problem. You should talk to your doctor about your headaches in these scenarios:

- You have several headaches per month and each lasts for several hours or days
- Your headaches disrupt your home, work, or school life
- You have nausea, vomiting, or vision or other sensory problems (such as numbness or tingling)
- You have pain around the eye or ear
- You have a severe headache with a stiff neck
- You have a headache with confusion or loss of alertness
- You have a headache with convulsions
- You have a headache after a blow to the head
- You used to be headache-free, but now have headaches a lot

What tests are used to find out if I have migraine?

If you think you get migraine headaches, talk with your doctor. Before your appointment, write down these items:

- How often you have headaches
- Where the pain is
- How long the headaches last
- When the headaches happen, such as during your period
- Other symptoms, such as nausea or blind spots
- Any family history of migraine
- All the medicines that you are taking for all your medical problems
- All the medicines you have taken in the past that you can recall

Your doctor may also do an exam and ask more questions about your health history. Your doctor may be able to diagnose migraine just from the information you provide. You may get a blood test or other tests if your doctor thinks that something else is causing your headaches.

Are migraine headaches more common in women than men?

Yes. About three out of four people who have migraines are women. Migraines are most common in women between the ages of 20 and 45. At this time of life women often have more job, family, and social duties. Women tend to report more painful and longer lasting headaches and more symptoms, such as nausea and vomiting.

I get migraines right before my period. Could they be related to my menstrual cycle?

More than half of migraines in women occur right before, during, or after a woman has her period. This often is called "menstrual migraine." But just a small fraction of women only have migraine at this time. Most have migraine headaches at other times of the month as well.

How the menstrual cycle and migraine are linked is still unclear. We know that just before the cycle begins, levels of the female hormones, estrogen and progesterone, go down sharply. This drop in hormones may trigger a migraine because estrogen controls chemicals in the brain that affect a woman's pain sensation.

Can migraine be worse during menopause?

If your migraine headaches are closely linked to your menstrual cycle, menopause may make them less severe. About two-thirds of women with migraines report that their symptoms improve with menopause.

But for some women, menopause worsens migraine or triggers them to start. It is not clear why this happens. In general, though, the worsening of migraine symptoms goes away once menopause is complete.

Can using birth control pills make my migraines worse?

In some women, birth control pills improve migraine. But in other women, the pills may worsen their migraines. In still other women, taking birth control pills has no effect on their migraines.

Talk with your doctor if you think birth control pills are making your migraines worse. Switching to a pill pack in which all the pills for the entire month contain hormones and using that for three months in a row can improve headaches.

611

Can stress cause migraines?

Yes. Stress can trigger both migraine and tension-type headache. Studies show that everyday stresses—not major life changes—cause most headaches. Making time for yourself and finding healthy ways to deal with stress are important. Some things you can do to help prevent or reduce stress include the following:

- Eating healthy foods
- Being active (at least 30 minutes most days of the week is best)
- Doing relaxation exercises
- Getting enough sleep

How are migraines treated?

Migraine has no cure. But your migraines can be managed with your doctor's help. Together, you will find ways to treat migraine symptoms when they happen, as well as ways to help make your migraines less frequent and severe. Your treatment plan may include some or all of these methods.

Medicine: There are two ways to approach the treatment of migraines with drugs: stopping a migraine in progress (called "abortive" or "acute" treatment) and prevention. Many people with migraine use both forms of treatment.

- **Acute treatment:** Over-the-counter pain-relief drugs relieve mild migraine pain for some people. If these drugs don't work for you, your doctor might want you to try a prescription drug. Most acute drugs for migraine work best when taken right away, when symptoms first begin.

- **Prevention:** Some medicines used daily can help prevent attacks. Many of these drugs were designed to treat other health conditions, such as epilepsy and depression. Some examples are antidepressants, anticonvulsants, beta-blockers, and calcium channel blockers.

These drugs may not prevent all migraines, but they can help a lot. Hormone therapy may help prevent attacks in women whose migraines seem to be linked to their menstrual cycle.

Lifestyle changes: Practicing these habits can reduce the number of migraine attacks:

- Avoid or limit triggers.

- Get up and go to bed the same time every day.

- Eat healthy foods and do not skip meals.

- Engage in regular physical activity.

- Limit alcohol and caffeine intake.

- Learn ways to reduce and cope with stress.

What are rebound migraines?

Women who use acute pain-relief medicine more than two or three times a week or more than 10 days out of the month can set off a cycle called rebound. As each dose of medicine wears off, the pain comes back, leading the patient to take even more. This overuse causes your medicine to stop helping your pain and actually start causing headaches. Rebound headaches can occur with both over-the-counter and prescription pain-relief medicines. Talk to your doctor if you're caught in a rebound cycle.

I'm pregnant or breastfeeding. Can my migraines still be treated?

Some migraine medicines should not be used when you are pregnant because they can cause birth defects and other problems. This includes over-the-counter medicines, such as aspirin and ibuprofen. Talk with your doctor if migraine is a problem while you are pregnant or if you are planning to become pregnant.

Ask your doctor about what migraine medicines are safe to take while breastfeeding. Some medicines can be passed through breast milk and might be harmful to your baby.

What are some ways I can prevent migraine?

The best way to prevent migraine is to find out what triggers your attacks and avoid or limit these triggers. Finding healthy ways to cut down on and cope with stress might help. Talk with your doctor if you need to take your pain-relief medicine more than twice a week. If your doctor has prescribed medicine for you to help prevent migraine, take them exactly as prescribed.

Chapter 56

Osteoporosis

What is osteoporosis?

Osteoporosis is a disease of the bones. People with osteoporosis have bones that are weak and break easily. A broken bone can cause severe pain and disability. It can make it harder to do daily tasks on your own, such as walking.

What bones does osteoporosis affect?

Osteoporosis affects all bones in the body. However, breaks are most common in the hip, wrist, and spine, also called vertebrae. Vertebrae support your body, helping you to stand and sit up.

Osteoporosis in the vertebrae can cause serious problems for women. A fracture in this area occurs from day-to-day activities like climbing stairs, lifting objects, or bending forward. Signs of osteoporosis are the following:

- Sloping shoulders
- Height loss
- Hunched posture
- Curve in the back
- Back pain
- Protruding abdomen

Excerpted from "Osteoporosis Fact Sheet," U.S. Department of Health and Human Services Office on Women's Health (www.womenshealth.gov), January 31, 2011.

What increases my chances of getting osteoporosis?

There are several risk factors that raise your chances of developing osteoporosis. Factors that you can't control are the following:

- Being female

- Getting older

- Menopause

- Having a small, thin body (under 127 pounds)

- Having a family history of osteoporosis

- Being white or Asian, but African American women and Latinas are also at risk

- Not getting your period (if you should be getting it)

- Having a disorder that increases your risk of getting osteoporosis (such as rheumatoid arthritis, type 1 diabetes, premature menopause, anorexia nervosa)

- Not getting enough exercise

- Long-term use of certain medicines, including glucocorticoids, some antiseizure medicines, gonadotropin-releasing hormone used to treat endometriosis, antacids with aluminum, some cancer treatments, or too much replacement thyroid hormone

Factors that you can control are as follows:

- Smoking

- Drinking too much alcohol (experts recommend no more than one drink a day for women)

- A diet low in dairy products or other sources of calcium and vitamin D

- Not getting enough exercise

You may also develop symptoms that are warning signs for osteoporosis. If you develop the following, you should talk to your doctor about any tests or treatment you many need:

- Loss in height, developing a slumped or hunched posture, or onset of sudden unexplained back pain

- You are over age 45 or postmenopausal and you break a bone

How can I find out if I have weak bones?

There are tests you can get to find out your bone density. This is related to how strong or fragile your bones are. One test is called dual-energy X-ray absorptiometry (DXA or dexa). A DXA scan takes X-rays of your bones. Screening tools also can be used to predict the risk of having low bone density or breaking a bone.

When should I get a bone density test?

If you are age 65 or older, you should get a bone density test to screen for osteoporosis. If you are younger than 65 and have risk factors for osteoporosis, ask your doctor or nurse if you need a bone density test. Bone density testing is recommended for older women whose risk of breaking a bone is the same or greater than that of a 65-year-old white woman with no risk factors other than age. To find out your fracture risk and whether you need early bone density testing, your doctor will consider certain factors:

- Your age and whether you have reached menopause
- Your height and weight
- Whether you smoke
- Your daily alcohol use
- Whether your mother or father has broken a hip
- Medicines you use
- Whether you have a disorder that increases your risk of getting osteoporosis

How can I prevent weak bones?

The best way to prevent weak bones is to work on building strong ones. Building strong bones during childhood and the teen years is one of the best ways to keep from getting osteoporosis later. As you get older, your bones don't make new bone fast enough to keep up with the bone loss. And after menopause, bone loss happens more quickly. But there are steps you can take to slow the natural bone loss with aging and to prevent your bones from becoming weak and brittle.

1. **Get enough calcium each day:** Bones contain a lot of calcium. It is important to get enough calcium in your diet. You can get calcium through foods and/or calcium pills. Getting calcium through food is definitely better since the food provides other nutrients that keep you healthy. Talk with your doctor or nurse before taking

617

calcium pills to see which kind is best for you. Taking more calcium pills than recommended doesn't improve your bone health. So try to reach these goals through a combination of food and supplements. Here's how much calcium you need each day:

- **Ages 9–18:** 1,300 mg (milligrams)
- **Ages 19–50:** 1,000 mg
- **Ages 51 and older:** 1,200 mg

2. **Get enough vitamin D each day:** It is also important to get enough vitamin D, which helps your body absorb calcium from the food you eat. Vitamin D is produced in your skin when it is exposed to sunlight. You need 10 to 15 minutes of sunlight to the hands, arms, and face, two to three times a week, to make enough vitamin D. The amount of time depends on how sensitive your skin is to light. It also depends on your use of sunscreen, your skin color, and the amount of pollution in the air. You can also get vitamin D by eating foods, such as milk, or by taking vitamin pills. Vitamin D taken in the diet by food or pills is measured in international units (IU). Here's how much vitamin D you need each day:

- **Ages 19–70:** 600 IU
- **Ages 71+:** 800 IU

3. **Eat a healthy diet:** Other nutrients (like vitamin K, vitamin C, magnesium, and zinc, as well as protein) help build strong bones too. Milk has many of these nutrients. So do foods like lean meat, fish, green leafy vegetables, and oranges.

4. **Get moving:** Being active helps your bones in these ways:

- Slows bone loss
- Improves muscle strength
- Helps your balance

Bone strength is built by doing weight-bearing physical activity, which is any activity in which your body works against gravity. There are many things you can do.

5. **Don't smoke:** Smoking raises your chances of getting osteoporosis. It harms your bones and lowers the amount of estrogen in your body. Estrogen is a hormone made by your body that can help slow bone loss.

6. **Drink alcohol moderately:** If you drink, don't drink more than one alcoholic drink per day. Alcohol can make it harder

for your body to use the calcium you take in. And, importantly, too much at one time can affect your balance and lead to falls.

7. **Make your home safe:** Reduce your chances of falling by making your home safer. Use a rubber bath mat and grab bars in the shower or tub. Keep your floors free from clutter. Remove throw rugs that may cause you to trip.

8. **Think about taking medicines to prevent or treat bone loss:** Talk with your doctor or nurse about the risks and benefits of medicines for bone loss.

What if dairy foods make me sick or I don't like to eat them? How can I get enough calcium?

If you're lactose intolerant, it can be hard to get enough calcium. Lactose is the sugar that is found in dairy products like milk. Lactose intolerance means your body has a hard time digesting foods that contain lactose. You may have symptoms like gas, bloating, stomach cramps, diarrhea, and nausea.

Lactose-reduced and lactose-free products are sold in food stores. There's a great variety, including milk, cheese, and ice cream. You can also take pills or liquids before eating dairy foods to help you digest them. Please note: If you have symptoms of lactose intolerance, see your doctor or nurse. These symptoms could also be from a different, more serious illness.

People who are lactose intolerant or who are vegans (eat only plant-based foods) can choose from other food sources of calcium, including canned salmon with bones, sardines, Chinese cabbage, bok choy, kale, collard greens, turnip greens, mustard greens, broccoli, and calcium-fortified orange juice. Some cereals also have calcium added. You can also take calcium pills.

Do men get osteoporosis?

Yes. In the United States, over two million men have osteoporosis. Men over age 50 are at greater risk. So keep an eye on the men in your life, especially if they are over 70 or have broken any bones.

How will pregnancy affect my bones?

To grow strong bones, a baby needs a lot of calcium. The baby gets his or her calcium from what you eat (or the supplements you take). In some cases, if a pregnant woman isn't getting enough calcium, she may lose a little from her bones, making them less strong. So, pregnant women should make sure they are getting the recommended amounts of calcium and vitamin D.

Will I suffer bone loss during breastfeeding?

Although bone density can be lost during breastfeeding, this loss tends to be temporary. Several studies have shown that when women have bone loss during breastfeeding, they recover full bone density within six months after weaning.

How is osteoporosis treated?

If you have osteoporosis, you may need to make some lifestyle changes and also take medicine to prevent future fractures. A calcium-rich diet, daily exercise, and drug therapy are all treatment options.

These different types of drugs are approved for the treatment or prevention of osteoporosis:

- **Bisphosphonates:** Bisphosphonates are approved for both prevention and treatment of postmenopausal osteoporosis. Drugs in this group also can treat bone loss and, in some cases, can help build bone mass.

- **SERMs:** A class of drugs called estrogen agonists/antagonists, commonly referred to as selective estrogen receptor modulators, are approved for the prevention and treatment of postmenopausal osteoporosis. They help slow the rate of bone loss.

- **Calcitonin:** Calcitonin is a naturally occurring hormone that can help slow the rate of bone loss.

- **Menopausal hormone therapy (MHT):** These drugs, which are used to treat menopausal symptoms, also are used to prevent bone loss. But recent studies suggest that this might not be a good option for many women. The Food and Drug Administration (FDA) has made the following recommendations for taking MHT:

  - Take the lowest possible dose of MHT for the shortest time to meet treatment goals.

  - Talk about using other osteoporosis medications instead.

- **Parathyroid hormone or teriparatide:** Teriparatide is an injectable form of human parathyroid hormone. It helps the body build up new bone faster than the old bone is broken down.

Chapter 57

Thyroid Disorders in Women

What is the thyroid?

Your thyroid is a small gland found at the base of your neck, just below your Adam's apple. The thyroid produces two main hormones called T3 and T4. These hormones travel in your blood to all parts of your body. The thyroid hormones control the rate of many activities in your body. These include how fast you burn calories and how fast your heart beats. All of these activities together are known as your body's metabolism. A thyroid that is working right will produce the right amounts of hormones needed to keep your body's metabolism working at a rate that is not too fast or too slow.

What kinds of thyroid problems can affect women?

Women are more likely than men to develop thyroid disorders. Thyroid disorders that can affect women include the following:

- Disorders that cause hyperthyroidism
- Disorders that cause hypothyroidism
- Thyroid nodules
- Thyroiditis

Excerpted from "Thyroid Disease Fact Sheet," U.S. Department of Health and Human Services Office on Women's Health (www.womenshealth.gov), January 14, 2010.

- Thyroid cancer
- Goiter

What is hyperthyroidism?

Some disorders cause the thyroid to make more thyroid hormones than the body needs. This is called hyperthyroidism, or overactive thyroid. The most common cause of hyperthyroidism is Graves disease. Graves disease is an autoimmune disorder, in which the body's own defense system, called the immune system, stimulates the thyroid. This causes it to make too much of the thyroid hormones. Hyperthyroidism can also be caused by thyroid nodules that prompt excess thyroid hormones to be made.

What are the symptoms of hyperthyroidism?

At first, you might not notice symptoms of hyperthyroidism. They usually begin slowly. But over time, a speeded up metabolism can cause symptoms such as these:

- Weight loss, even if you eat the same or more food
- Eating more than usual
- Rapid or irregular heartbeat or pounding of your heart
- Anxiety
- Irritability
- Trouble sleeping
- Trembling in your hands and fingers
- Increased sweating
- Increased sensitivity to heat
- Muscle weakness
- More frequent bowel movements
- Less frequent menstrual periods with lighter than normal menstrual flow

In addition to these symptoms, people with hyperthyroidism may have osteoporosis, or weak, brittle bones. In fact, hyperthyroidism might affect your bones before you have any of the other symptoms of the disorder. This is especially true of postmenopausal women, who are already at high risk of osteoporosis.

What is hypothyroidism?

Hypothyroidism is when your thyroid does not make enough thyroid hormones. It is also called underactive thyroid. The most common cause of hypothyroidism in the United States is Hashimoto disease. Hashimoto disease is an autoimmune disease, in which the immune system mistakenly attacks the thyroid. This attack damages the thyroid so that it does not make enough hormones. Hypothyroidism also can be caused by the following:

- Treatment of hyperthyroidism

- Radiation treatment of certain cancers

- Thyroid removal

In rare cases, problems with the pituitary gland can cause the thyroid to be less active.

What are the symptoms of hypothyroidism?

Symptoms of hypothyroidism tend to develop slowly, often over several years. At first, you may just feel tired and sluggish. Later, you may develop other symptoms of a slowed down metabolism:

- Weight gain, even though you are not eating more food

- Increased sensitivity to cold

- Constipation

- Muscle weakness

- Joint or muscle pain

- Depression

- Fatigue (feeling very tired)

- Pale dry skin

- A puffy face

- A hoarse voice

- Excessive menstrual bleeding

In addition to these symptoms, people with hypothyroidism may have high blood levels of LDL cholesterol. This is the so-called "bad" cholesterol, which can increase your risk for heart disease.

What are thyroid nodules?

A thyroid nodule is a swelling in one section of the thyroid gland. The nodule can be solid or filled with fluid or blood. You can have just one thyroid nodule or many.

Most thyroid nodules do not cause symptoms. But some thyroid nodules make too much of the thyroid hormones, causing hyperthyroidism. Sometimes, nodules get to be big enough to cause problems with swallowing or breathing. In fewer than 10% of cases, thyroid nodules are cancerous.

Thyroid nodules are quite common. By the time you reach the age of 50, you have a 50% chance of having a thyroid nodule larger than a half inch wide. We do not know why nodules form in otherwise normal thyroids.

You can sometimes see or feel a thyroid nodule yourself. Try standing in front of a mirror and raise your chin slightly. Look for a bump on either side of your windpipe below your Adam's apple. If the bump moves up and down when you swallow, it may be a thyroid nodule. Ask your doctor to look at it.

What is thyroiditis?

Thyroiditis is inflammation, or swelling, of the thyroid. There are several types of thyroiditis, one of which is Hashimoto thyroiditis. Other types of thyroiditis include the following:

Postpartum thyroiditis: Like Hashimoto disease, postpartum thyroiditis seems to be caused by a problem with the immune system. In the United States, postpartum thyroiditis occurs in about 5% to 10% of women. The first phase starts 1 to 4 months after giving birth. In this phase, you may get symptoms of hyperthyroidism because the damaged thyroid is leaking thyroid hormones out into the bloodstream. The second phase starts about 4 to 8 months after delivery. In this phase, you may get symptoms of hypothyroidism because, by this time, the thyroid has lost most of its hormones. Not everyone with postpartum thyroiditis goes through both phases. In most women who have postpartum thyroiditis, thyroid function returns to normal within 12 to 18 months after symptoms start.

Risk factors for postpartum thyroiditis include having the following:

- An autoimmune disease, like type 1 diabetes

- A personal history or family history of thyroid disorders

- Having had postpartum thyroiditis after a previous pregnancy

Silent or painless thyroiditis: Symptoms are the same as in postpartum thyroiditis, but they are not related to having given birth.

Subacute thyroiditis: Symptoms are the same as in postpartum and silent thyroiditis, but the inflammation in the thyroid leads to pain in the neck, jaw, or ear. Unlike the other types of thyroiditis, subacute thyroiditis may be caused by an infection.

What are the symptoms of thyroid cancer?

Most people with thyroid cancer have a thyroid nodule that is not causing any symptoms. If you have a thyroid nodule, there is a small chance it may be thyroid cancer. To tell if the nodule is cancerous, your doctor will have to do certain tests. A few people with thyroid cancer may have symptoms. If the cancer is big enough, it may cause swelling you can see in the neck. It may also cause pain or problems swallowing. Some people get a hoarse voice.

Thyroid cancer is rare compared with other types of cancer. It is more common in people with the following risk factors:

- Have a history of exposure of the thyroid to radiation (but not routine X-ray exposure, as in dental X-rays or mammograms)

- Have a family history of thyroid cancer

- Are older than 40 years of age

What is a goiter?

A goiter is an abnormally enlarged thyroid gland. Causes of goiter include the following:

- Iodine deficiency (Iodine is a mineral that your thyroid uses for making thyroid hormones, and not getting enough iodine in your food and water can cause your thyroid to get bigger; this cause of goiter is uncommon in the United States because iodine is added to table salt)

- Hashimoto disease

- Graves disease

- Thyroid nodules

- Thyroiditis

- Thyroid cancer

Usually, the only symptom of a goiter is a swelling in your neck. But a very large or advanced goiter can cause a tight feeling in your throat, coughing, or problems swallowing or breathing.

Having a goiter does not always mean that your thyroid is not making the right amount of hormones. Depending on the cause of your goiter, your thyroid could be making too much, not enough, or the right amount of hormones.

How are thyroid disorders diagnosed?

Thyroid disorders can be hard to diagnose because their symptoms can be linked to many other health problems. Your doctor will start by taking a medical history and asking if any of your family members has a history of thyroid disorders. Your doctor will also give you a physical exam and check your neck for thyroid nodules. Depending on your symptoms, your doctor may also do other tests:

Blood tests: Testing the level of thyroid stimulating hormone (TSH) in your blood can help your doctor figure out if your thyroid is overactive or underactive. TSH tells your thyroid to make thyroid hormones. Depending on the results, your doctor might order another blood test to check levels of one or both thyroid hormones in your blood. If your doctor suspects an immune system problem, your blood may also be tested for signs of this.

Radioactive iodine uptake test: For this test, you swallow a liquid or capsule containing a small dose of radioactive iodine (radio-iodine). The radioiodine collects in your thyroid because your thyroid uses iodine to make thyroid hormones. Then, a probe placed over your thyroid measures the amount of radioiodine in your thyroid. A high uptake of radioiodine means that your thyroid is making too much of the thyroid hormones. A low uptake of radioiodine means that your thyroid is not making enough of the thyroid hormones.

Thyroid scan: A thyroid scan usually uses the same radioiodine dose that was given by mouth for your uptake test. You lie on a table while a special camera creates an image of your thyroid on a computer screen. This test may be helpful in showing whether a thyroid nodule is cancerous. Three types of nodules show up in this test:

- Thyroid nodules that take up excess radioiodine are making too much of the thyroid hormones, causing hyperthyroidism. These nodules show up brightly on the scan and are called "hot" nodules.

- Thyroid nodules that take up the same amount of radioiodine as normal thyroid cells are making a normal amount of thyroid hormones. These are called "warm" nodules.

- Thyroid nodules that do not take up radioiodine are not making thyroid hormones. They appear as defects or holes in the scan and are called "cold" nodules.

Hot nodules are almost never cancerous. A small percentage of warm and cold nodules are cancerous.

Thyroid fine needle biopsy: This test is used to see if thyroid nodules have normal cells in them. Local anesthetic may be used to numb an area on your neck. Then, a very thin needle is inserted into the thyroid to withdraw some cells and fluid. The withdrawal of cells and fluid is called a biopsy. A special type of doctor called a pathologist examines the cells under a microscope to see if they are abnormal. Abnormal cells could mean thyroid cancer.

Thyroid ultrasound: The thyroid ultrasound uses sound waves to create a computer image of the thyroid. This test can help your doctor tell what type of nodule you have and how large it is. Ultrasound may also be helpful in detecting thyroid cancer, although by itself it cannot be used to diagnose thyroid cancer. You may have repeat thyroid ultrasounds to see if your nodule is growing or shrinking.

How is hyperthyroidism treated?

Your doctor's choice of treatment will depend on the cause of your hyperthyroidism and how severe your symptoms are. Treatments include the following:

- Antithyroid medicines block the thyroid's ability to make new thyroid hormones. These drugs do not cause permanent damage to the thyroid.

- Radioiodine damages or destroys the thyroid cells that make thyroid hormones. For this treatment, your doctor will give you a higher dose of a different type of radioiodine than is used for the radioiodine uptake test or the thyroid scan.

- Surgery can be used to remove most of the thyroid.

- Beta-blockers are medicines that block the effects of thyroid hormones on the body. These medicines can be helpful in slowing your heart rate and reducing other symptoms until one of the other forms of treatment can take effect. Beta-blockers do not reduce the amount of thyroid hormones that are made.

If your thyroid is destroyed by radioiodine or removed through surgery, you must take thyroid hormone pills for the rest of your life. These pills give your body the thyroid hormones that your thyroid would normally make.

How is hypothyroidism treated?

Hypothyroidism is treated with medicine to supply the body with the thyroid hormones it needs to function right. The most commonly used medicine is levothyroxine. This is a man-made form of T4. It is exactly the same as the T4 that your thyroid makes. When you take T4, your body makes the T3 it needs from the T4 in the pills. A man-made form of T3, called liothyronine, is also available. Some doctors and patients prefer a combination of T4 and T3 or T3 by itself. Most patients with hypothyroidism will need to be on thyroid hormone treatment for the rest of their lives.

How are thyroid nodules treated?

Treatment depends on the type of nodule or nodules that you have. Treatments include the following:

- **Watchful waiting:** If your nodule is not cancerous, your doctor may decide to simply watch your condition. This involves giving you regular physical exams, blood tests, and perhaps thyroid ultrasound tests. If your nodule does not change, you may not need further treatment.

- **Radioiodine:** If you have nodules that are making too much of the thyroid hormones, radioiodine treatment may be used. The radioiodine is absorbed by the thyroid nodules, and it causes them to shrink and make smaller amounts of thyroid hormones.

- **Alcohol ablation:** In this procedure, your doctor injects alcohol into thyroid nodules that make too much of the thyroid hormones. The alcohol shrinks the nodules and they make smaller amounts of thyroid hormones.

- **Surgery:** All nodules that are cancerous are surgically removed. Sometimes, nodules that are not cancerous but are big enough to cause problems breathing or swallowing are also surgically removed.

How is thyroid cancer treated?

- **Surgery:** The main treatment for thyroid cancer is to remove the entire thyroid gland, or as much of it as can be safely removed. Often, surgery alone will cure the thyroid cancer, especially if the cancer is small.

- **Radioiodine:** A large dose of radioiodine will destroy thyroid cancer cells with little or no damage to other parts of the body.

How is goiter treated?

The treatment for goiter depends on the cause of the goiter. If your goiter is caused by not getting enough iodine, you may be given an iodine supplement to swallow and T4 hormone, if need be. Other treatments include these:

- Radioiodine to shrink the goiter, especially if parts of the goiter are overactive

- Surgery to remove part or almost all of the thyroid

Can thyroid disorders cause problems with pregnancy?

Both hyperthyroidism and hypothyroidism can make it more difficult for you to become pregnant.

Hyperthyroidism that is not properly treated during pregnancy can cause the following:

- Early labor and premature babies

- Preeclampsia, a serious condition starting after 20 weeks of pregnancy that causes high blood pressure and problems with the kidneys and other organs

- Fast heart rate of the developing baby

- Smaller babies

- Stillbirths

Women who have hypothyroidism that is not diagnosed or properly treated during pregnancy may be at increased risk for these symptoms:

- Anemia (lower than normal number of healthy red blood cells)

- Preeclampsia

- Low-birth-weight babies

- Problems with brain development in the baby

- Abnormal bleeding after giving birth

If you are pregnant or are thinking about becoming pregnant, ask your doctor if you need a thyroid test. This is especially true if you or a family member has a history of thyroid problems or conditions related to thyroid disorders, including the following:

- Prematurely gray hair

- White patches on the skin

- Type 1 diabetes

Can I exercise if I have a thyroid problem?

Some people with thyroid problems may find exercise difficult. It is important to talk to your doctor about the right amount of physical activity for you.

Should I get tested for thyroid diseases?

Ask your doctor or nurse if you need to have a thyroid test. This is especially important if you are of childbearing age, have already had a thyroid problem, or have had surgery or radiotherapy affecting the thyroid gland. You may also be at higher risk if you have the following:

- Goiter

- Pernicious anemia

- Type 1 diabetes

- Vitiligo

- Prematurely gray hair

At any age, be sure to ask your doctor about any thyroid disorder symptoms you might have.

Chapter 58

Urinary Tract Disorders

Chapter Contents

Section 58.1

Interstitial Cystitis (Painful Bladder Syndrome)

Excerpted from "Interstitial Cystitis/Bladder Pain Syndrome Fact Sheet,"
U.S. Department of Health and Human Services Office on Women's
Health (www.womenshealth.gov), April 14, 2010.

What is interstitial cystitis/bladder pain syndrome (IC/BPS)?

Interstitial cystitis (IC) is a chronic pain condition that affects the
bladder. Many experts now call it bladder pain syndrome (BPS). Symptoms of IC/BPS include the following:

- Pain or discomfort believed to be related to the bladder, which
  often gets worse as the bladder fills

- Feeling like you need to urinate right away (urgency), often (frequency), or both (most people urinate between 4 and 7 times a
  day, yet with IC/BPS, the bladder may hold less urine; people
  with severe IC/BPS urinate as often as 30 times a day)

- Pain, pressure, or tenderness in the pelvic area and/or genitals

- Pain during sexual intercourse, or pain during ejaculation for men

- Ulcers and/or bleeding in the bladder

The symptoms of IC/BPS vary from person to person and can change
over time. Women's symptoms often get worse during their menstrual
periods. Some people with IC/BPS feel only mild discomfort. Others
have severe pain and symptoms.

IC/BPS can greatly affect a person's quality of life. Severe cases of
IC/BPS can keep people from going to work or school and being socially
active. It can affect a person's sex life and relationships. Living with a
chronic condition can increase your risk of depression.

Who gets IC/BPS?

More than 1.3 million Americans have IC/BPS, but some studies
suggest that millions more may have symptoms of IC/BPS. About 8 in

10 people with IC/BPS are women, although more men might have IC/BPS than we think. Men who actually have IC/BPS may be diagnosed with conditions that have similar symptoms, such as some prostate conditions. Most people with IC/BPS are diagnosed in middle age, but it may be diagnosed in teenagers and senior citizens as well.

What are the causes of IC/BPS?

No one knows what causes IC/BPS. The following factors may play a role in IC/BPS:

- A defect in the bladder wall that allows substances in the urine to irritate the bladder
- A specific type of cell that releases histamine (chemical released during an allergic reaction) and other chemicals, which lead to symptoms of IC/BPS
- Something in the urine that damages the bladder
- Changes in the nerves that carry bladder sensations, making normal events, such as bladder filling, painful
- The body's immune system attacks the bladder

It's hard to know if some of these factors actually cause IC/BPS or are part of the process that leads to IC/BPS. Also, the causes of IC/BPS in some people may be different than the causes in other people with IC/BPS. Studies of people who have IC/BPS suggest that it sometimes develops after an injury to the bladder, such as an infection. Genes also may play a role in some forms of IC/BPS. In some cases, IC/BPS affects both a mother and daughter or sisters. Still, IC/BPS does not commonly run in families.

Recently, researchers have identified a substance found almost only in the urine of people with IC/BPS. This substance appears to block the normal growth of the cells that line the wall of the bladder. Learning more about this substance might help researchers better understand the causes of IC/BPS and possible treatments.

Many women with IC/BPS have other conditions, such as irritable bowel syndrome and fibromyalgia. Allergies also are common in people with IC/BPS. Learning about these conditions also might provide clues on the cause of IC/BPS.

How can I tell if I have IC/BPS?

No single test can tell if you have IC/BPS, which can make it hard to diagnose. Your doctor will ask you lots of questions about your symptoms. Your doctor also will need to rule out other health problems that may be causing your symptoms, such as the following:

• Urinary tract infection (UTI)

• Bladder cancer

• Endometriosis

• Sexually transmitted infections (STIs)

• Kidney stones

Some tests used to help rule out other health problems that can cause bladder pain include these:

• **Urine test:** Your doctor will insert a catheter, which is a thin tube, to drain urine. Or you may be asked to give a urine sample using the "clean catch" method. For a clean catch, you will wash your genital area before collecting urine midstream in a sterile container. Your urine will be looked at under a microscope or sent to a lab to see if you have germs that cause UTIs or STIs.

• **Cystoscopy with or without bladder distention:** Your doctor may use a cystoscope, which is a thin tube with a tiny camera, to see inside the bladder. Further testing may include slowly stretching the bladder, called bladder distention, by filling it with liquid. This helps the doctor get a better look inside the bladder. The doctor can look for signs of cancer, bladder stones, or other problems. It can show whether your bladder wall is swollen, thick, or stiff and can measure how much urine the bladder can hold. It can also find bleeding or ulcers in the bladder. This test is often done as an outpatient surgery.

• **Biopsy:** A biopsy is when a tissue sample is removed and looked at under a microscope. Samples of the bladder and urethra may be removed during cystoscopy. A biopsy helps your doctor rule out bladder cancer.

Is there a cure for IC/BPS?

Doctors have not yet found a cure for IC/BPS. They cannot predict who will respond best to the different treatment options. Sometimes, symptoms may go away for no reason or after a change in diet or treatment. Even when symptoms do go away, they may return after days, weeks, months, or years.

How is IC/BPS treated?

There are treatments available to help ease the symptoms of IC/BPS. Doctors usually start with a conservative approach and progress to other therapies as needed. Although no one treatment helps everyone, over time many women are able to find a treatment plan that helps them to feel better. Some of these include the following:

Self-help strategies: Some people with IC/BPS find relief with self-care methods, such as these:

- Bladder retraining (this helps the bladder hold more urine before signaling the urge to urinate)
- Dietary changes
- Wearing loose clothing
- Quitting smoking
- Reducing stress (stress cannot cause IC/BPS, but it can trigger flare-ups)
- Pelvic exercises (a doctor or physical therapist can teach you how to do these)
- Low-impact physical activity, such as stretching and walking

Oral medicines: Several types of medicine might help with symptoms of IC/BPS. Over-the-counter pain relievers, such as aspirin and ibuprofen, might help with mild bladder pain. Talk to your doctor if you feel you need stronger pain medicine.

A prescription medicine called pentosan polysulfate sodium (Elmiron) can help ease symptoms in about one-third of patients. Because Elmiron has not been tested in pregnant women, it's not recommended for use during pregnancy, except in severe cases. Doctors aren't sure how it works, but it may restore the inner surface of the bladder and protect the bladder wall from irritating substances. You may have to take this medicine for up to six months before you start to feel better. Other oral medicines for IC/BPS include amitriptyline, an antidepressant that can help increase bladder capacity and block pain, and antihistamines.

Bladder distention: The doctor slowly stretches the bladder by filling it with liquid. Doctors aren't sure why, but this procedure eases pain for some patients.

Bladder instillation (a bladder wash or bath): The bladder is filled with a liquid medicine that is held for different periods of time before being emptied. Treatments are given every week or two in about six- or eight-week cycles. Some people are able to do this at home.

Nerve stimulation: Wires send mild electric pulses to the nerves that control the bladder. Scientists don't know exactly how nerve stimulation works, but it helps ease urgency and urinary frequency in some people.

Surgery: If other treatments have failed and the pain is disabling, surgery may be an option. Surgery may or may not ease symptoms.

Keep in mind, these treatments do not cure IC/BPS. But you may find that these treatments help to ease your IC/BPS symptoms. Researchers continue to study new treatments for IC/BPS. Talk to your doctor to find out if taking part in a clinical trial might be right for you.

Can consuming certain foods and drinks bring on symptoms or make them worse?

Studies have not proven a link between diet and IC/BPS. Yet some people find that that their symptoms begin or get worse after consuming certain foods or drinks, such as the following:

- Alcohol
- Tomatoes
- Spices
- Chocolate
- Caffeinated and citrus drinks
- High-acid foods
- Artificial sweeteners

Keeping a food diary might reveal a link, if there is one, between certain foods or drinks and the onset of symptoms. Or you can avoid foods or drinks you think might bring on your symptoms or make them worse. Then you can start eating or drinking these products again one at a time to see if any affect your symptoms. Some people with IC/BPS find no link between symptoms and what they eat.

If you decide to avoid certain foods or drinks, make sure that your meals are still well-balanced and healthy.

Does IC/BPS affect pregnancy?

Doctors do not have much information about pregnancy and IC/BPS. IC/BPS is not thought to affect fertility or the health of the unborn baby. Some women find that their IC/BPS symptoms get better during pregnancy. Others find their symptoms get worse. If you are thinking about becoming pregnant, talk to your doctor about your IC/BPS and any medicines you might be using to treat IC/BPS or other conditions. Some medicines and treatments are not safe to use during pregnancy.

I just found out I have IC/BPS. What else can I do to cope?

Learn as much as you can about IC/BPS and play an active role in your treatment and self-care. Adopt a healthy lifestyle, so you can feel your best. Try to live life as normally as possible. Reach out to loved ones and trusted friends for support. Think about joining a support group for people with IC/BPS, which can help you to cope with symptoms and stress.

Section 58.2

Urinary Incontinence in Women

Excerpted from "Urinary Incontinence Fact Sheet,"
U.S. Department of Health and Human Services Office on
Women's Health (www.womenshealth.gov), March 18, 2010.

What is urinary incontinence (UI)?

UI is also known as "loss of bladder control" or "urinary leakage." UI is when urine leaks out before you can get to a bathroom. If you have UI, you are not alone. Millions of women have this problem, especially as they get older.

Some women may lose a few drops of urine when they cough or laugh. Others may feel a sudden urge to urinate and cannot control it. Urine loss can also occur during sexual activity and can cause great emotional distress.

What causes UI?

UI is usually caused by problems with muscles and nerves that help to hold or pass urine.

Urine is stored in the bladder. It leaves the body through a tube that is connected to the bladder called the urethra. Muscles in the wall of the bladder contract to force urine out through the urethra. At the same time, sphincter muscles around the urethra relax to let the urine pass out of the body.

Incontinence happens if the bladder muscles suddenly contract or the sphincter muscles are not strong enough to hold back urine.

UI is twice as common in women as in men. Pregnancy, childbirth, and menopause are major factors. But both women and men can become incontinent from brain injury, birth defects, stroke, diabetes, multiple sclerosis, and physical changes associated with aging.

- **Pregnancy:** Unborn babies push down on the bladder, urethra (tube that you urinate from), and pelvic floor muscles. This pressure may weaken the pelvic floor support and lead to leaks or problems passing urine.

- **Childbirth:** Many women leak urine after giving birth. Labor and vaginal birth can weaken pelvic floor support and damage nerves that control the bladder. Most problems with bladder control during pregnancy and childbirth go away after the muscles have time to heal. Talk to your doctor if you still have bladder problems six weeks after childbirth.

- **Menopause:** Some women have bladder control problems after they stop having periods. After menopause, the body stops making the female hormone estrogen. Some experts think this loss of estrogen weakens the urethral tissue.

Other causes of UI that can affect women and men are the following:

- **Constipation:** Problems with bladder control can happen to people with long-term (chronic) constipation.

- **Medicines:** UI may be a side effect of medicines such as diuretics ("water pills" used to treat heart failure, liver cirrhosis, hypertension, and certain kidney diseases). Hormone replacement has been shown to cause worsening UI.

- **Caffeine and alcohol:** Drinks with caffeine, such as coffee or soda, cause the bladder to fill quickly and sometimes leak.

- **Infection:** Infections of the urinary tract and bladder may cause incontinence for a short time. Bladder control returns when the illness goes away.

- **Nerve damage:** Damaged nerves may send signals to the bladder at the wrong time, or not at all. Trauma or diseases such as diabetes and multiple sclerosis can cause nerve damage. Nerves may also become damaged during childbirth.

- **Excess weight:** Being overweight is also known to put pressure on the bladder and make incontinence worse.

What are the types of UI?

- **Stress incontinence:** Leakage happens with coughing, sneezing, exercising, laughing, lifting heavy things, and other movements that put pressure on the bladder. This is the most common type of incontinence in women. It is often caused by physical changes from pregnancy, childbirth, and menopause. It can be treated and sometimes cured.

- **Urge incontinence:** This is sometimes called "overactive bladder." Leakage usually happens after a strong, sudden urge to urinate. This may occur when you don't expect it, such as during sleep, after drinking water, or when you hear or touch running water.

- **Functional incontinence:** People with this type of incontinence may have problems thinking, moving, or speaking that keep them from reaching a toilet. For example, a person with Alzheimer disease may not plan a trip to the bathroom in time to urinate. A person in a wheelchair may be unable to get to a toilet in time.

- **Overflow incontinence:** Urine leakage happens because the bladder doesn't empty completely. Overflow incontinence is less common in women.

- **Mixed incontinence:** This is two or more types of incontinence together (usually stress and urge incontinence).

- **Transient incontinence:** Urine leakage happens for a short time due to an illness (such as a bladder infection or pregnancy). The leaking stops when the illness is treated.

How do I talk to my doctor about UI?

Many women do not want to talk to their doctor about such a personal topic. But UI is a common medical problem. Millions of women have the same problem. Many have been treated successfully.

Even if you feel shy, it is up to you to take the first step. Some doctors don't treat bladder control problems, so they may not think to ask about it. They might expect you to bring up the subject.

Family practitioners and internists can treat bladder problems. If your doctor does not treat such problems, ask for help finding a doctor who does, such as a urologist, OB/GYN, or urogynecologist.

Here are some questions to ask your doctor:

- Could what I eat or drink cause bladder problems?

- Could my medicines (prescription and over-the-counter) cause bladder problems?

- Could other medical conditions cause loss of bladder control?

- What are the treatments to regain bladder control? Which one is best for me?

- What can I do about the odor and rash caused by urine?

It also helps to keep a bladder diary. This means you write down when you leak urine. Be sure to note what you were doing at the time, such as sneezing, coughing, laughing, stepping off a curb, or sleeping. Take this log with you when you visit your doctor.

How do I find out if I have UI?

Schedule a visit with your doctor. Your doctor will ask you about your symptoms and take a medical history, including the following:

- How often you empty your bladder

- How and when you leak urine

- How much urine you leak

Your doctor will do a physical exam to look for signs of health problems that can cause incontinence. Your doctor also will do a test to figure out how well your bladder works and how much it can hold. For this test, you will drink water and urinate into a measuring pan. The doctor will then measure any urine still in the bladder. Your doctor also may order other tests:

- **Bladder stress test:** During this test, you will cough or bear down as the doctor watches for loss of urine.

- **Urinalysis:** A urinalysis tests your urine for signs of infection or other causes of incontinence.

- **Ultrasound:** Sound waves are used to take a picture of the kidneys, bladder, and urethra.

- **Cystoscopy:** A doctor places a thin tube connected to a tiny camera in the urethra to look at the inside of the urethra and bladder.

- **Urodynamics:** A doctor places a thin tube into your bladder and your bladder is filled with water. The doctor then measures the pressure in the bladder.

Your doctor may ask you to write down when you empty your bladder and how much urine you produce for a day or a week.

How is UI treated?

There are many ways to treat UI. Your doctor will work with you to find the best treatment for you.

Types of treatments include the following:

Behavioral treatments: By changing some basic behaviors, you may be able to improve your UI. Behavioral treatments include these:

- **Pelvic muscle exercises (Kegel exercises):** Exercising your pelvic floor muscles regularly can help reduce or cure stress leakage. To do Kegel exercises:

  - First, try practicing these exercises while lying down.

  - Squeeze the muscles in your genital area as if you were trying to stop the flow of urine or trying to stop from passing gas. Try to squeeze only the pelvic muscles. Be extra careful not to tighten your stomach, legs, or buttocks.

  - Relax. Squeeze the muscles again and hold for three seconds. Then relax for three seconds. Work up to three sets of 10 repeats.

  - When your muscles get stronger, try doing your exercises while sitting or standing. You can do these exercises any time, while sitting at your desk, in the car, waiting in line, doing the dishes, etc.

See your doctor, nurse, or physical therapist to learn how to do these exercises correctly. Kegel exercises are most effective when the patient has received proper instruction from a health care professional.

- **Bladder retraining:** You may regain bladder control by going to the bathroom at set times, before you get the urge to urinate. You can slowly increase the time between set bathroom trips as you gain control.

- **Weight loss:** Extra weight puts more pressure on your bladder and nearby muscles. This can cause bladder control problems. Work with your doctor to plan a diet and exercise program if you are overweight.

- **Dietary changes:** Some foods and beverages are thought to contribute to bladder leakage. While doctors do not know if these foods really do cause UI, it is reasonable to see if stopping one or all of these items is helpful:

  - Alcoholic beverages

  - Carbonated beverages (with or without caffeine)

  - Coffee or tea (with or without caffeine)

  Other changes include drinking fewer fluids after dinner and eating enough fiber to avoid constipation. Also, avoid drinking too much. Six eight-ounce glasses of fluid a day is enough for most people.

- **Quitting smoking:** Researchers are still looking at the link between incontinence and cigarette smoking. Studies show that smokers have more frequent and severe urine leaks.

Medicines for bladder control: Medications can reduce some types of leakage. Some medicines, for example, help relax the bladder muscles and prevent bladder spasms. Talk to your doctor to see if medication is right for you.

It is always important to take your medicine exactly as your doctor tells you to. Also, all drugs have side effects and may affect people differently. Always tell your doctor about any over-the-counter medicines you are taking.

Devices: A pessary is the most common device used to treat stress incontinence. It is a stiff ring that a doctor or nurse inserts into the vagina. The device pushes up against the wall of the vagina and the urethra. This helps reposition the urethra to reduce stress leakage.

Nerve stimulation: Some people with urge incontinence may not respond to behavioral treatments or medicine. In this case, electrical stimulation of the nerves that control the bladder may help.

You will be tested to see if this treatment, called neuromodulation, can work for you. The doctor will first place a device outside your body to deliver a pulse. If it works well, a surgeon will implant the device.

Biofeedback: Biofeedback helps you learn how your body works. A therapist puts an electrical patch over your bladder and urethral muscles. A wire connected to the patch is linked to a TV screen. You and your therapist watch the screen to see when these muscles contract, so you can learn to control these muscles.

Biofeedback can be used with pelvic muscle exercises and electrical stimulation to help control stress incontinence and urge incontinence.

Surgery: Surgery is most effective for people with stress UI who have not been helped by other treatments. Talk to your doctor about whether surgery would help you, and what type of surgery is best for you.

Catheterization: The doctor may suggest a catheter if you are incontinent because your bladder never empties completely (overflow incontinence). This is also an option if your bladder cannot empty because of poor muscle tone, past surgery, or a spinal cord injury. A catheter is a thin tube that is placed in the bladder by a doctor or by you. It drains the bladder into a bag that you can attach to your leg.

Section 58.3

Urinary Tract Infections in Women

Excerpted from "Urinary Tract Infection Fact Sheet,"
U.S. Department of Health and Human Services Office on
Women's Health (www.womenshealth.gov), May 1, 2008.

What is a urinary tract infection (UTI)?

A UTI is an infection anywhere in the urinary tract. The urinary
tract makes and stores urine and removes it from the body. Parts of
the urinary tract include the following:

- **Kidneys:** Collect waste from blood to make urine

- **Ureters:** Carry the urine from the kidneys to the bladder

- **Bladder:** Stores urine until it is full

- **Urethra:** A short tube that carries urine from the bladder out of
  your body when you pass urine

What causes UTIs?

Bacteria, a type of germ that gets into your urinary tract, cause a
UTI. This can happen in many ways:

- Wiping from back to front after a bowel movement (BM), which
  can cause germs to get into your urethra

- Having sexual intercourse, which can cause germs in the vagina
  to be pushed into the urethra

- Waiting too long to pass urine, which causes more germs to be
  made and a UTI to become worse

- Using a diaphragm for birth control, or spermicides (creams that
  kill sperm) with a diaphragm or on a condom

- Anything that makes it hard to completely empty your bladder,
  like a kidney stone

- Having diabetes, which makes it harder for your body to fight
  other health problems

- Loss of estrogen (a hormone) and changes in the vagina after menopause
- Having had a catheter in place

What are the signs of a UTI?

If you have an infection, you may have some or all of these signs:

- Pain or stinging when you pass urine
- An urge to pass urine a lot, but not much comes out when you go
- Pressure in your lower belly
- Urine that smells bad or looks milky, cloudy, or reddish in color; if you see blood in your urine, tell a doctor right away
- Feeling tired or shaky or having a fever

How does a doctor find out if I have a UTI?

To find out if you have a UTI, your doctor will need to test a clean sample of your urine. The doctor or nurse will give you a clean plastic cup and a special wipe. Wash your hands before opening the cup. When you open the cup, don't touch the inside of the lid or inside of the cup. Clean the genital area with the wipe. Wipe from front to back. Hold the labia open and pass a little bit of urine into the toilet. Then, catch the rest in the cup. This is called a "clean-catch" sample.

If you are prone to UTIs, your doctor may want to take pictures of your urinary tract with an X-ray or ultrasound. These pictures can show swelling, stones, or blockage. Your doctor also may want to look inside your bladder using a cystoscope, a small tube that's put into the urethra to see inside of the urethra and bladder.

How is a UTI treated?

UTIs are treated with antibiotics, medicines that kill the bacteria that cause the infection. Your doctor will tell you how long you need to take the medicine. Make sure you take all of your medicine, even if you feel better!

If you don't take medicine for a UTI, the UTI can hurt other parts of your body. Also, if you're pregnant and have signs of a UTI, see your doctor right away. A UTI could cause problems in your pregnancy, such as having your baby too early or getting high blood pressure. Also, UTIs in pregnant women are more likely to travel to the kidneys.

Will a UTI hurt my kidneys?

If treated right away, a UTI is not likely to damage your kidneys or urinary tract. But UTIs that are not treated can cause serious problems in your kidneys and the rest of your body.

How can I keep from getting UTIs?

These are steps you can take to try to prevent a UTI. But you may follow these steps and still get a UTI. If you have symptoms of a UTI, call your doctor.

- Urinate when you need to. Don't hold it. Pass urine before and after sex. After you pass urine or have a bowel movement, wipe from front to back.

- Drink water every day and after sex. Try for six to eight glasses a day.

- Clean the outer lips of your vagina and anus each day.

- Don't use douches or feminine hygiene sprays.

- If you get a lot of UTIs and use spermicides, talk to your doctor about using other forms of birth control.

- Wear underpants with a cotton crotch. Don't wear tight-fitting pants, which can trap in moisture.

- Take showers instead of tub baths.

I get UTIs a lot. Can my doctor do something to help?

About one in five women who get UTIs will get another one. Some women get three or more UTIs a year. If you are prone to UTIs, ask your doctor about your treatment options. Your doctor may ask you to take a small dose of medicine every day to prevent infection. Or your doctor might give you a supply of antibiotics to take after sex or at the first sign of infection. "Dipsticks" can help test for UTIs at home. They are useful for some women with repeat UTIs. Ask your doctor if you should use dipsticks at home to test for UTI. Your doctor may also want to do special tests to see what is causing repeat infections.

Part Seven

Additional Help and Information

Chapter 59

Glossary of Women's Health Terms

allergies: Allergies are disorders that involve an immune response in the body. Allergies are reactions to allergens such as plant pollen, other grasses and weeds, certain foods, rubber latex, insect bites, or certain drugs.

Alzheimer disease: Alzheimer disease is a brain disease that cripples the brain's nerve cells over time and destroys memory and learning. It usually starts in late middle age or old age and gets worse over time. Symptoms include loss of memory, confusion, problems in thinking, and changes in language, behavior, and personality.

anemia: Anemia occurs when the amount of red blood cells or hemoglobin (the substance in the blood that carries oxygen to organs) becomes reduced, causing fatigue that can be severe.

bacterial vaginosis (BV): BV is the most common vaginal infection in women of childbearing age, which happens when the normal bacteria (germs) in the vagina get out of balance, such as from douching or from sexual contact. Symptoms include vaginal discharge that can be white, gray, or thin and can have an odor; burning or pain when urinating; or itching around the outside of the vagina. There also may be no symptoms.

The terms in this glossary were excerpted from the glossary at the U.S. Department of Health and Human Services Office on Women's Health at www.womens health.gov/glossary.

blood pressure: Blood pressure is the force of blood against the walls of arteries. Blood pressure is noted as two numbers—the systolic pressure (as the heart beats) over the diastolic pressure (as the heart relaxes between beats). The numbers are written one above or before the other, with the systolic number on top and the diastolic number on the bottom. For example, a blood pressure reading of 120/80 mmHg (millimeters of mercury) is called 120 over 80.

diabetes: Diabetes is a disease in which blood glucose (blood sugar) levels are above normal. There are two main types of diabetes. Type 1 diabetes is caused by a problem with the body's defense system, called the immune system. This form of diabetes usually starts in childhood or adolescence. Type 2 diabetes is the most common form of diabetes. It starts most often in adulthood.

eating disorder: Eating disorders, such as anorexia nervosa, bulimia nervosa, and binge-eating disorder, involve serious problems with eating. This could include an extreme decrease of food or severe overeating, as well as feelings of distress and concern about body shape or weight.

ectopic pregnancy: This is a pregnancy that is not in the uterus. It happens when a fertilized egg settles and grows in a place other than the inner lining of the uterus. Most happen in the fallopian tube but can happen in the ovary, cervix, or abdominal cavity.

endometriosis: Endometriosis is a condition in which tissue that normally lines the uterus grows in other areas of the body, usually inside the abdominal cavity, but acts as if it were inside the uterus. Blood shed monthly from the misplaced tissue has no place to go, and tissues surrounding the area of endometriosis may become inflamed or swollen. This can produce scar tissue. Symptoms include painful menstrual cramps that can be felt in the abdomen or lower back, or pain during or after sexual activity, irregular bleeding, and infertility.

estrogen: Estrogen is a group of female hormones that are responsible for the development of breasts and other secondary sex characteristics in women. Estrogen is produced by the ovaries and other body tissues. Estrogen, along with progesterone, is important in preparing a woman's body for pregnancy.

genetic counseling: This type of counseling is a communication process between a specially trained health professional and a person concerned about the genetic risk of disease. The person's family and personal medical history may be discussed, and counseling may lead to genetic testing.

glandular tissue: This is body tissue that produces and releases one or more substances for use in the body. Some glands produce fluids that affect tissues or organs. Others produce hormones or participate in blood production. In the breast, glandular tissue is involved in the production of milk.

heart disease: Heart disease involves a number of abnormal conditions affecting the heart and the blood vessels in the heart. The most common type of heart disease is coronary artery disease, which is the gradual buildup of plaques in the coronary arteries, the blood vessels that bring blood to the heart. This disease develops slowly and silently, over decades. It can go virtually unnoticed until it produces a heart attack.

hormone: A hormone is a substance produced by one tissue and conveyed by the bloodstream to another to effect a function of the body, such as growth or metabolism.

immune system: The immune system is a complex system in the body that recognizes and responds to potentially harmful substances, like infections, in order to protect the body.

immunization: Also called vaccination, an immunization is a shot that contains germs that have been killed or weakened. When given to a healthy person, it triggers the immune system to respond and build immunity to a disease.

infertility: Infertility refers to a condition in which a couple has problems conceiving, or getting pregnant, after one year of regular sexual intercourse without using any birth control methods. If a woman keeps having miscarriages, it's also called infertility. Infertility can be caused by a problem with the man or the woman, or both.

inflammation: This term is used to describe an area on the body that is swollen, red, hot, and in pain.

inflammatory bowel disease (IBD): IBD is a long-lasting problems that cause irritation and ulcers in the gastrointestinal tract. The most common disorders are ulcerative colitis and Crohn disease.

influenza: Also called the flu, influenza is a respiratory infection caused by multiple viruses. The viruses pass through the air and enter the body through the nose or mouth. The flu can be serious or even deadly for elderly people, newborn babies, and people with certain chronic illnesses. Symptoms may include body or muscle aches, chills, cough, fever, headache, and sore throat.

menopausal hormone therapy (MHT): MHT replaces the hormones that a woman's ovaries stop making at the time of menopause, easing symptoms like hot flashes and vaginal dryness. It involves using man-made estrogen alone or estrogen with progestin, often in the form of a pill or skin patch. MHT used to be called hormone replacement therapy, or HRT. (A recent, large study found that use of MHT poses some serious risks, such as increasing some women's risk for breast cancer, heart disease, stroke, and pulmonary embolism, a blood clot in the lung. Women who choose to use MHT should use the lowest dose that helps for the shortest time needed. Talk with your doctor to find out if MHT is right for you and discuss other ways to relieve menopause symptoms.)

menopause: Menopause is the transition in a woman's life when production of the hormone estrogen in her body falls permanently to very low levels, the ovaries stop producing eggs, and menstrual periods stop for good.

menstrual cycle: The menstrual cycle is a recurring cycle in which the lining of the uterus thickens in preparation for pregnancy and then is shed if pregnancy does not occur.

migraine: Migraine is a medical condition that usually involves a very painful headache, usually felt on one side of the head. Besides intense pain, migraine also can cause nausea and vomiting and sensitivity to light and sound. Some people also may see spots or flashing lights or have a temporary loss of vision.

nerves: Nerves are cells in the human body that are the building blocks of the nervous system (the system that records and transmits information chemically and electrically within a person). Nerve cells, or neurons, are made up of a nerve cell body and various extensions from the cell body that receive and transmit impulses from and to other nerves and muscles. For example, nerve tissue in the breast makes breasts sensitive to touch, allowing the baby's sucking to stimulate the let-down or milk-ejection reflex and milk production.

obesity: Obesity means having too much body fat. People with a body mass index (BMI) of 30 or higher are obese.

osteoarthritis (OA): OA is a joint disease that mostly affects cartilage, the slippery tissue that covers the ends of bones in a joint. The top layer of cartilage breaks down and wears away. This allows bones under the cartilage to rub together, which causes pain, swelling, and loss of motion of the joint.

osteoporosis: Osteoporosis is a bone disease that is characterized by progressive loss of bone density and thinning of bone tissue, causing bones to break easily.

ovarian cancer: This is cancer of the ovary or ovaries, which are organs in the female reproductive system that make eggs and hormones. Most ovarian cancers develop from the cells that cover the outer surface of the ovary, called epithelial cells.

ovary (ovaries): Part of a woman's reproductive system, the ovaries produce her eggs. Each month, through the process called ovulation, the ovaries release eggs into the fallopian tubes, where they travel to the uterus, or womb. If an egg is fertilized by a man's sperm, a woman becomes pregnant and the egg grows and develops inside the uterus. If the egg is not fertilized, the egg and the lining of the uterus are shed during a woman's monthly menstrual period.

ovulation: Ovulation is the release of a single egg from a follicle that developed in the ovary. It usually occurs regularly, around day 14 of a 28-day menstrual cycle.

Pap test: The Pap test is a test that finds changes in the cells of the cervix. The test can find cancer or cells that can turn into cancer. To perform a Pap test, a health care provider uses a small brush to gently scrape cells from the cervix for examination under a microscope.

pelvic exam: During this exam, the doctor or nurse practitioner looks for redness, swelling, discharge, or sores on the outside and inside of the vagina. A Pap test tests for cell changes on the cervix. The doctor or nurse practitioner will also put two fingers inside the vagina and press on the abdomen with the other hand to check for cysts or growths on the ovaries and uterus. Sexuality transmitted disease (STD) tests may also be done.

pelvic inflammatory disease (PID): PID is an infection of the female reproductive organs that are above the cervix, such as the fallopian tubes and ovaries. It is the most common and serious problem caused by sexually transmitted diseases. PID can cause ectopic pregnancies, infertility, chronic pelvic pain, and other serious problems. Symptoms include fever, foul-smelling vaginal discharge, extreme pain, and vaginal bleeding.

perimenopause: This is the phase in a woman's reproductive life-cycle leading up to menopause. Menopause is reached when a woman hasn't had a period for 12 months in a row. Before that point, during perimenopause, a woman's body slowly makes less of the hormones estrogen and progesterone. This causes some women to have symptoms such as hot flashes and changes in their periods. Many women go through it in their forties and fifties.

perinatal depression: Perinatal depression occurs during pregnancy or within a year after delivery.

polycystic ovary syndrome (PCOS): PCOS is a health problem that can affect a woman's menstrual cycle, ability to have children, hormones, heart, blood vessels, and appearance. With PCOS, women typically have high levels of androgens or male hormones, missed or irregular periods, and many small cysts in their ovaries.

postpartum depression (PPD): Postpartum depression is a serious condition that requires treatment from a health care provider. With this condition, feelings of the baby blues (feeling sad, anxious, afraid, or confused after having a baby) do not go away or get worse.

preconception health: This involves a woman's health before she becomes pregnant. It involves knowing how health conditions and risk factors could affect a woman or her unborn baby if she becomes pregnant.

preeclampsia: Also known as toxemia, preeclampsia is a syndrome occurring in a pregnant woman after her 20th week of pregnancy that causes high blood pressure and problems with the kidneys and other organs. Symptoms include sudden increase in blood pressure, too much protein in the urine, swelling in a woman's face and hands, and headache.

premenstrual syndrome (PMS): PMS is a group of symptoms linked to the menstrual cycle that occur in the week or two weeks before menstruation. The symptoms usually go away after menstruation begins and can include acne, breast swelling and tenderness, feeling tired, having trouble sleeping, upset stomach, bloating, constipation or diarrhea, headache or backache, appetite changes or food cravings, joint or muscle pain, trouble concentrating or remembering, tension, irritability, mood swings or crying spells, and anxiety or depression.

preterm birth: Also called premature birth, it is a birth that occurs before the 37th week of pregnancy.

progesterone: Progesterone is a female hormone produced by the ovaries. Progesterone, along with estrogen, prepares the uterus (womb) for a possible pregnancy each month and supports the fertilized egg if conception occurs. Progesterone also helps prepare the breasts for milk production and breastfeeding.

progestin: Progestin is a hormone that works by causing changes in the uterus. When taken with the hormone estrogen, progestin works to prevent thickening of the lining of the uterus. This is helpful for women who are in menopause and are taking estrogen for their symptoms. Progestins also are prescribed to regulate the menstrual cycle, treat unusual stopping of the menstrual periods, help a pregnancy occur or maintain a pregnancy, or treat unusual or heavy bleeding of the uterus. They also can be used to prevent pregnancy, help treat cancer of the breast, kidney, or uterus, and help treat loss of appetite and severe weight or muscle loss.

puberty: Puberty is the time when the body is changing from the body of a child to the body of an adult. This process begins earlier in girls than in boys, usually between ages 8 and 13, and lasts two to four years.

thyroid: The thyroid is a small gland in the neck that makes and stores hormones that help regulate heart rate, blood pressure, body temperature, and the rate at which food is converted into energy.

tumor: A tumor is an abnormal mass of tissue that results when cells divide more than they should or do not die when they should. Tumors can be benign or malignant. Benign tumors are not cancer. Malignant tumors are cancer.

ultrasound: This is a painless, harmless test that uses sound waves to produce images of the organs and structures of the body on a screen. Also called sonography.

urinary tract infection (UTI): A UTI is an infection anywhere in the urinary tract, or organs that collect and store urine and release it from your body (the kidneys, ureters, bladder, and urethra). An infection occurs when microorganisms, usually bacteria from the digestive tract, cling to the urethra (opening to the urinary tract) and begin to multiply.

uterine fibroids: Fibroids are common, benign (noncancerous) tumors that grow in the muscle of the uterus, or womb. Fibroids often cause no symptoms and need no treatment, and they usually shrink after menopause. But sometimes fibroids cause heavy bleeding or pain, and require treatment.

uterus: The uterus is a woman's womb, or the hollow, pear-shaped organ located in a woman's lower abdomen between the bladder and the rectum.

yeast infections: Yeast infections are common infections in women caused by an overgrowth of the fungus *Candida*. It is normal to have some yeast in your vagina, but sometimes it can overgrow because of hormonal changes in your body, such as during pregnancy, or from taking certain medications, such as antibiotics. Symptoms include itching, burning, and irritation of the vagina; pain when urinating or with intercourse; and cottage cheese–looking vaginal discharge.

Chapter 60

Directory of Women's Health Resources and Organizations

General Women's Health Resources

Agency for Healthcare Research and Quality Clearinghouse
Office of Communications and Knowledge Transfer
540 Gaither Road, Suite 2000
Rockville, MD 20850
Toll-Free: 800-358-9295
Toll-Free TDD: 888-586-6340
Phone: 301-427-1104
Website: www.ahrq.gov/research/womenix.htm

American Academy of Family Physicians
P.O. Box 11210
Shawnee Mission, KS 66207-1210
Toll-Free: 800-274-2237
Phone: 913-906-6000
Fax: 913-906-6075
Website: www.aafp.org (main website) and www.familydoctor.org (health information)

American College of Obstetricians and Gynecologists
P.O. Box 70620
Washington, DC 20024-9998
Toll-Free: 800-673-8444
Phone: 202-638-5577
Website: www.acog.org
E-mail: resources@acog.org

MedlinePlus
MedlinePlus provides health information from the National Institutes of Health and other trusted sources. The website

---

The information in this chapter was compiled from various sources deemed accurate. All contact information was verified and updated. Inclusion does not imply endorsement. This list is not comprehensive.

also has a medical encyclopedia, information on prescription and nonprescription drugs, and the latest health news.
Website: www.medlineplus.gov

National Center for Complementary and Alternative Medicine (NCCAM)
NCCAM Clearinghouse
P.O. Box 7923
Gaithersburg, MD 20898
Toll-Free: 888-644-6226
Toll-Free TTY: 866-464-3615
Toll-Free Fax: 866-464-3616
Phone: 301-519-3153
Website: nccam.nih.gov
E-mail: info@nccam.nih.gov

National Institute of Allergy and Infectious Diseases (NIAID)
Office of Communications and Government Relations
6610 Rockledge Drive, MSC 6612
Bethesda, MD 20892-6612
Toll-Free: 866-284-4107
Toll-Free TDD: 800-877-8339
Phone: 301-496-5717
Fax: 301-402-3573
Website: www.niaid.nih.gov
E-mail: ocpostoffice@niaid.nih.gov

National Institute of Diabetes and Digestive and Kidney Diseases (NIDDK)
Office of Communications and Public Liaison
NIDDK, NIH
Building 31, Room 9A06
31 Center Drive, MSC 2560

Bethesda, MD 20892-2560
Phone: 301-496-3583
Website: www.niddk.nih.gov

National Institute on Aging (NIA)
Building 31, Room 5C27
31 Center Drive, MSC 2292
Bethesda, MD 20892
Toll-Free: 800-222-2225
Toll-Free TTY: 800-222-4225
Phone: 301-496-1752
Fax: 301-496-1072
Website: www.nia.nih.gov

National Women's Health Network
1413 K Street NW, 4th Floor
Washington, D.C. 20005
Phone: 202-628-2640
or 202-682-2646
(Women's Health Voice)
Fax: 202-682-2648
Website: www.nwhn.org
E-mail: nwhn@nwhn.org

National Women's Health Resource Center
157 Broad Street, Suite 200
Red Bank, NJ 07701
Toll-Free: 877-986-9472
Fax: 732-530-3347
Website: www.healthywomen.org
E-mail: info@healthywomen.org

Office of Minority Health Resource Center
P.O. Box 37337
Washington, DC 20013-7337
Toll-Free: 800-444-6472
Phone: 240-453-2882
TDD: 301-251-1432

Fax: 240-453-2883
Website: minorityhealth.hhs.gov
E-mail:
info@minorityhealth.hhs.gov

Office of Research on Women's Health, National Institutes of Health (NIH)
6707 Democracy Boulevard
Suite 400
Bethesda, MD 20892-5484
Phone: 301-402-1770
Fax: 301-402-1798
Website: orwh.od.nih.gov

Office of Women's Health, Centers for Disease Control and Prevention (CDC)
1600 Clifton Road, MS E-89
Atlanta, GA 30333
Toll-Free: 800-CDC-INFO
(800-232-4636)
Toll-Free TTY: 888-232-6348
Website: www.cdc.gov/women
E-mail: cdcinfo@cdc.gov

Office of Women's Health, U.S. Food and Drug Administration (FDA)
10903 New Hampshire Avenue
WO32-2333
Silver Spring, MD 20993
Toll-Free: 888-INFO-FDA
(888-463-6332)
Phone: 301-796-9440
Fax: 301-847-8604
Website: www.fda.gov/womens

Office on Women's Health, U.S. Department of Health and Human Services (HHS)
200 Independence Avenue SW

Room 712E
Washington, DC 20201
Toll-Free: 800-994-9662
Toll-Free TDD: 888-220-5446
Phone: 202-690-7650
Fax: 202-205-2631
Website:
www.womenshealth.gov

Society for Women's Health Research
1025 Connecticut Avenue NW
Suite 601
Washington, DC 20036
Phone: 202-223-8224
Fax: 202-833-3472
Website:
www.womenshealthresearch.org
E-mail: info@swhr.org

Weight-Control Information Network (WIN)
1 WIN Way
Bethesda, MD 20892-3665
Toll-Free: 877-946-4627
Phone: 202-828-1025
Fax: 202-828-1028
Website:
www.win.niddk.nih.gov
E-mail: win@info.niddk.nih.gov

Allergies and Asthma

Asthma and Allergy Foundation of America
8201 Corporate Drive
Suite 1000
Landover, MD 20785
Toll-Free: 800-7-ASTHMA
(800-727-8462)
Website: www.aafa.org
E-mail: info@aafa.org

Arthritis and Musculoskeletal Diseases

American College of Rheumatology
2200 Lake Boulevard NE
Atlanta, GA 30319
Phone: 404-633-3777
Fax: 404-633-1870
Website: www.rheumatology.org
E-mail: acr@rheumatology.org

Arthritis Foundation
1330 West Peachtree Street
Suite 100
Atlanta, GA 30309
Toll-Free: 800-283-7800
Phone: 404-872-7100
Website: www.arthritis.org

National Institute of Arthritis and Musculoskeletal and Skin Diseases (NIAMS)
1 AMS Circle
Bethesda, MD 20892-3675
Toll-Free: 877-22-NIAMS
(877-226-4267)
Phone: 301-495-4484
TYY: 301-565-2966
Fax: 312-718-6366
Website: www.niams.nih.gov
E-mail: NIAMSinfo@mail.nih.gov

National Osteoporosis Foundation
1150 17th Street NW, Suite 850
Washington, DC 20036
Toll-Free: 800-231-4222
Phone: 202-223-2226
Fax: 202-223-2237
Website: www.nof.org

Cancer

American Cancer Society
250 Williams Street NW
Atlanta, GA 30303
Toll-Free: 800-227-2345
Toll-Free TTY: 866-228-4327
Website: www.cancer.org

Foundation for Women's Cancer
230 West Monroe, Suite 2528
Chicago, IL 60606
Toll-Free: 800-444-4441 (hotline)
Phone: 312-578-1439
Fax: 312-578-9769
Website: www.foundationfor womenscancer.org
E-mail: info@ foundationforwomenscancer.org

National Cancer Institute
6116 Executive Boulevard
Suite 300
Bethesda, MD 20892-8322
Toll-Free: 800-4-CANCER
(800-422-6237)
Toll-Free TTY: 800-332-8615
Website: www.cancer.gov

National Ovarian Cancer Coalition, Inc.
2501 Oak Lawn Avenue
Suite 435
Dallas, Texas 75219
Toll-Free: 888-OVARIAN
(888-682-7426)
Fax: 214-273-4201
Website: www.ovarian.org

Skin Cancer Foundation
149 Madison Avenue, Suite 901

New York, NY 10016
Phone: 212-725-5176
Website: www.skincancer.org

Susan G. Komen for the Cure
5005 LBJ Freeway, Suite 250
Dallas, TX 75244
Toll-Free: 877-GO-KOMEN
(877-465-6636)
Website: www.komen.org

Children and Young Adults

Eunice Kennedy Shriver National Institute of Child Health and Human Development (NICHD) Information Resource Center
P.O. Box 3006
Rockville, MD 20847
Toll-Free: 800-370-2943
Toll-Free TTY: 888-320-6942
Toll-Free Fax: 866-760-5947
Website: www.nichd.nih.gov
E-mail: NICHDInformation
ResourceCenter@mail.nih.gov

GirlsHealth.gov
200 Independence Avenue SW
Room 712E
Washington, DC 2020
Toll-Free: 800-994-9662
Toll-Free TDD: 888-220-5446
Website: www.girlshealth.gov

KidsHealth
Website: www.kidshealth.org

Safe and Healthy Kids
4770 Buford Highway, MS E-89
Atlanta, GA 30341

Toll-Free: 800-CDC-INFO
(800-232-4636)
Toll-Free TTY: 888-232-6348
Phone: 770-488-8190
Website: www.cdc.gov/family
E-mail: cdcinfo@cdc.gov

Diabetes

American Diabetes Association
Attention: Center for Information
1701 North Beauregard Street
Alexandria, VA 22311
Toll-Free: 800-DIABETES
(800-342-2383)
Website: www.diabetes.org
E-mail: AskADA@diabetes.org

National Diabetes Education Program (NDEP)
1 Diabetes Way
Bethesda, MD 20814-9692
Toll-Free: 888-693-NDEP
(888-693-6337
to order materials)
Phone: 301-496-3583
Website: www.ndep.nih.gov
E-mail: ndep@mail.nih.gov

National Diabetes Information Clearinghouse (NDIC)
1 Information Way
Bethesda, MD 20892-3560
Toll-Free: 800-860-8747
Toll-Free TTY: 866-569-1162
Fax: 703-738-4929
Website: diabetes.niddk.nih.gov
E-mail: ndic@info.niddk.nih.gov

Eating Disorders

National Association of Anorexia Nervosa and Associated Disorders
750 East Diehl Road #127
Naperville, IL 60563
Helpline: 630-577-1330
(9 a.m. to 5 p.m. CST, Mon.–Fri.)
Phone: 630-577-1333
Website: www.anad.org
E-mail: anadhelp@anad.org

National Eating Disorders Association
165 West 46th Street
New York, NY 10036
Phone: 212-575-6200
Toll-Free Hotline: 800-931-2237
(9 a.m. to 5 p.m. EST)
Fax: 212-575-1650
Website: www.
nationaleatingdisorders.org
E-mail: info@
nationaleatingdisorders.org

Gastrointestinal and Digestive Disorders

Academy of Nutrition and Dietetics
120 South Riverside Plaza
Suite 2000
Chicago, IL 60606-6995
Toll-Free: 800-877-1600
Phone: 312-899-0040
Website: www.eatright.org
E-mail: knowledge@eatright.org

American Celiac Disease Alliance
2504 Duxbury Place
Alexandria, VA 22308
Phone: 703-622-3331
Website:
www.americanceliac.org
E-mail: info@americanceliac.org

American College of Gastroenterology
6400 Goldsboro Road, Suite 200
Bethesda, MD 20817
Phone: 301-263-9000
Website: gi.org
E-mail: info@acg.gi.org

American Gastroenterological Association
4930 Del Ray Avenue
Bethesda, MD 20814
Phone: 301-654-2055
Fax: 301-654-5920
Website: www.gastro.org
E-mail: member@gastro.org

Celiac Disease Foundation
20350 Ventura Boulevard
Suite 240
Woodland Hills CA 91364
Phone: 818-716-1513
Fax: 818-267-5577
Website: www.celiac.org
E-mail: cdf@celiac.org

Crohn's and Colitis Foundation of America (CCFA)
386 Park Avenue South
17th Floor
New York, NY 10016
Toll-Free: 800-932-2423
Phone: 212-685-3440
Fax: 212-779-4098

Website: www.ccfa.org
E-mail: info@ccfa.org

National Digestive Diseases Information Clearinghouse (NDDIC)
2 Information Way
Bethesda, MD 20892-3570
Toll-Free: 800-891-5389
Toll-Free TTY: 866-569-1162
Fax: 703-738-4929
Website:
www.digestive.niddk.nih.gov
E-mail: nddic@info.niddk.nih.go

Immunizations

National Center for Immunization and Respiratory Diseases, CDC
1600 Clifton Road NE, MS E-05
Atlanta, GA 30333
Toll-Free: 800-CDC-INFO
(800-232-4636)
Toll-Free TTY: 888-232-6348
Website: www.cdc.gov/vaccines

Immunization Action Coalition
1573 Selby Avenue, Suite 234
St Paul, MN 55104
Phone: 651-647-9009
Fax: 651-647-9131
Website: www.immunize.org
E-mail: admin@immunize.org

Heart and Lung Health

American Heart Association
7272 Greenville Avenue
Dallas, TX 75231
Toll-Free: 800-AHA-USA-1

(800-242-8721)
Website: www.americanheart.org

American Lung Association
1301 Pennsylvania Avenue NW
Suite 800
Washington, DC 20004
Toll-Free: 800-LUNGUSA
(800-586-4872)
Toll-Free Helpline: 800-548-8252
Phone: 212-315-8700
or 202-785-3355
Fax: 202-452-1805
Website: www.lungusa.org

National Heart, Lung, and Blood Institute (NHLBI)
NHLBI Health Information Center
P.O. Box 30105
Bethesda, MD 20824-0105
Phone: 301-592-8573
TTY: 240-629-3255
Fax: 240-629-3246
Website: www.nhlbi.nih.gov
E-mail: nhlbiinfo@nhlbi.nih.gov

WomenHeart: The National Coalition for Women with Heart Disease
818 18th Street NW, Suite 1000
Washington, DC 20006
Toll-Free: 877-771-0030
Phone: 202-728-7199
Fax: 202-728-7238
Website: www.womenheart.org
E-mail: mail@womenheart.org

Mental Health

National Institute of Mental Health
6001 Executive Boulevard

663

Room 6200, MSC 9663
Bethesda, MD 20892-9663
Toll-Free: 866-615-NIMH
(866-615-6464)
Toll-Free TTY: 866-415-8051
Phone: 301-443-4513
TTY: 301-443-8431
Fax: 301-443-4279
Website: www.nimh.nih.gov
E-mail: nimhinfo@nih.gov

Substance Abuse and Mental Health Services Administration (SAMHSA)
SAMHSA's Health Information Network
P.O. Box 2345
Rockville, MD 20847-2345
Toll-Free: 877-SAMHSA-7
(877-726-4727)
Toll-Free Suicide Prevention Lifeline: 800-273-TALK (800-273-8255)
Toll-Free 24/7 Treatment Referral Line: 800-622-HELP
(800-622-4357)
Toll-Free TTY: 800-487-4889
Toll-Free TDD: 866-889-2647
Website: samhsa.gov
E-mail:
SAMHSAInfo@samhsa.hhs.gov

Reproductive Health

American Pregnancy Association
1425 Greenway Drive, Suite 440
Irving, TX 75038
Phone: 972-550-0140
Fax: 972-550-0800
Website: americanpregnancy.org
E-mail: Questions@
AmericanPregnancy.org

March of Dimes
1275 Mamaroneck Avenue
White Plains, NY 10605
Phone: 914-997-4488
Website: www.marchofdimes.com

Planned Parenthood Federation of America
New York Office:
434 West 33rd Street
New York, NY 10001
Toll-Free: 800-230-PLAN
(800-230-7526)
Phone: 212-541-7800
DC Office: 202-973-4800
Fax: 212-245-1845
Website:
www.plannedparenthood.org

Urologic Health

American Urological Association Foundation
1000 Corporate Boulevard
Linthicum, MD 21090
Toll-Free: 800-828-7866
Phone: 410-689-3700
Fax: 410-689-3998
Website: www.urologyhealth.org
E-mail:
info@urologycarefoundation.org

National Kidney and Urologic Diseases Information Clearinghouse
3 Information Way
Bethesda, MD 20892-3580
Toll-Free: 800-891-5390
Toll-Free TTY: 866-569-1162
Fax: 703-738-4929
Website: www.kidney.niddk.nih.gov
E-mail: nkudic@info.niddk.nih.gov

Index

Index

Page numbers followed by 'n' indicate a footnote. Page numbers in *italics* indicate a table or illustration.

Health Reference Series